# Critical Cases in Electrocardiography

An Annotated Atlas of Don't-Miss ECGs for Emergency
Medicine and Critical Care

**Steven R. Lowenstein**
University of Colorado School of Medicine

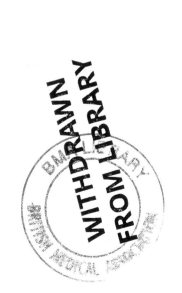

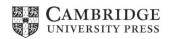
**CAMBRIDGE**
UNIVERSITY PRESS

# CAMBRIDGE
## UNIVERSITY PRESS

University Printing House, Cambridge CB2 8BS, United Kingdom

One Liberty Plaza, 20th Floor, New York, NY 10006, USA

477 Williamstown Road, Port Melbourne, VIC 3207, Australia

314–321, 3rd Floor, Plot 3, Splendor Forum, Jasola District Centre, New Delhi – 110025, India

79 Anson Road, #06–04/06, Singapore 079906

Cambridge University Press is part of the University of Cambridge.

It furthers the University's mission by disseminating knowledge in the pursuit of education, learning, and research at the highest international levels of excellence.

www.cambridge.org
Information on this title: www.cambridge.org/9781107535916
DOI: 10.1017/9781316336106

© Cambridge University Press 2018

First published 2018

Printed in the United Kingdom by Clays, St Ives plc

A catalogue record for this publication is available from the British Library.

Library of Congress Cataloging-in-Publication Data
Names: Lowenstein, Steven, 1950– author.
Title: Critical cases in electrocardiography : an annotated atlas of don't miss ECGs for emergency and critical care / Steven R. Lowenstein.
Description: Cambridge, United Kingdom ; New York, NY : Cambridge University Press, 2018. | Includes bibliographical references and index.
Identifiers: LCCN 2017045846 | ISBN 9781107535916 (paperback)
Subjects: | MESH: Electrocardiography | Myocardial Infarction – diagnosis | Critical Care | Emergency Service, Hospital | Case Reports | Atlases
Classification: LCC RC683.5.E5 | NLM WG 17 | DDC 616.1/207547–dc23
LC record available at https://lccn.loc.gov/2017045846

ISBN 978-1-107-53591-6 Paperback

........................................................................................................

All of the cases in this atlas represent real patients who were seen by physicians in various hospitals. In some cases, ages and other details were changed to protect personal health information.

# Contents

# Foreword

For my entire career as a cardiologist I have worked for organizations that provided time and money each year for me to attend any medical education conference of my choosing. Unlike most of my colleagues, I did not use those resources to attend the annual meetings sponsored by the American College of Cardiology or the European Society of Cardiology. I decided that it would be better for my patients and me if I attended a conference focused on a particular theme. I would choose a meeting on echocardiography, heart failure or another specific topic.

Several years ago I attended a meeting focused on what I thought was the diagnosis and treatment of cardiac dysrhythmias. At the opening of the conference the hosting cardiologist said, "I know we're all here because of our love of electricity." Being deeply clinically oriented, I related not at all to what he said. As I looked at the titles of the morning's lectures, though, it became clear that the meeting was for electrophysiologists rather than general cardiologists like me. The hosting physician then declared that the conference was the first electrophysiology board review in the United States!

For the duration of the course I sat through hour-long lectures discussing physics, electrophysiologic principles and invasive catheter-based treatments of which I would have no part. A small portion of each lecture covered something relevant to a general cardiologist. It was a long week.

This story comes to mind because, having been asked to write the foreword for Dr. Steven Lowenstein's *Critical Cases in Electrocardiography* – and having the privilege of reading it beforehand – it is gratifyingly clear that Dr. Lowenstein did not write the book because he loves electricity. He wrote it because he loves *electrocardiography* and especially the sharing of it with clinicians in an effort to have us not only better understand the genesis and identification of various waveforms but, by doing so, arrive at correct diagnoses and treatments in complicated cases.

Dr. Lowenstein's enthusiasm for teaching is apparent throughout the book. He does us the favor of approaching ECG tracings from the sharing of patient stories – which makes the reading more appealing, easier to remember, sometimes amazing and often fun. Have you seen an image of a suspension bridge in any other medical text? To help us recognize a certain pathologic ST-segment waveform – similar to the curvature of the cables of a suspension bridge – Dr. Lowenstein incorporates one here!

This atlas is also made more interesting because of not only *what* is written but also *how* it is written. Dr. Lowenstein includes insightful and often lyrical historical comments from pioneers in electrocardiography. Both the historical sages and he at times offer philosophical comments about the deeper meanings of what an electrocardiogram can tell us to remind us of why we want to know all we can about a tracing – to perhaps spare suffering or prolong a life.

I have learned more from Dr. Lowenstein and his fascinating book than I did spending that tedious week with electrophysiology – or from any other book on electrocardiography I have read. I suspect that you will learn a lot from his book, too, and will have a good time doing so.

*Lawrence J. Hergott, M.D.*
*Emeritus Professor of Medicine*
*Center for Bioethics and Humanities*
*University of Colorado School of Medicine*

# Preface

*There is a need in any worthwhile human endeavor for substantive engagement. In biology, the engagement is with the processes of life; in medicine, with the problems of the sick. In electrocardiography, it is with the electrical outpourings of the heart.*
—*Horan (1978)*

This atlas deals solely with the electrocardiogram (ECG) and its applications in emergency medicine and critical care practice. Despite advances in diagnosis and therapeutics, the ECG remains an indispensable tool in emergency care. The ECG is painless and noninvasive. It is quick. It is reproducible. And it has no known risks.

It is self-evident that the ECG plays a pivotal role in patient care. The information contained in the ECG cannot be duplicated by even the most painstaking patient history nor by palpation, percussion or auscultation. Nor is the same information readily obtainable through blood work, radiographs, sonograms or high-tech body imaging. The electrocardiogram is, according to Horan, "a form of nonverbal communication from the patient's heart to the physician" (Horan, 1978). The ECG is "where the money is" for a wide variety of chief complaints, including chest pain, dyspnea, syncope, electrolyte abnormalities, shock, cardiac arrest, arrhythmias, poisonings and other critical emergencies. More often than not, the ECG rules in or out one or more life-threatening conditions and changes management. As Sir Zachary Pope wrote in his introduction to *Early Diagnosis of the Acute Abdomen*, "There is little need to labour the truism that earlier diagnosis means better prognosis" (Cope, 1972).

I have prepared this atlas with two simple objectives in mind. The first is to help readers advance beyond the stage of "competent" electrocardiographer, since basic competence is not sufficient. Emergency physicians must be *expert electrocardiographers*. Referring colleagues, consultants, hospital administrators and, most importantly, patients expect that front-line emergency physicians can recognize all the common electrolyte abnormalities, decipher complex tachycardias, distinguish among various causes of "nonspecific ST-T changes" and detect acute myocardial infarctions in their early, subtle stages. It is not enough that the emergency physician is able to recognize an acute inferior wall myocardial infarction when there are 7 mm "tombstone" ST-segment elevations in the inferior leads. Readers of this atlas will learn that ST-segment straightening in lead III may be the only abnormality that warns of an impending infarction and that isolated depression of the ST-segment in lead aVL may also herald the development of an inferior wall ST-elevation myocardial infarction (STEMI). Therefore, one critical goal of this atlas is to enable emergency physicians to make lifesaving diagnoses before others can. As Zoneraich and Spodick wrote, "Identification of subtle changes in the ECG ... remains the privilege of the well-informed" (Zoneraich and Spodick, 1995).

My second goal in preparing this atlas is to help emergency physicians develop a sense of excitement about reading ECGs. This is possible, I believe, by emphasizing clinically relevant topics, by presenting examples of obvious and not-so-obvious disease, by integrating electrocardiography with bedside clinical practice and by focusing squarely on situations where interpretation of the ECG contributes to clinical decision-making. I have also included numerous examples of ECG "misses" – cases where the computer or the clinicians (or both) got it wrong.

Interest and excitement in ECG reading are also reinforced by paying close attention to the anatomic and electrophysiologic origins of various ECG abnormalities. Therefore, wherever relevant, each chapter includes a brief "basic sciences" or "coronary anatomy" section, which attempts to explain the surface ECG tracings by describing clearly their anatomic or electrophysiologic correlations. The ECG is a remarkably true reflection of anatomy and electrophysiology, and in most cases we are better served by learning these connections than by relying solely on pattern memorization.

It seems surprising that there are no accepted standards for measuring physician competency in ECG interpretation in the emergency department setting. No one has defined the essential electrocardiographic skills or experience that are necessary for safe practice. In 2003 the majority of emergency medicine residency program directors voiced opposition to establishing a national ECG competency examination or even a national model curriculum (Ginde and Char, 2003). Thus, for emergency medicine trainees and practitioners, self-study remains the only game in town. I will accept at face value the argument that ECG interpretative skills improve with study and practice. They have for me.

Some clinicians have warned that interest and expertise in ECG interpretation are waning as new procedures and technologies "compete for the attention of the bright young clinician and clinical investigator" (Fisch, 1989). More than 30 years ago, Wellens lamented that "invasive procedures, with their diagnostic (and financial) rewards, have stolen the interest of the younger generation" (Wellens, 1986). Horan warned, "We may program computers to read electrocardiograms, [but] we must not deprogram doctors" (Horan, 1978). Fye, Fisch and others have also argued that computer-assisted ECGs have led to complacency, are "an obstacle to acquisition of electrocardiographic skills" and have "hastened the decline of clinical electrocardiography" (Fisch, 1989; Fye, 1994). This is debatable. I will grant that computer-assisted electrocardiograms and alternative technologies have captured the attention of cardiologists and other specialists, but I do not sense that interest in electrocardiography is waning in emergency medicine, although systematic instruction has not always kept pace.

In reference to computer-assisted ECG interpretation, we should remember that computer algorithms are notoriously insensitive for the diagnosis of acute STEMIs and many other critical emergencies. As highlighted throughout this atlas, computers often miss subtle STEMIs; early STEMIs; anterior, posterior and lateral STEMIs and STEMIs hiding under the cover of a bundle branch block or left ventricular hypertrophy with "strain" (Massel et al., 2000; Elko et al., 1992; Kudenchuk et al., 1991; Southern and Arnsten, 2009; Kligfield et al., 2007; Ayer and Terkelsen, 2014). Computer algorithms miss all manner of "STEMI equivalents," such as widespread ST-segment depressions with ST-elevation in lead aVR, which may signify acute left main coronary artery obstruction. Practice and confidence are needed to overrule the computer's missteps. As Marriott wrote, "Marvelous as the computer is, it has not yet achieved glory in ECG interpretation . . . [and] sometimes the computer is dangerously deficient" (Marriott, 1997).

A final word about the organization of this book: *Critical Cases in Electrocardiography* is an atlas, not a comprehensive textbook. The emphasis is on "don't-miss" ECG tracings. *Critical Cases in Electrocardiography* emphasizes the subtle and the advanced, if this knowledge is critical to the practice of emergency medicine or critical care. For example, the Brugada syndrome is included in the chapter on nonischemic causes of ST-segment elevation (coronary mimics); Brugada is rare statistically. But in young patients with syncope, its presence is unmistakable to the trained eye. Recognition of the Brugada pattern in syncope patients is an opportunity to prevent sudden cardiac death.

This atlas also differs from other ECG textbooks, which devote more attention to standard ECG criteria for topics such as left ventricular hypertrophy, p-mitrale, right bundle branch block and the like. Some of the chapters in this textbook cover conventional topics, such as inferior, anterior or posterior wall myocardial infarction. But other chapters in *Critical Cases* are quite different from most ECG textbooks because they are organized according to patients' presenting problems. Thus, there is a chapter on the electrocardiography of shortness of breath, where pulmonary embolism, myocarditis and

pericardial tamponade are covered. Several of the chapters highlight STEMI equivalents, while other chapters focus on deciphering nondiagnostic ST-T changes that can masquerade as myocardial ischemia, such as LVH with strain, early repolarization, electrolyte abnormalities and digitalis effect. For the most part, it is assumed that readers already have a strong understanding of the normal ECG, although the genesis of the normal ECG is reviewed in Chapter 1.

In preparing this atlas, I have been inspired by some of the great textbooks and manuals of electrocardiography, some of which have also focused specifically on the diagnosis of acute myocardial ischemia and infarction (Wagner and Strauss, 2014; Goldberger et al., 2013; Chan et al., 2005; Smith et al., 2002; Surawicz and Knilans, 2008). Perhaps most of all, I have been inspired by Marriott's *Emergency Electrocardiography*, which the author called "a vademecum for every caretaker of cardiac crises" (Marriott, 1997). Marriott was one of the first to spell out the importance of the ECG changes that routinely "escape the eye of the unwary." And Marriott's *Emergency Electrocardiography* is also the book where I was first introduced to his many wonderful words and phrases, such as T-waves that are "humble," "bulky," "noble" or "spread eagle," and also the "wishbone" effect, ST-elevations in "indicative leads," "milking the QRS complex" and "fishhooks" in the J-point.

A final disclaimer: in this atlas, there is no mention, even in passing, of Einthoven's triangle, summed action potentials or vectorcardiograms. These concepts may be interesting to some, and they represented fundamental discoveries in the early days of cardiac electrophysiology and electrocardiography. However, they are not necessary for an in-depth understanding of normal and abnormal electrocardiograms. Einthoven's triangle is seldom mentioned in the emergency department, the catheterization laboratory or the intensive care unit. As Marriott wrote in the preface to the first edition of his classic textbook, *Practical Electrocardiography*, too often, introductory chapters are "so intricate and longwinded that the reader's interest is easily drowned in a troubled sea of vectors, axes and gradients" (Marriott, 1988).

My goal in this atlas, in the tradition of Marriott and other classic electrocardiographers and teachers, is to emphasize "the concepts required for everyday ECG interpretation" (Wagner and Strauss, 2014). The focus is clinical diagnosis, late at night in the emergency department or critical care unit, in the service of seriously ill patients.

Almost a century ago, cardiologist Calvin Smith cautioned:

> The person who undertakes to make a success of electrocardiography . . . must be prepared to devote all his time to acquiring and understanding of [the] art . . . [which] must be practiced regularly, systematically and faithfully, day after day, week after week, before proficiency is obtained. The mere possession of electrocardiographic equipment no more makes a person a cardiologist than the possession of Shakespeare's volume makes the owner a litterateur."
>
> (Smith, 1923)

I do not agree, necessarily, that a lifetime of devotion is required to learn to interpret electrocardiograms. No one can practice reading ECGs "systematically and faithfully, day after day." *Critical Cases in Electrocardiography* was written so that emergency and critical care physicians can learn to recognize electrocardiographic "life threats" and strengthen their electrocardiographic skills – over a much shorter time.

# References

Ayer A., Terkelsen C. J. Difficult ECGs in STEMI: Lessons learned from serial sampling of pre- and in-hospital ECGs. *J Electrocardiol.* 2014; **47**:448–458.

Chan T. C., Brady W. J., Harrigan R. A. et al. *ECG in emergency medicine and acute care.* Philadelphia, PA: Elsevier Mosby, 2005.

Cope Z. *The early diagnosis of the acute abdomen.* Fourteenth edition. London: Oxford University Press, 1972 (Quotation from the preface to the first edition, 1921).

Elko P. P., Weaver W. D., Kudenchuk P., Rowlandson I. The dilemma of sensitivity versus specificity in computer-interpreted acute myocardial infarction. *J Electrocardiol.* 1992; **24**(Suppl.):2–7.

Fisch C. Evolution of the clinical electrocardiogram. *J Am Coll Cardiol.* 1989; **14**:1127–1128.

Fye W. B. A history of the origin, evolution and impact of electrocardiography. *Am J Cardiol.* 1994; **73**:937–949.

Ginde A. A., Char D. M. Emergency medicine residency training in electrocardiogram interpretation. *Acad Emerg Med.* 2003; **10**:738–742.

Goldberger A. L., Goldberger Z. D., Shvilkin A. *Goldberger's clinical electrocardiography: A simplified approach.* Eighth edition. Philadelphia, PA: Elsevier Saunders, 2013.

Horan L. G. The quest for optimal electrocardiography. *Am J Cardiol.* 1978; **41**:126–129.

Kligfield P., Gettes L. S., Bailey J. J. et al. Recommendations for the standardization and interpretation of the electrocardiogram. Part I: The electrocardiogram and its technology. A scientific statement from the American Heart Association Electrocardiography and Arrhythmias Committee, Council on Clinical Cardiology; the American College of Cardiology Foundation; and the Heart Rhythm Society. *J Am Coll Cardiol.* 2007; 491109–491127.

Kudenchuk P. J., Ho M. T., Weaver W. D. et al. Accuracy of computer-interpreted electrocardiography in selecting patients for thrombolytic therapy. MITI Project Investigators. *J Am Coll Cardiol.* 1991; **17**:1486–1491.

Marriott H. J. L. *Practical electrocardiography.* Preface to the first edition. Eighth edition. Baltimore, MD: Williams & Wilkins, 1988.

Marriott H. J. L. *Emergency electrocardiography.* Naples, FL: Trinity Press, 1997.

Massel D., Dawdy J. A., Melendez L. J. Strict reliance on a computer algorithm or measurable ST segment criteria may lead to errors in thrombolytic therapy eligibility. *Am Heart J.* 2000; **140**:221–226.

Smith S. C. *Heart records: Their interpretation and preparation.* Philadelphia,

PA: FA Davis, 1923. Cited in: Fye WB. A history of the origin, evolution and impact of electrocardiography. *Am J Cardiol.* 1994; 73: 937–949.

Smith S. W., Zvosec D. L., Sharkey S. W., Henry T. W. *The ECG in acute MI. An evidence-based manual of reperfusion therapy.* Philadelphia, PA: Lippincott Williams & Wilkins, 2002.

Southern W. N., Arnsten J. H. The effect of erroneous computer interpretation of ECGs on resident decision making. *Med Decis Making.* 2009; **29**:372–376.

Surawicz B., Knilans T. K. *Chou's electrocardiography in clinical practice.* Sixth edition. Philadelphia, PA: Elsevier Saunders, 2008.

Wagner G. S., Strauss D. G. *Marriott's practical electrocardiography.* Twelfth edition. Philadelphia, PA: Lippincott, Williams & Wilkins, 2014.

Wellens H. J. J. The electrocardiogram 80 years after Einthoven. *J Am Coll Cardiol.* 1986; 7:484–491. Cited in: Fye WB. A history of the origin, evolution and impact of electrocardiography. *Am J Cardiol.* 1994; 73: 937–949.

Zoneraich S., Spodick D. H. Bedside science reduces laboratory art: Appropriate use of physical findings to reduce reliance on sophisticated and expensive methods. *Circulation.* 1995; **91**:2089–2092.

# Acknowledgments

I am indebted to my friends and colleagues in the emergency departments where I have worked and to all my colleagues on the faculty at the University of Colorado School of Medicine. Many of you have sent me challenging ECG tracings over the years; you have generously shared your expertise, often pointing out important ECG abnormalities that we may have missed in the emergency department.

In preparing this atlas, I have also been helped by a generation of emergency medicine residents. I am inspired by your intelligence, your dedication to the care of our patients and your humanity. Thank you for everything you have taught me.

I am indebted and grateful to my wife, Elaine, and to our sons, Adam and Chris, most of all. I am certain that ECGs are not the focus of your existence. I am just as certain that you are the focus of mine.

# The Normal Electrocardiogram
## A Brief Review

**Chapter 1**

Chapter 1 reviews the genesis and inherent logic of the normal 12-lead electrocardiogram (ECG). This chapter explains, electrophysiologically and anatomically, "normal sinus rhythm," junctional rhythms, normal and abnormal q-waves and cardiac axis. This chapter also reviews several common (albeit non-life-threatening) abnormalities, such as poor R-wave progression, atrial enlargement, old anterior, septal and inferior myocardial infarctions and common ECG artifacts (for example, limb lead reversal and misplacement of the chest leads).

## The Basics

The electrophysiologic principles that underlie the normal 12-lead ECG are more than a century old. Here are the basics:

- The ECG recording represents an electrical current (a depolarization wave) flowing between myocardial cells. The depolarization current is possible because the myocardial cells are coupled to one another through electrical gap junctions ("electrical synapses"). The ECG records the summed electrical currents of millions of myocytes, depolarizing in a synchronous fashion (Surawicz and Knilans, 2008; Wagner and Strauss, 2014).
- The standard ECG includes 12 different leads located in different positions; these permit us to record depolarization currents flowing toward or away from specific monitoring leads. The leads are labeled in Figure 1.1 *according to their positive poles.* We can refer to them as "monitoring" or "exploring" leads because they record electrical activity in the myocardial segment right beneath them.
- "Depolarization" represents electrical activation of the myocardium. Depolarization is followed by contraction of the chamber (the process of excitation-contraction coupling). "Repolarization" represents restoration of the original electrical potential of the myocardial cells.
- If there is greater myocardial mass (more electrically active myocytes), the depolarization wave (R-wave or P-wave) is taller. That is, there is greater voltage in the leads facing that portion of the heart. Taller R-waves in the left-facing leads may be a sign of left ventricular enlargement, while loss of R-wave voltage often indicates old myocardial infarction (electrical silence). In later chapters, we examine other life-threatening conditions, such as pericardial tamponade and myocarditis, that may present as "low-voltage" QRS complexes.

## The Cardiac Depolarization Current Is *Directional*

This is the most important concept of all. Understanding the direction of the depolarization current, and also the position of

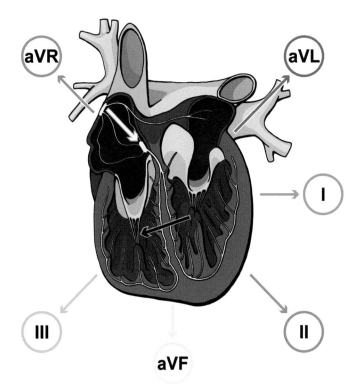

**Figure 1.1** The normal electrical conduction pathways through the heart.

the ECG leads, will help explain not only normal sinus rhythm but also junctional rhythms, the "regional changes" of ST-elevation myocardial infarctions (STEMIs), most "STEMI equivalents," old myocardial infarctions, atrial enlargement and numerous other conditions.

- The depolarization current originates in the sinus (SA, or sino-atrial) node, which is a collection of spontaneously firing pacemaker cells located in the upper reaches ("ceiling") of the right atrium (Surawicz and Knilans, 2008; University of Minnesota, 2014).
- The impulse then travels through the atria on its way to the AV node. Although this is controversial, the depolarization wave appears to proceed through the right and left atria via semi-specialized (or "preferential") pathways, known as internodal tracts, leading to activation of the right and left atria and inscription of the P-wave (Surawicz and Knilans, 2008; University of Minnesota, 2014).
- Not surprisingly, given the location of the SA node in the right atrium, the P-waves are often slightly notched in the limb leads (and they may be biphasic in lead V1), as the right atrium is depolarized slightly before the left atrium.

Even when the P-wave is smooth and rounded, we know that the first one-third of the P-wave represents right atrial depolarization, while the terminal third represents left atrial depolarization. Both atria contribute to the middle third of the P-wave (Wagner and Strauss, 2014). The duration, "notching" and biphasic shape of the P-wave are more pronounced if the left atrium is enlarged. (See the discussion and the self-study ECG tracings later in this chapter for examples of left and right atrial enlargement.)

## The Six Limb Leads

Figure 1.1 shows the "locations" of the six limb leads.

- The six limb leads are labeled according to their *positive poles*.[1] When we say that lead III "points to the right and inferiorly" (toward the right leg), we mean that this is the location of the positive pole of lead III.
- The ECG circuitry is configured so that a positive (upright) deflection – a P-wave or R-wave – is inscribed if the depolarization wave is traveling toward the positive pole of that lead.
- A negative deflection – a negative P-wave or (for the QRS complexes) a Q-wave if it is the first deflection or an S-wave – is inscribed if the depolarization wave is moving away from the positive pole.

Leads II, III and aVF are the inferior leads; leads I and aVL, which point toward the upper left side and the left shoulder, are the "high lateral" leads. Lead aVL is electrically "reciprocal" to lead III, since their positive poles point in nearly opposite directions. It is no surprise that an acute inferior STEMI is usually characterized not only by ST-segment elevations in leads II, III and aVF but also by *ST-segment depressions* in the "reciprocal leads (I and, especially, aVL). For additional discussion of the importance of ST-segment depressions in lead aVL, see Chapter 2, Inferior Wall Myocardial Infarction.

## Normal Sinus Rhythm: The Complete Definition

Most introductory textbooks and lectures insist that a rhythm is "normal sinus" if there is a P-wave before every QRS and a QRS after every P-wave. However, this definition is unsatisfactory and incomplete. Because the sinus node, which initiates the depolarization wave, resides in the upper portion of the right atrium, the atrial depolarization wave begins at the "right shoulder" (beneath lead aVR); then it moves away from aVR toward lead II. Therefore, in normal sinus rhythm not only must there be a P-wave before every QRS, but *the P-wave must be negative in lead AVR, and it must be upright in lead II*. This is the complete definition of "normal sinus rhythm." Refer again to Figure 1.1 and ECG 1.1 (which demonstrates normal sinus rhythm).

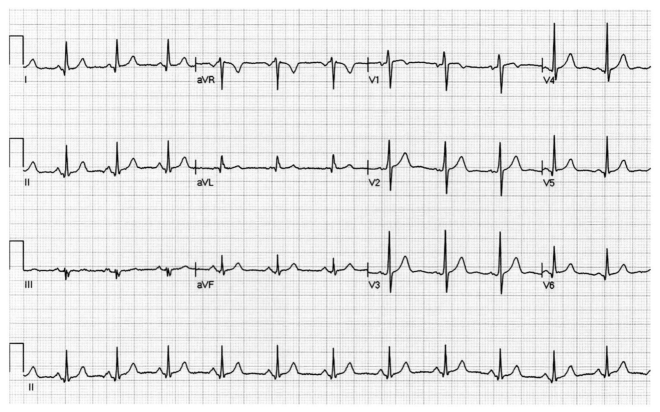

**ECG 1.1** The normal electrocardiogram.

[1] Each ECG lead monitors a specific region of the heart (for example, the inferior or high lateral wall of the left ventricle). Although limb leads I, II and III are "bipolar" while the "augmented" limb leads aVR, aVL and aVF are said to be unipolar, this distinction just introduces confusion. In fact, all the ECG leads are bipolar. Even the three "unipolar" leads have a "reference electrode that is constructed electrically from the other limb electrodes" (Gorgels et al., 2001; Wagner and Strauss, 2014; Kligfield et al., 2007). What is critical is that each lead is labeled according to its positive pole.

As an aside, in normal sinus rhythm the P-wave is often flat or indistinct in lead aVL. This is not surprising, as the atrial depolarization vector proceeds in a direction that is approximately 90 degrees perpendicular to the positive pole of aVL. Refer again to Figure 1.1 and ECG 1.1.

## Conduction through the AV Node

- As noted previously, after leaving the SA node, the depolarization wave travels through the atria, along semi-specialized pathways (internodal tracks), until it arrives at the AV node (Surawicz and Knilans, 2008; University of Minnesota, 2014). It takes approximately 30 msec for the impulse to travel from the SA node through the internodal bundles to the AV node. It takes an additional 130–150 msec to travel through the AV node and His bundle. Thus, the normal PR interval (which includes the P-wave and the PR segment) ranges from 120–200 msec.
- The PR interval is not static; rather, AV nodal conduction is highly sensitive to the balance of sympathetic and parasympathetic tone. The PR interval is often shorter during tachycardias and when there is heightened sympathetic tone and longer when parasympathetic tone predominates. Interestingly, some young, healthy individuals may develop first-degree AV block or even Mobitz Type 1 second-degree heart block during sleep, when parasympathetic tone is high.
- After emerging from the AV node, the depolarization wave travels through the short His bundle, which pierces the interventricular septum. The AV node and the His bundle, together, constitute the "AV junction."

## The Three Functions of the AV Node

The AV node serves three electrophysiologic functions:

- The principal function of the AV node is to generate a pause; this enables the atria to contract and optimizes filling of the ventricles prior to ventricular systole.
- A second function of the AV node is to block rapid or ultra-rapid atrial impulses from reaching the ventricles (for example, during atrial fibrillation or flutter). The ability of the AV node to slow rapid impulses from the atria – and, thus, the "ventricular response" during atrial flutter or fibrillation – is exquisitely sensitive to the balance of sympathetic and parasympathetic tone. Of course, AV nodal conduction is also slowed in the presence of AV nodal blocking drugs and in the presence of sclerodegenerative conduction system disease, a condition primarily of elderly patients.
- Third, the AV junction can serve as a pacemaker, either when excited or when serving as an escape pacemaker. Acceleration of junctional pacemaker activity (accelerated junctional rhythm or nonparoxysmal junctional tachycardia) is commonly seen in patients with digitalis toxicity or acute inferior wall myocardial infarction, in the setting of cardiac surgery, during therapy with calcium channel blocking agents, and (years ago) in patients with acute rheumatic carditis (Surawicz and Knilans, 2008; Wagner and Strauss, 2014).

## Junctional Rhythms

Junctional rhythms arise from a discrete pacemaker within the AV node or His bundle. They are characterized by inverted P-waves in the inferior leads and an upright P-wave in lead aVR, reflecting retrograde atrial depolarization (toward aVR and away from lead II). The inverted P-waves in the inferior leads may appear before or after the QRS complex; or, commonly, if atrial and ventricular depolarization occur concurrently, the inverted P-waves are hidden in the QRS complex.

Negative P-waves in the inferior leads may also represent an ectopic pacemaker originating in the low right or left atrium. It is more likely that the inverted P-wave represents a junctional pacemaker if the PR interval is short (< 120 msec). Conversely, if the PR interval is normal (≥ 120 msec), the origin of the inverted P-wave is more likely to be within the atria (ectopic or low atrial rhythm) (Surawicz and Knilans, 2008; Wagner and Strauss, 2014; Mirowski, 1966). The important point is that negative P-waves in II, III and aVF and upright P-waves in aVR signify that the atria are being activated from the junctional or low atrial tissue, with the atrial activation wave moving upward and to the patient's right shoulder (aVR).

ECG 1.2 is an example of a junctional rhythm.

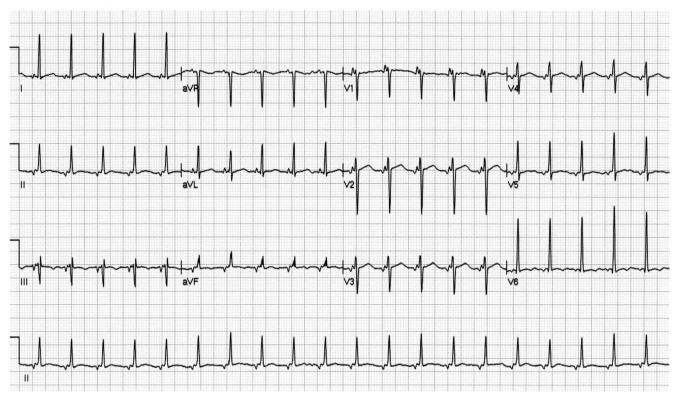

**ECG 1.2** A 21-year-old female with end-stage renal disease, systemic lupus and severe vasculitis presented because of lethargy and general weakness.

## The Electrocardiogram

The ECG demonstrates a junctional tachycardia (accelerated junctional rhythm) with a heart rate of 122. The P-waves are inverted in the inferior leads and upright in lead aVR. This unusual, superiorly directed P-wave axis is indicative of a junctional pacemaker. Also, since the PR interval is short (90 msec), we are reasonably confident that this is a junctional, rather than an ectopic atrial, tachycardia. The ECG also demonstrates nonspecific ST- and T-wave flattening.

Accelerated junctional rhythms (also referred to as "nonparoxysmal junctional tachycardias") typically have a heart rate of 60–100 beats per minute.[2]

## Clinical Course

No cause for her junctional tachycardia was identified, and it resolved spontaneously after treatment with antibiotics, intravenous fluids, stress-dose corticosteroids and other supportive care.

---

[2] The usual rate for a junctional escape rhythm is approximately 40–60 beats per minute. If the rate is < 40, it is a junctional bradycardia. When the rate is 60–100, the rhythm is usually referred to as an "accelerated junctional rhythm." Common etiologies of accelerated junctional rhythms include digitalis excess, inferior myocardial infarction, cardiac surgery and (in years past) acute rheumatic carditis. Junctional tachycardias that exceed 100–120 beats per minute are called "accelerated junctional tachycardias" (Surawicz and Knilans, 2008).

ECG 1.3, from a young man with chest pain, is an example of an ectopic atrial rhythm.

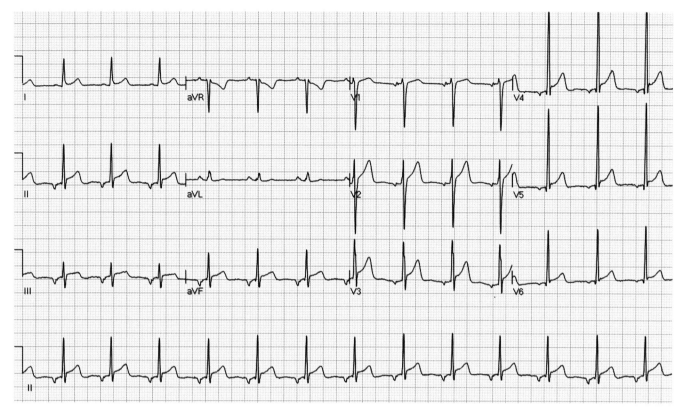

**ECG 1.3**  A 29-year-old man presented with sharp left-sided chest pain that was "better when he rode his bicycle."

## The Electrocardiogram

The P-waves are inverted in the inferior leads and are upright in lead aVR. Although there is a "P-wave before every QRS and a QRS after every P-wave," this cannot be normal sinus rhythm. The P-wave (atrial depolarization) vector is directed superiorly and to the patient's right. The PR interval is normal (164 msec). Therefore, this is an ectopic atrial rhythm. There are borderline voltage criteria for left ventricular hypertrophy (LVH), although this is likely a nonspecific finding in a patient under age 35. There are diffuse ST-segment elevations involving all the precordial and limb leads (notably, except aVR).

## Clinical Course

His eventual diagnosis was acute pericarditis. He recovered uneventfully.

## Ventricular Depolarization (the QRS Complexes)

Once the cardiac action potential has traversed the His bundle, it moves antegrade through the left and right bundle branches and spreads to the contractile myocytes via the ultra-rapidly conducting purkinje fibers.

- The purkinje fibers reside in the bundle branches and fascicles, and their principal function is to conduct impulses rapidly to all the cardiac myocytes, allowing for orderly and synchronous ventricular excitation.
- The overall direction (electrical vector) of the ventricular depolarization wave is downward and to the patient's left. Thus, the QRS axis points downward and to the left (and also posteriorly). See Figure 1.1.
- The initial deflection of the QRS complex (approximately 0.03 seconds) represents depolarization of the interventricular septum, in a left-to-right direction (Figure 1.1; also discussed later).
- The normal ECG produces predominantly upright, tall-amplitude QRS complexes in the left-facing leads (leads I, aVL and V5–V6). The ECG records mostly negative deflections (S-waves) in leads that are right-sided and anterior (for example, lead aVR, lead III and precordial leads V1 and V2).

## Cardiac Axis

"Cardiac axis" refers to the overall electrical direction of the QRS complexes. As highlighted earlier, the normal direction of ventricular depolarization is downward and to the patient's left, producing upright QRS complexes in limb leads I and aVF. This represents a normal cardiac axis. If the QRS complex is upright in lead I but negative in aVF, the axis has shifted leftward. Conversely, if the QRS complex is negative in lead I (a larger than normal S-wave) but upright in aVF, there is right axis deviation. Infants, children, adolescents and young adults often have a right axis, but the axis generally shifts leftward with age. Significant S-waves in lead I (right axis deviation) are rarely normal in middle-aged or older adults, and their sudden appearance may signify pulmonary embolism or another cause of acute right heart strain.

Left axis deviation is a common ECG abnormality, which often reflects left anterior fascicular block, left ventricular hypertrophy, left bundle branch block or prior inferior myocardial infarction. As noted previously, modest degrees of left axis deviation also occur commonly with advancing age. Right axis deviation is common in children and young adults; after middle age, it usually suggests right ventricular hypertrophy, acute right heart strain or left posterior fascicular block. In older patients with chest pain, dizziness or shortness of breath, the simple finding of an S-wave in lead I should raise the suspicion of acute pulmonary embolism.[3]

## The Six Precordial (Chest) Leads

Figure 1.2 depicts the six precordial (chest) leads.

- Lead V1, which is placed in the fourth intercostal space just to the right of the sternum, monitors the septum and is

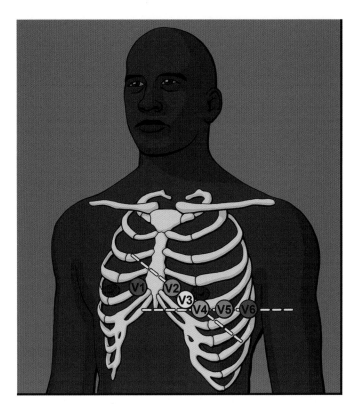

**Figure 1.2** The precordial leads. Note that lead V1 is placed just to the right of the sternum (in the fourth intercostal space); it "monitors" the interventricular septum and is referred to as the "septal lead." V1 also monitors the right ventricle; in the setting of an acute inferior wall STEMI (caused by a right coronary artery occlusion), concomitant ST-segment elevation in precordial lead V1 usually signifies a right ventricular infarction. As highlighted in chapter 2, lead V1 is also a "right ventricular lead."

referred to as the "septal" lead. ST-segment elevation in V1 usually signifies an acute septal infarction.

- Lead V1 also monitors the right ventricle. Therefore, when an acute inferior wall STEMI is present, ST-segment elevation in V1 usually indicates a concomitant right ventricular infarction. (See Chapter 2.)
- Leads V2–V4 are the anterior (or "anteroapical") precordial leads, whereas leads V5 and V6 are the lateral precordial leads. A STEMI that involves V2–V4 is referred to as an anterior wall infarction; if ST-segment elevations are present in leads V1–V4, an anteroseptal myocardial infarction is present.
- ST-elevations in V5 and V6 usually represent a lateral wall infarction. Limb leads I and aVL are also lateral-facing electrodes. (In this atlas, they are called the "high lateral" leads.)

## R-Wave Progression

Refer to Figure 1.3 and the normal ECG (ECG 1.1). In the normal heart, the R-wave amplitude should increase steadily (while the depth of the S-wave decreases) across the precordium from V1 to V5. The *precordial transition* zone – where the R-wave and S-wave voltages are equal – should occur no later than lead V4 (Surawicz and Knilans, 2008). If the precordial transition zone is delayed until V5 or V6 or if it never occurs (the R-wave height never exceeds the depth of the S-wave), the pattern is termed

---

[3] The other causes of an abnormal right axis deviation include: left posterior fascicular block; chronic hypoxic pulmonary disease; prior, extensive lateral wall myocardial infarction; and other causes of right ventricular hypertrophy (Surawicz and Knilans, 2008).

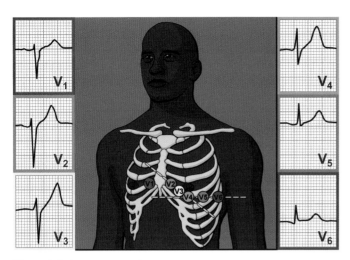

**Figure 1.3**  R-wave progression.

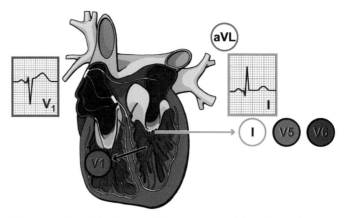

**Figure 1.4**  Septal depolarization: The initial phase of the QRS complex.

"poor R-wave progression" (Surawicz and Knilans, 2008; Wagner and Strauss, 2014).

The most common causes of poor R-wave progression are old anterior wall myocardial infarction, left ventricular hypertrophy, left bundle branch block, emphysema, dextrocardia or misplacement of the precordial electrodes (typically, 1–2 rib interspaces too high) (Rosen et al., 2014). Reverse R-wave progression (any decrement in the amplitude of the R-wave across the precordial leads moving from V1 to V5) may also occur, indicating a prior anterior wall myocardial infarction. These conditions are illustrated in the self-study ECGs.

V5 frequently has the highest amplitude because it is roughly situated at the apex of the left ventricle. If V6 is taller than V5, it may indicate left ventricular hypertrophy, as the enlarged LV pulls the depolarization vector in a more leftward and posterior direction. This corresponds to the bedside physical examination finding of a "laterally displaced point-of-maximal impulse" (PMI).

## The Two Phases of the Normal QRS Complex – and the Concept of "Septal Q- and R-Waves"

As illustrated in Figures 1.1 and 1.4, depolarization of the ventricles – the QRS complex – actually consists of two distinct phases, which are readily detected on the ECG. The first phase (or "vector"), lasting 0.03 seconds or less, represents depolarization of the interventricular septum from left to right. The interventricular septum is depolarized from left to right simply because the depolarization wave, after exiting the His bundle, travels slightly faster down the left bundle branch (and more slowly down the right). This simple electrical fact explains the appearance of the normal, septal Q-waves that typically appear in the left-sided leads of the ECG (limb leads I and aVL and precordial leads V5 and V6). These R-waves are narrow (<.03 seconds) because the septum itself is so thin (Thygesen et al., 2012).

The small, leading R-wave in the septal lead (V1) is also easily explained: V1 is placed in the fourth intercostal space, just to the right of the sternum, an ideal position to record the left-to-right depolarization of the septum as a positive deflection. In ECG 1.1, and in almost every other normal tracing, the QRS complex in lead V1 begins with a small, narrow R-wave, representing normal left-to-right septal depolarization. If the

initial R-wave is absent in V1, the patient has probably sustained a septal infarction (although faulty placement of the chest leads is an alternate explanation). Limb lead aVR also monitors the right side of the heart, and therefore aVR also begins with a small, initial septal R-wave. Because septal Q-waves (in the left-sided leads) and septal R-waves (in lead V1) represent depolarization of the septum from left to right, they are often absent if the patient has a left bundle branch block.

The second and longer phase of the QRS complex represents the simultaneous depolarization of the left and right ventricles, with the mass of the left ventricle predominating. Depolarization of the ventricles typically inscribes large R-waves in leads that monitor the left ventricle (V4, V5, V6 and leads I, II and aVF), since the impulse is traveling toward these leads; deep S-waves appear in right-sided leads (aVR, V1 and V2).

## Abnormal Q-Waves Signifying Old Myocardial Infarction

As noted earlier, "septal" Q-waves are normal, thin, narrow Q-waves seen in the left-facing leads (limb leads I and aVL and precordial leads V5 and V6). Q-waves can, of course, also signal that the patient has sustained a prior myocardial infarction (variably labeled as "old," "remote" or "indeterminate age" myocardial infarction). These pathologic Q-waves reflect the absence of electrical activity (that is, absence of a normal transmural depolarization wave) in the zone of the infarction, beneath the exploring electrode. Stated differently, the upright QRS complex changes into a Q-wave or simply an S-wave (called a QS) beneath the electrode, reflecting electrical forces moving away from the lead. Old myocardial infarction can also be suspected if there is loss of R-wave voltage (a "Q-wave equivalent").

It is usually not difficult to distinguish normal from pathologic Q-waves. The distinction depends on duration, depth and location of the Q-waves. "Pathologic" Q-waves, signifying old infarction, typically include: (a) Q-waves involving contiguous leads in a defined region of the heart (for example, leads II, III and aVF); (b) any Q-wave in precordial leads V1–V3; (c) Q-waves in any leads that are >.04 seconds in duration (1 small box wide); or (d) Q-waves of a depth > 1 mm (1 small box) deep or deeper than 25 percent of the R-wave amplitude (Wagner and Strauss, 2014; Thygesen et al., 2012).

ECG 1.4 was obtained from a 70-year-old man.

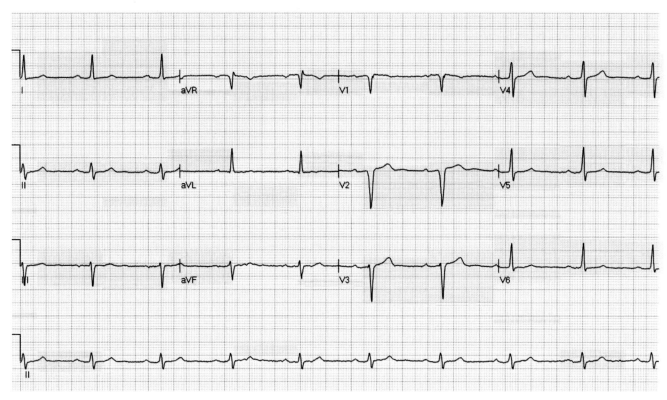

**ECG 1.4** A 70-year-old man reported a history of esophageal reflux disease, coronary artery disease, hypertension and hyperlipidemia. He underwent coronary artery bypass grafting 15 years earlier. He presented to the emergency department with chest pressure.

## The Electrocardiogram

The ECG demonstrates sinus bradycardia and a first-degree AV block (PR interval = 212 msec). The ECG also demonstrates a left axis deviation along with absent R-waves in precordial leads V1–V3. The ECG is consistent with this patient's old anteroseptal myocardial infarction.

## Clinical Course

In the hospital, serial troponins were all negative, and his ECG was stable. His antihypertensive medications were adjusted, and he had no further chest pain. A recent coronary angiogram showed patent saphenous vein grafts. He was discharged in stable condition.

# Right and Left Atrial Enlargement

Conceptually, it is important to remember that the right atrium is activated first because atrial depolarization begins in the SA node, located in the upper portion of the right atrium. The left atrium is activated second. Thus, the normal P-wave may be slightly notched, although the duration of the P-wave should not exceed 0.12 seconds. The initial portion of the P-wave represents right atrial depolarization, while the terminal portion of the P-wave represents left atrial depolarization (Surawicz and Knilans, 2008; Wagner and Strauss, 2014; Hancock et al., 2009).

As illustrated in Figure 1.5, right atrial enlargement (RAE) does not prolong the duration of the P-wave; rather, RAE is characterized by an increase in the amplitude of the initial P-wave deflection – and loss of the normal, rounded contour of the P-wave. In RAE, the P-wave becomes taller and "peaked," "gothic" or "steeple-like" (Surawicz and Knilans, 2008). RAE is best seen in leads II and III. To meet strict criteria for RAE, the P-waves should be at least 2.5 mm (small boxes) tall in the inferior limb leads (Surawicz and Knilans, 2008; Wagner and Strauss, 2014; Hancock et al., 2009).

In the past, RAE was called "P-pulmonale," a logical term since RAE is most often caused by chronic hypoxic lung disease in association with pulmonary hypertension and right ventricular enlargement (cor pulmonale). Commonly, RAE on the ECG is associated with right ventricular enlargement, right axis deviation and other features of chronic lung disease. RAE is also commonly caused by congenital heart disease (for example, tetralogy of Fallot or pulmonic stenosis), primary pulmonary hypertension and other causes of chronic hypoxemia.

In left atrial enlargement (LAE), the P-wave is classically broad and often notched ("double humped") in leads I and II (and sometimes aVL). The most important lead for diagnosing LAE is precordial lead V1, which is located on the right side of the chest, in an anterior position. LAE typically inscribes a biphasic P-wave in lead V1. The terminal portion of the P-wave represents the left atrium because the enlarged left atrium is depolarized later and for a longer time (Wagner and Strauss, 2014). The terminal portion of the P-wave is negative in the anterior-facing precordial lead V1. This is because the left atrium is normally located in a posterior position, almost abutting the esophagus.

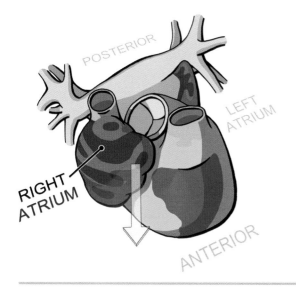
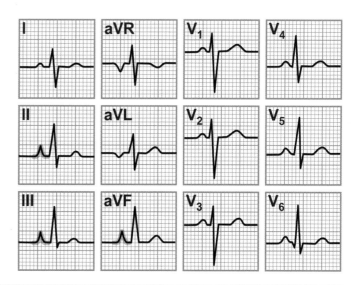
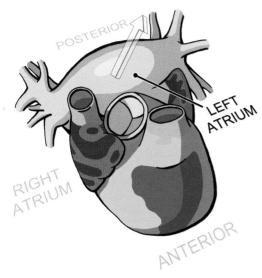
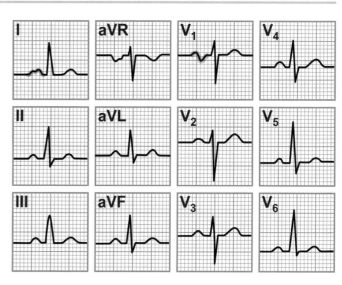

**Figure 1.5** Right and left atrial enlargement.

Historically, the pattern of broad and notched P-waves was referred to as "P-mitrale" because mitral stenosis was the most common etiology of left atrial enlargement.

Because atrial chamber enlargement cannot always be distinguished from atrial fibrosis, distention, strain or conduction delay, the less specific terms "right atrial abnormality" and "left atrial abnormality" are frequently used (Hancock et al., 2009; Wagner and Strauss, 2014). Bi-atrial enlargement can often be recognized on the ECG as a hybrid of the two patterns described previously. Examples of atrial enlargement are included in the self-study electrocardiograms.

## Left and Right Arm Lead Reversal

Reversal of the left and right arm leads is a relatively common technical error. It is easily detected by finding a negative P-QRS-T in lead I *in the presence of normal R-wave progression.* Thus, arm lead reversal represents a spurious cause of right axis deviation on the ECG. Not surprisingly, the P-QRS-T waves are all upright in aVR, a clear signal that the 12-lead is abnormal. That is, the patterns in lead I and lead aVR are reversed (Surawicz and Knilans, 2008; Wagner and Strauss, 2014; Rosen et al., 2014; Hancock et al., 2009; Kligfield et al., 2007; Harrigan et al., 2012).

Finding net negative P-waves and QRS complexes in lead I is sometimes referred to as the "lead 1 alerting sign" (ECGpedia.org, 2016). As a general rule, the most likely diagnosis is limb lead reversal. The "lead 1 alerting sign" (predominantly negative P-waves, QRS complexes and T-waves in lead I) is also seen with dextrocardia, but in dextrocardia there is loss of (actually, reverse) R-wave progression in the left chest leads. (See ECGs 1.5 and 1.6.)

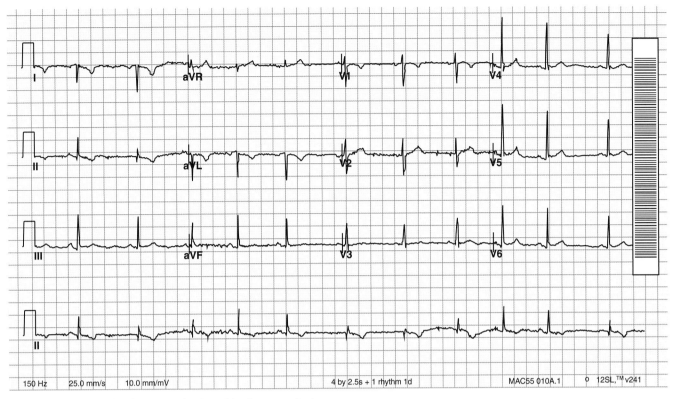

I  aVR  V1  V4

II  aVL  V2  V5

III  aVF  V3  V6

II

| 150 Hz | 25.0 mm/s | 10.0 mm/mV | | | 4 by 2.5s + 1 rhythm 1d | | MAC55 010A.1 | 0  12SL,™ v241 |

**ECG 1.5** A 28-year-old female presented with a mild asthma exacerbation.

## The Electrocardiogram

The P-wave, QRS complex and T-wave are inverted in lead I (the "alerting sign"); in lead aVR, the main QRS and T-wave deflections are positive. The ECG suggests a right axis deviation, but this too is an artifact. The right and left arm leads have been reversed. The precordial R-wave progression is normal, ruling out dextrocardia as the explanation for these abnormal patterns. This ECG was repeated 4 minutes later (after correcting the left and right arm lead cable connections), and it was completely normal.

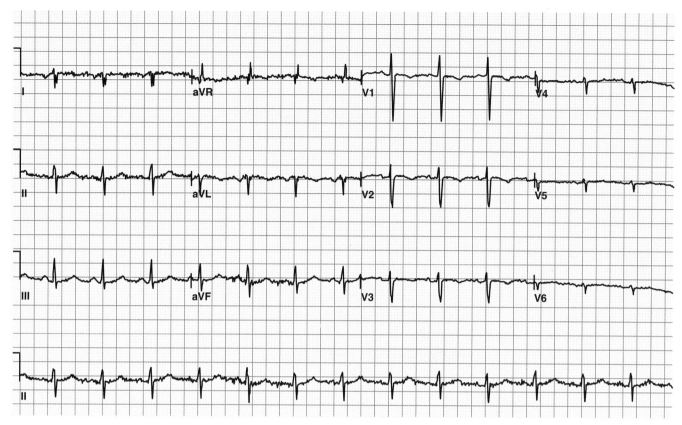

**ECG 1.6**   A 58-year-old woman with diabetes and hypertension presented with altered mentation and weakness.

## The Electrocardiogram

Her electrocardiogram is technically unsatisfactory; however, it demonstrates at least two findings: First, the P-wave and QRS complex are negative in lead I (the "lead 1 alerting sign"). Conversely, the main QRS deflection appears to be upright in lead aVR. This is also abnormal. Usually, the "lead 1 alerting sign" (and reversal of the expected patterns in leads I and aVR) indicates reversal of the right and left arm leads. But that is not the diagnosis in this case. She has complete absence of R-wave progression; in fact, the precordial leads show reverse R-wave progression. This suggests that she has dextrocardia. Her chest radiograph (Figure 1.6) confirms this diagnosis.

## Clinical Course

This patient was evaluated first for a possible stroke. However, her bedside glucose reading was 50, and she had complete resolution of her symptoms after receiving intravenous glucose.

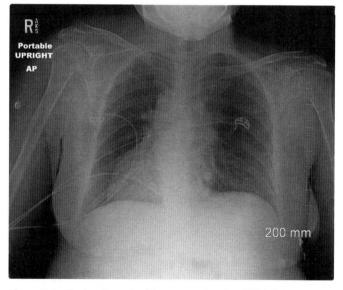

**Figure 1.6**   Chest radiograph of the same patient (see ECG 1.6).

# Self-Study Electrocardiograms

**Case 1.1** A 27-year-old female presented with abdominal pain.

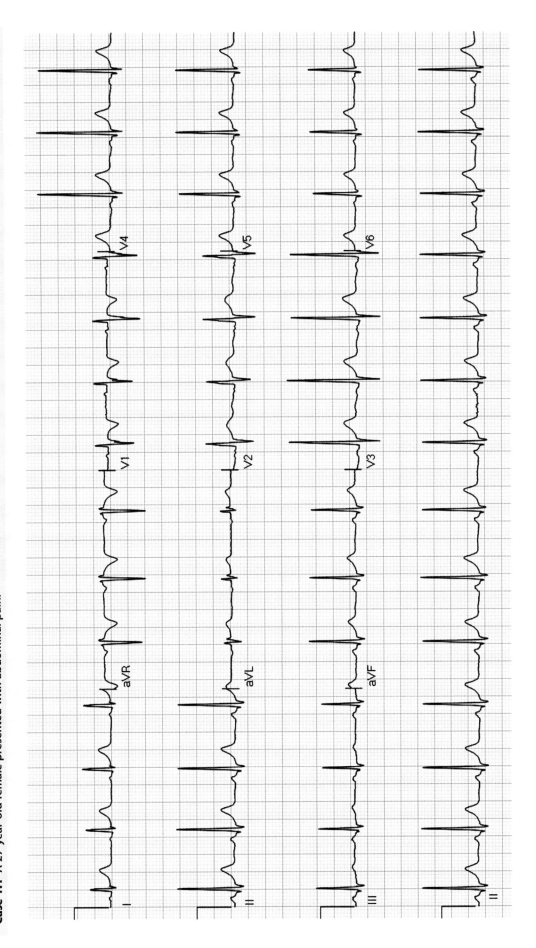

**Case 1.2** A 57-year-old man presented with intermittent episodes of left-sided chest pain.

Male

Room: S51

Opt:

| Vent. rate | 91 bpm |
| PR interval | 144 ms |
| QRS duration | 82 ms |
| QT/QTc | 366/450 ms |
| P-R-T axes | 58 35 41 |

Normal sinus rhythm
Possible Lateral infarct, age undetermined
Abnormal eCG

Technician: 26770
Test ind:

Reference

Order no.: 71673550
Unconfirmed

Y:

Y:

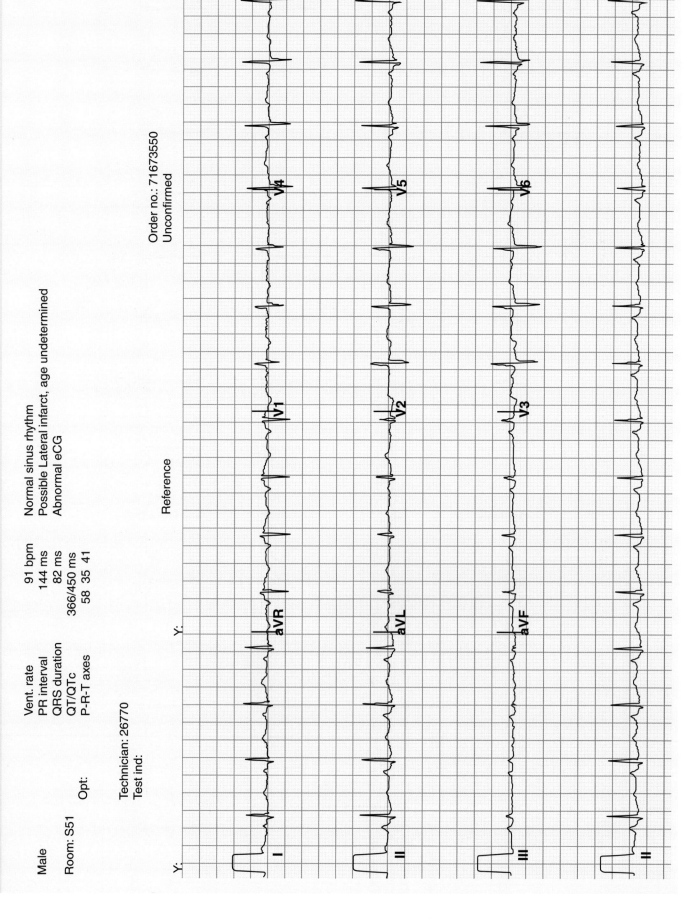

**Case 1.3** A 61-year-old man presented with fatigue and shortness of breath; he had moderate, bilateral rales on lung examination.

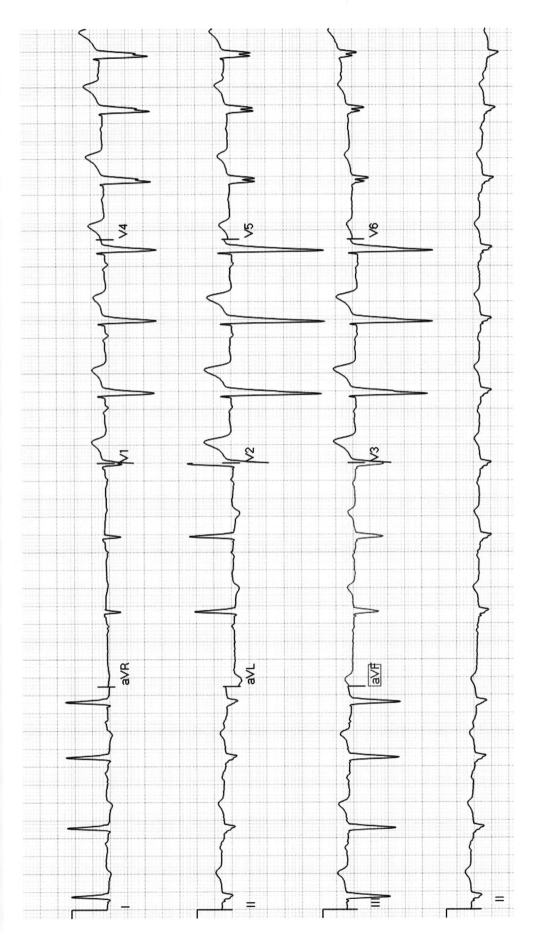

**Case 1.4** An 84-year-old female with a history of kidney stones, hypertension and coronary artery disease presented with fever and dysuria.

**Case 1.5** A 38-year-old man presented with sharp, right-sided, atypical chest pain. He denied chest pressure or shortness of breath, and he had no history of coronary artery or other heart disease.

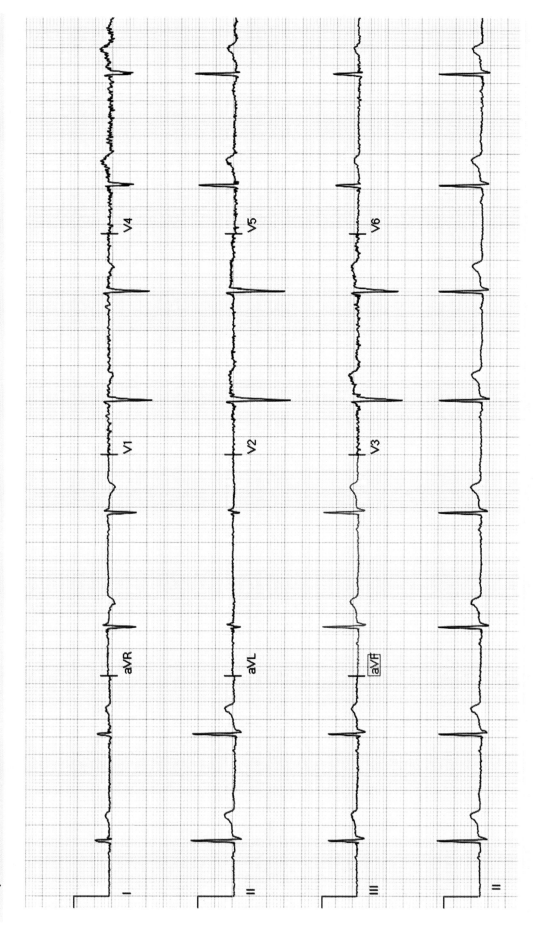

**Case 1.5 (Continued)** Same patient with proper placement of the chest leads (two interspaces lower).

**Case 1.6** A healthy 25-year-old man endorsed nausea, vomiting and crampy abdominal pain.

**Case 1.6 (Continued)** Same patient – prehospital rhythm strip.

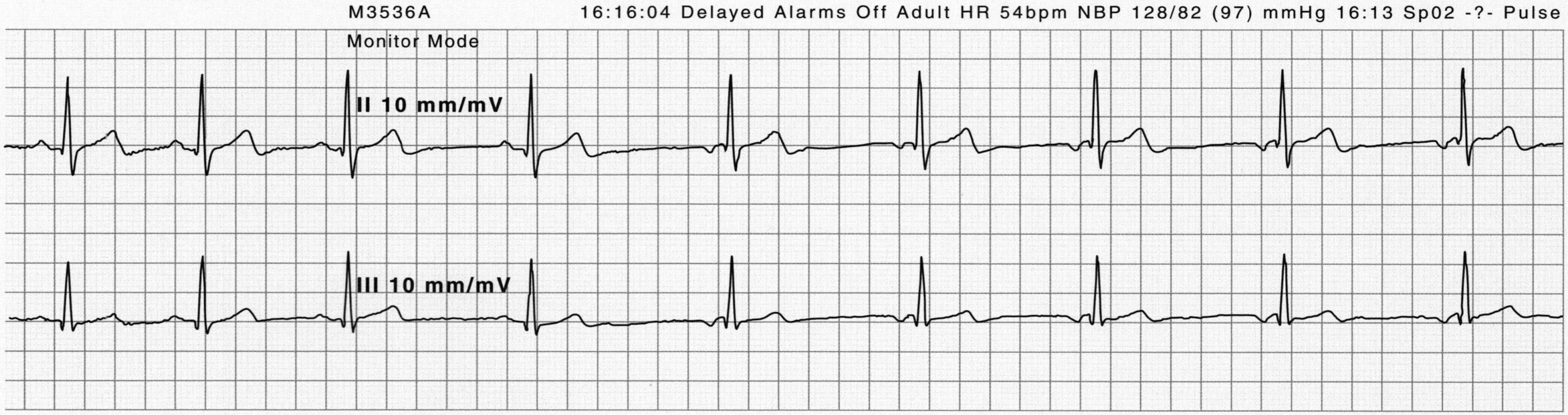

M3536A          16:16:04 Delayed Alarms Off Adult HR 54bpm NBP 128/82 (97) mmHg 16:13 SpO2 -?- Pulse

Monitor Mode

II 10 mm/mV

III 10 mm/mV

**Case 1.7** A 68-year-old female with a prior coronary artery bypass (revascularization of the left anterior descending and right coronary arteries) presented with gradually worsening palpitations. She also reported mild nausea and shortness of breath.

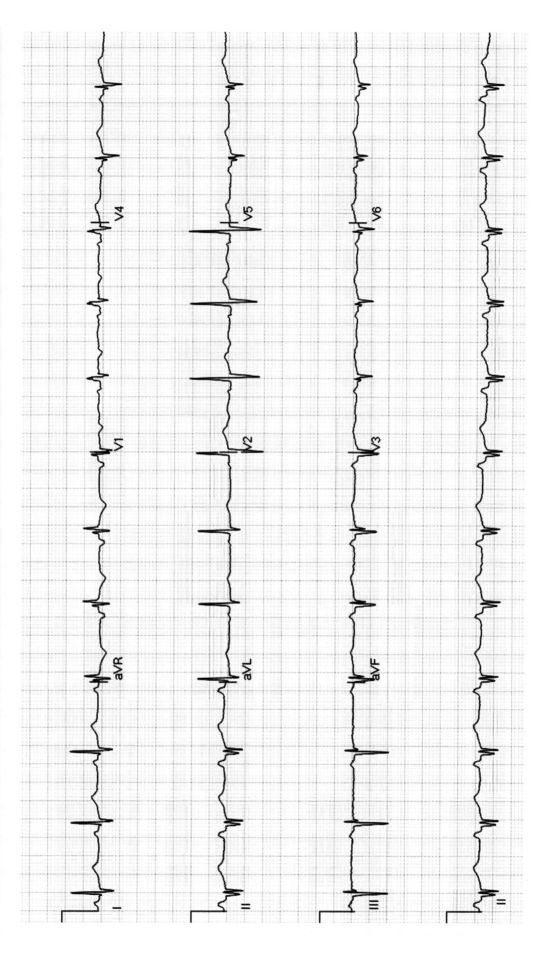

**Case 1.8** A 50-year-old female with a history of developmental delay, chronic aspiration and lung infections, and chronic obstructive pulmonary disease.

**Case 1.9** A 33-year-old female presented with shortness of breath. She had a history of severe cardiomyopathy and recently worsening hypotension, renal insufficiency and volume overload.

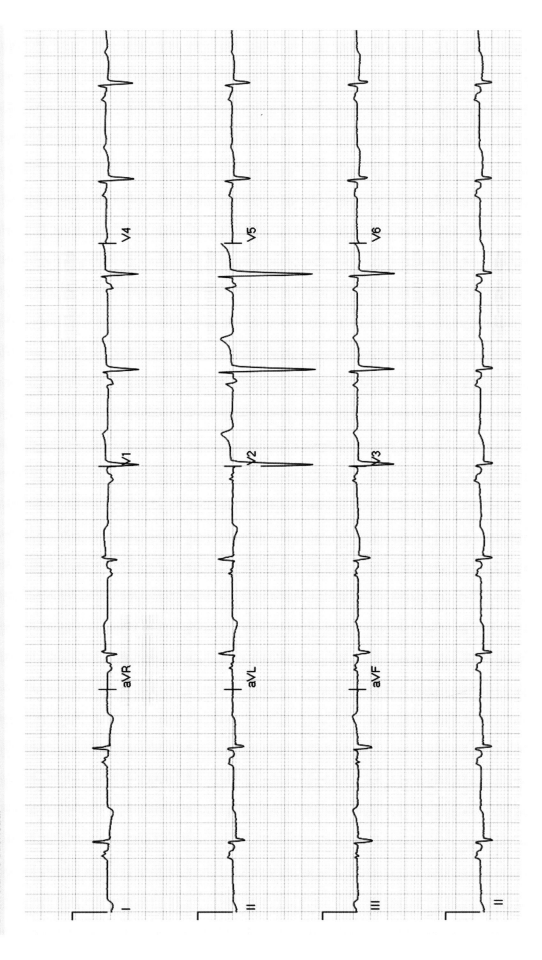

**Case 1.10** A 79-year-old female had a history of coronary artery disease and ischemic cardiomyopathy, congestive heart failure and chronic obstructive pulmonary disease. She presented with an exacerbation of her COPD.

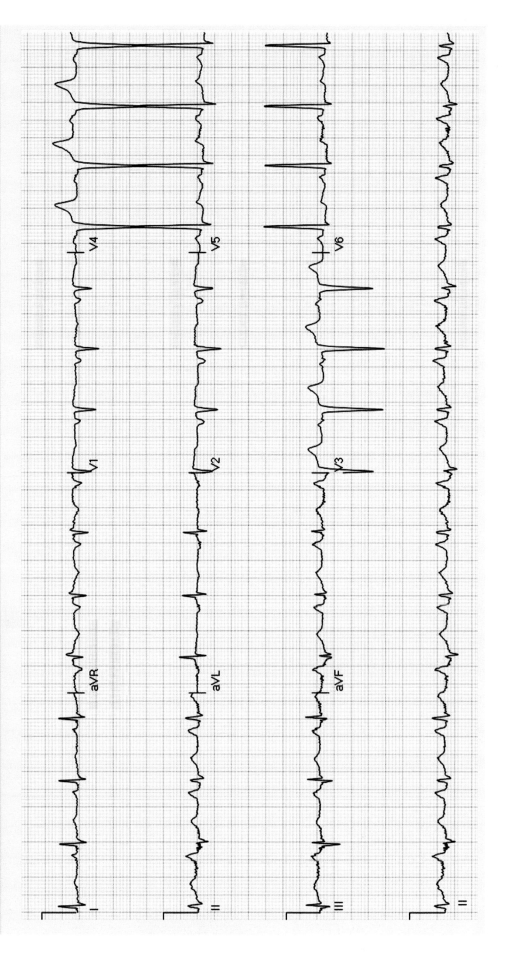

**Case 1.11** A 75-year-old female with diabetes, dementia and end-stage renal disease presented with a cough.

| Vent. rate | 68 | BPM | Normal sinus rhythm |
|---|---|---|---|
| PR interval | 174 | ms | Left axis deviation |
| QRS duration | 88 | ms | Abnormal ECG |
| QT/QTc | 422/448 | ms | When compared with ECG of |
| P-R-T axes | * -45 | 51 | Minimal criteria for Septal infarct are no longer Present |

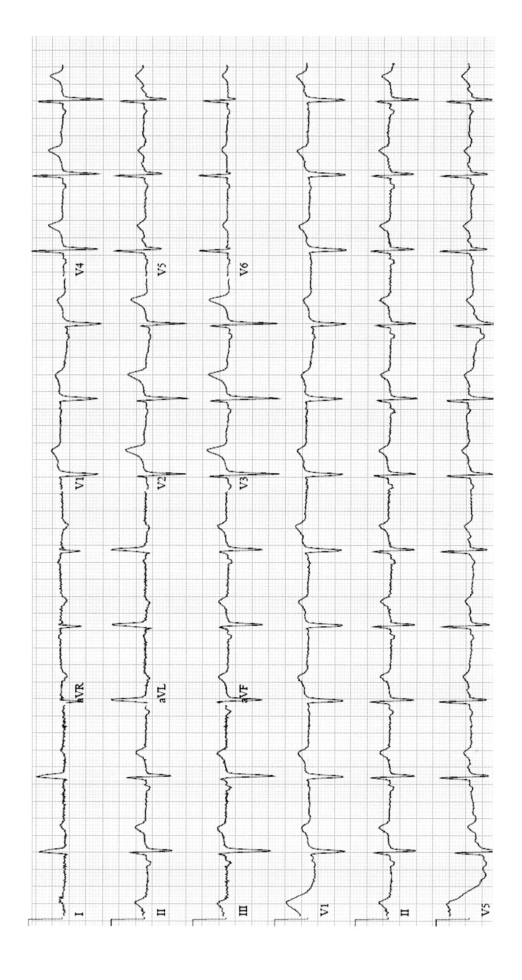

**Case 1.12** A 49-year-old woman presented with chest pain and cough. She reported a history of prior cocaine use, hypertension and hyperthyroidism.

**Case 1.13** A 60-year-old female with a history of non-insulin-dependent diabetes presented with chest pain that radiated to her back.

**Case 1.14** A 48-year-old man had a history of coronary artery disease and a recent myocardial infarction that was complicated by development of cardiogenic shock.

**Case 1.15** A 44-year-old man with frequent bouts of alcohol intoxication presented after a mechanical fall.

**Case 1.15 (Continued)** Same patient, now with the chest leads placed one interspace lower.

**Case 1.16** A 65-year-old man with a history of severe emphysema and a recent hospitalization for pneumonia presented with worsening shortness of breath, cough and purulent sputum. At home, he used 3 liters oxygen 24 hours per day. On presentation to the ED, he had marked hypoxemia and hypercarbia.

om: 0216
c: 100

| Vent. rate | 94 BPM |
| PR interval | 116 ms |
| QRS duration | 76 ms |
| QT/QTc | 332/415 ms |
| P-R-T axes | * 84  61 |

Normal sinus rhythm with short PR
Nonspecific ST abnormality
Abnormal ECG
When compared with ECG of 01-JAN-2012 05:26,
PVCs no longer present

Reviewed & Interpreted by:

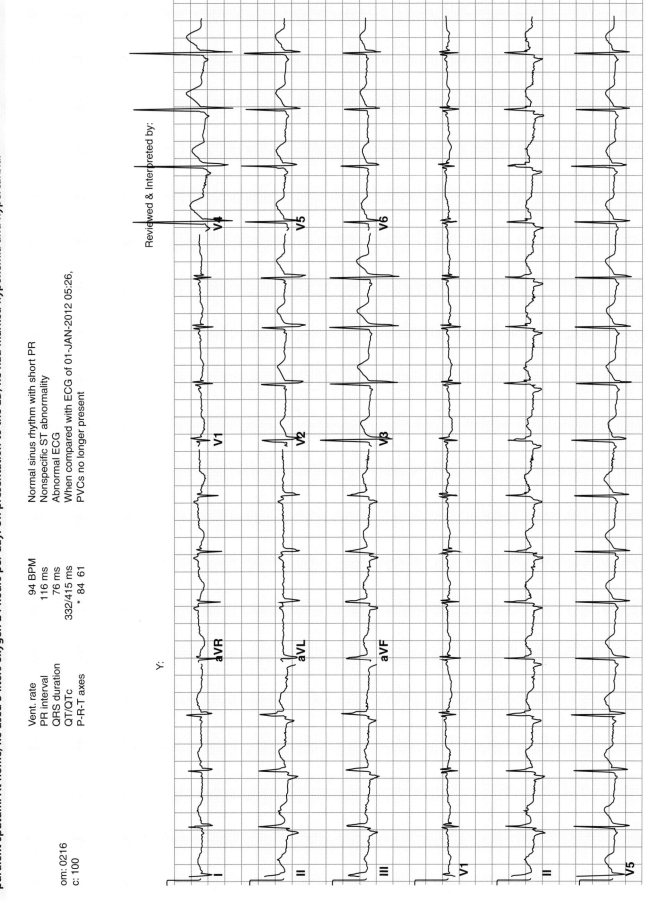

**Case 1.16 (Continued)** Same patient, 24 hours later.

# Self-Study Notes

## Case 1.1   A 27-year-old female presented with abdominal pain.

### The Electrocardiogram

This ECG is normal. Review the normal pathways of conduction (Figure 1.1) and the descriptions earlier in this chapter so that you can explain the following features of this normal electrocardiogram:

- The ECG demonstrates normal sinus rhythm; that is, there is a P-wave before each QRS and a QRS after each P-wave, *and the P-waves are upright in lead II and negative in lead aVR.* Not surprisingly, the P-wave in aVL is indistinct (flat) because atrial conduction is proceeding antegrade along an electrical pathway that is, more or less, perpendicular to the positive pole of aVL.
- There are tiny, narrow, "septal" Q-waves in the lateral leads (leads V5–V6) because the QRS complex (ventricular depolarization) begins with left-to-right activation of the septum. Often, septal Q-waves are also present in the high lateral leads (limb leads I and aVL).
- The small, leading R-wave in precordial lead V1 also reflects left-to-right septal depolarization. Lead V1 is called the "septal lead." The deep S-wave in V1 represents activation of the dominant left ventricle.
- There is a normal QRS axis and normal R-wave progression. The R-wave in V2 is actually abnormally tall; this is suggestive of an "early precordial transition," a common finding in some young, healthy individuals.

### Clinical Course

This patient's eventual diagnosis was a normal 15-week intra-uterine pregnancy and a urinary tract infection.

## Case 1.2   A 57-year-old man presented with intermittent episodes of left-sided chest pain.

### The Electrocardiogram

The computer misread this 12-lead electrocardiogram. First, there is no evidence of old lateral wall infarction; the small, narrow Q-waves in the left lateral leads (leads I, aVL, V5 and V6) are normal septal Q-waves, representing depolarization of the interventricular septum from left to right.

Second, no mention was made of the subtle ST-segment depressions in the right precordial leads (V1, V2, V3). As emphasized in Chapter 6, the ST-segments are commonly *elevated* in precordial leads V1–V3; therefore, even these minor ST-segment depressions are significant. In patients with chest pain, the differential diagnosis for anterior precordial ST-segment depressions includes anterior wall ischemia, posterior wall STEMI, electrolyte abnormalities and acute right heart strain (acute pulmonary hypertension, which may be due to pulmonary embolism). The R-wave in V1 is also unusually tall, which could represent posterior wall STEMI.

### Clinical Course

The patient had recurrent episodes of chest pain while in the emergency department. Posterior leads showed no ST-segment elevation. He was admitted for evaluation of his chest pain. On hospital day 2, he complained of more severe chest pain, and his electrocardiogram showed new T-wave inversions in the anterior precordial leads. He was taken to the catheterization laboratory, where a discrete, 90 percent mid-LAD stenosis was found. A drug-eluting stent was placed. All his troponin measurements were negative; his discharge diagnosis was obstructive LAD coronary artery disease and unstable angina. The ST-T-wave abnormalities in the anterior precordial leads completely resolved.

## Case 1.3   A 61-year-old man presented with fatigue and shortness of breath; he had moderate, bilateral rales on lung examination.

### The Electrocardiogram

This patient presented with symptoms and signs consistent with congestive heart failure, and the ECG provides a clear reason: extensive coronary artery disease, with prior myocardial infarctions involving the inferior wall and the anterolateral walls.

In the inferior leads, Q-waves are usually "pathologic" (indicative of prior myocardial infarction) if they are: >.04 seconds wide; at least 4 mm deep; or at least 25 percent as deep as the height of the R-wave. These deep and wide "QS" waves are unmistakable evidence of an inferior MI of "indeterminate age."

There is also clear evidence of a prior anterolateral myocardial infarction. There is poor R-wave progression; in fact, this ECG demonstrates reverse R-wave progression (a decline in R-wave amplitude after lead V2), which is specific for old anterior wall infarction (unless there is a precordial lead misplacement). Leads V5–V6 also demonstrate deep Q-waves. Left ventricular hypertrophy with QRS widening is also present along with left axis deviation and possible left atrial enlargement.

## Case 1.4   An 84-year-old female with a history of kidney stones, hypertension and coronary artery disease presented with fever and dysuria.

### The Electrocardiogram

On her ECG, the expected leading septal R-wave in V1 is "missing." Instead, there is only a QS pattern. Absence of the septal R-wave in V1 usually signals that the septum is dead (electrically silent); that is, this patient has sustained an old (indeterminate age) septal infarction. The deep Q-wave in lead V2 (actually, a QS pattern) confirms the diagnosis of remote anteroseptal MI. Sinus bradycardia is also present. (She was taking Carvedilol and Lisinopril for management of hypertension and heart failure post–myocardial infarction.)

### Clinical Course

The patient was found to have mild pyelonephritis along with stable coronary artery disease and hypertension

## Case 1.5   A 38-year-old man presented with sharp, right-sided, atypical chest pain. He denied chest pressure or shortness of breath, and he had no history of coronary artery or other heart disease.

### The Electrocardiogram

This patient's ECG is normal, except for sinus bradycardia and obvious poor R-wave progression, which could signify a prior anterior wall myocardial infarction. In fact, the computer reading stated, "Cannot rule out anterior infarct, age undetermined."

### Clinical Course

The emergency physician doubted that this patient had sustained a prior anterior wall infarction. Instead, the physician suspected abnormal lead placement – that is, that the precordial leads were applied too high on this patient's chest and were not properly "exploring" the left ventricle. The ECG was repeated 40 minutes later, with the precordial leads placed two interspaces lower.

## Case 1.5   Same patient with proper placement of the chest leads (two interspaces lower).

Normal R-wave progression is now magically restored. It is relatively common to detect poor R-wave progression in the absence of structural heart or lung disease. This occurs when the heart is relatively "vertical" or low-lying in the thorax and the exploring precordial leads are placed relatively high (for example, in patients with emphysema). In fact, this patient did not have heart disease. The precordial leads were erroneously placed at the level of the second or third, rather than the fourth, intercostal space.

## Case 1.6   A healthy 25-year-old man endorsed nausea, vomiting and crampy abdominal pain.

### The Electrocardiogram

Is this "normal sinus rhythm?" There is a P-wave before every QRS and a QRS after every P-wave. But it cannot be normal sinus rhythm. The P-waves are upright in lead aVR, which is distinctly abnormal. Also, the P-waves are inverted in leads II, III and aVF. Therefore, this is a junctional rhythm; that is, there is retrograde activation of the atria from a pacemaker originating in or near the AV node (or in the low atrium). The atrial depolarization wave spreads retrograde – *toward* the right shoulder (aVR) and *away from* the inferior leads.

In junctional rhythms the P-waves are always upright in aVR and negative in II, III and aVF. Commonly, retrograde atrial and antegrade ventricular depolarization occur simultaneously, and the inverted P-waves will be buried within the QRS complex. If the inverted P-waves precede the QRS complex, the PR interval is usually short (<.12 seconds). If there are negative P-waves before each QRS complex with a normal PR interval (≥ 12 msec), the rhythm is usually labeled an "ectopic atrial rhythm."

Because the P-waves in this tracing are also inverted in lead V6, some electrocardiographers classify this rhythm as "left atrial." ECG computer algorithms may code these rhythms as "junctional," "ectopic atrial" or "left atrial" rhythms, although the precise origin of the pacemaker may not always be clear from the surface ECG.[4]

The lead II rhythm strip in Case 1.6 is from the same patient, taken in the field prior to arrival in the emergency department.

## Case 1.6  Same patient – prehospital rhythm strip.

### The Electrocardiogram

At the start of the tracing, there is marked sinus bradycardia, probably a reflection of excessive parasympathetic tone. (His symptoms included nausea, vomiting and abdominal pain.) Then the sinus rate slows even further, and the lead II P-waves suddenly become inverted. This change signals the emergence of an "escape" junctional rhythm.

### Clinical Course

This patient did not require hospital admission, a pacemaker or any other intervention (except for intravenous fluids and anti-emetics).

## Case 1.7  A 68-year-old female with a prior coronary artery bypass (revascularization of the left anterior descending and right coronary arteries) presented with gradually worsening palpitations. She also reported mild nausea and shortness of breath.

### The Electrocardiogram

The ECG is consistent with all of the following: an old (indeterminate age) inferior wall myocardial infarction (deep and wide Q-waves in leads II, III and aVF, with no R-wave voltage); an old posterior wall infarction (abnormally tall and broad R-waves in the right precordial leads V1 and V2); and an old anterolateral infarction (decreasing R-wave amplitude across the anterior and lateral precordial leads).

### Clinical Course

Review of her health records revealed that her most recent cardiac event was an acute inferior and posterior wall STEMI 5 months prior to this ECG. Remarkably, after revascularization and intensive outpatient care, serial cardiac echocardiograms showed normal left ventricular function.

## Case 1.8  A 50-year-old female with a history of developmental delay, chronic aspiration and lung infections, and chronic obstructive pulmonary disease.

### The Electrocardiogram

The ECG demonstrates marked right atrial enlargement (RAE). As noted earlier, RAE does not prolong the duration of the P-wave; rather, RAE is characterized by an increase in the amplitude of the initial P-wave deflection – and loss of the normal, rounded contour of the P-wave. In RAE, the P-wave becomes taller and more "peaked," "gothic," or "steepled," best seen in leads II and III.

To meet criteria for RAE, the P-waves should be at least 2.5 mm tall in the inferior limb leads (as they are on this tracing). The inverted P-waves in lead aVR are also remarkably deep.

RAE is most often caused by chronic hypoxic lung disease in association with pulmonary hypertension and right ventricular enlargement (cor pulmonale). Commonly, RAE on the ECG is associated with right ventricular enlargement, right axis deviation and other features of chronic lung disease. (See Chapter 5, The Electrocardiography of Shortness of Breath.)

---

[4] Many electrocardiographers (and most computer algorithms) distinguish between junctional and "ectopic" atrial rhythms in the following manner: (a) if there is no visible P-wave, it is labeled "junctional"; (b) the rhythm is also labeled "junctional" if there is an inverted P-wave in the inferior leads and the PR interval is short (<.12 seconds); (c) the rhythm is also called "junctional" if the inverted P-wave is inscribed after the QRS; and (d) if there is an inverted P-wave in the inferior leads and the PR interval is normal (≥.12 seconds), it is called an ectopic atrial rhythm. An older term, "coronary sinus rhythm," is now seldom used (Mirowski, 1966; Surawicz and Knilans, 2008; Wagner and Strauss, 2014).

## Case 1.9 A 33-year-old female presented with shortness of breath. She had a history of severe cardiomyopathy and recently worsening hypotension, renal insufficiency and volume overload.

### The Electrocardiogram

The electrocardiogram shows sinus bradycardia, low limb lead voltage, left axis deviation, poor R-wave progression and ST-segment depressions and T-wave flattening in precordial leads V3–V6 and limb leads II and aVF. Also, there is left atrial enlargement (LAE). The P-wave is abnormally broad and notched ("double-humped") in leads I and II; the second hump represents the delayed depolarization of the enlarged left atrium (delayed because the enlarged left atrium is activated after the right atrium). V1 demonstrates a biphasic P-wave that is also consistent with LAE. As noted earlier in this chapter, depolarization of the left atrium occurs after the right atrium because the SA node resides in the right atrium. Enlargement of the left atrium is reflected in the terminal, negative deflection of the P-wave in V1; the left atrium inscribes a negative deflection in V1 because the left atrium is located in a posterior position; lead V1 is located on the right side of the chest in an anterior position.

## Case 1.10 A 79-year-old female had a history of coronary artery disease and ischemic cardiomyopathy, congestive heart failure and chronic obstructive pulmonary disease. She presented with an exacerbation of her COPD.

### The Electrocardiogram

This ECG demonstrates P-wave abnormalities indicative of both right and left atrial enlargement. Given her chronic cardiomyopathy and COPD, bi-atrial enlargement is not surprising. Her ECG also demonstrates changes of an old (or indeterminate age) anteroseptal myocardial infarction (absence of R-waves in leads V1–V4).

## Case 1.11 A 75-year-old female with diabetes, dementia and end-stage renal disease presented with a cough.

This cannot be normal sinus rhythm despite the computer's insistence. The P-waves are inverted in the inferior leads and are upright in lead aVR. This may be a junctional rhythm, or the pacemaker may be originating in the low atrium ("ectopic atrial rhythm"). The latter (ectopic atrial pacemaker) is more likely, since the PR interval is normal (0.17 sec). There is also a left axis deviation, likely due to left anterior fascicular block.

## Case 1.12 A 49-year-old woman presented with chest pain and cough. She reported a history of prior cocaine use, hypertension and hyperthyroidism.

### The Electrocardiogram

The electrocardiogram does not explain her chest pain, but there are several important and interesting features. First, there is a normal sinus rhythm, interrupted by frequent premature junctional beats (easily recognized by the inverted P-waves in lead II and the upright P-waves in aVR). The lead II rhythm strip ends with five beats of an accelerated junctional rhythm. The QT interval is also prolonged (the measured QTc is 515 msec). Finally, there is evidence of an anteroseptal myocardial infarction of indeterminate age (lack of R-waves in V1, V2 and V3).

## Case 1.13 A 60-year-old female with a history of non-insulin-dependent diabetes presented with chest pain that radiated to her back.

### The Electrocardiogram

The lead I "alerting sign" is present. That is, the P-wave, QRS and T-wave in lead I are all inverted when they should normally be upright. And the reverse pattern is seen in aVR, where the P wave, QRS and T-wave are upright instead of the usual inverted pattern. As highlighted earlier, the "lead 1 alerting sign" (with pattern reversal in limb leads I and aVR) usually indicates a reversal of the right and left arm leads. The other possible etiology is dextrocardia. In this case, the clue to the correct diagnosis is the disappearing QRS amplitude across the anterior and lateral precordial leads, signifying dextrocardia. These decreasing R-waves could also be explained by an old anterolateral myocardial infarction; however, this patient had no history of infarction.

**Case 1.13** Same patient: Her chest x-ray.

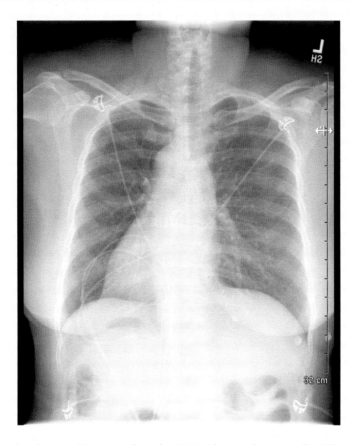

The chest x-ray helps explain the abnormalities noted on the ECG. There is dextrocardia. (The radiograph was repeated and compared with a prior study to confirm the correct orientation.) The chest x-ray also suggests a right-sided aortic arch. In addition, the stomach bubble is located beneath the right hemidiaphragm, and this, along with the elevated left hemidiaphragm, helps confirm that she has complete situs inversus.

### Clinical Course

She was admitted for observation and serial ECGs and troponin levels, which remained normal. There was no indication of an acute coronary syndrome. A CT angiogram of the chest showed no abnormality of the thoracic aorta. However, her CT and chest x-ray (shown in Case 1.13) confirmed the diagnosis of dextrocardia and complete situs inversus.

## Case 1.14  A 48-year-old man had a history of coronary artery disease and a recent myocardial infarction that was complicated by development of cardiogenic shock.

### The Electrocardiogram

This patient sustained a myocardial infarction about 1 week prior to this tracing. There is evidence of a right bundle branch block plus poor R-wave progression due to the recent anterior wall and septal infarction. The familiar rSR' pattern of the right bundle branch block is present in V1, with one exception: the initial R-wave is missing, a consequence of the earlier septal infarction.

Acute anteroseptal infarctions are frequently complicated by development of right bundle branch block, and it is not uncommon to see evidence of septal infarction and a bundle branch block on a single ECG tracing. This is not surprising, since the bundle branches course along the edges of the interventricular septum. As explained in Chapter 3, this pattern is usually caused by an obstructing thrombus in the left anterior descending artery (LAD) proximal to the septal perforator branches.

## Case 1.15 A 44-year-old man with frequent bouts of alcohol intoxication presented after a mechanical fall.

### The Electrocardiogram

The computer interpretation stated "sinus tachycardia, with anteroseptal infarct, age undetermined." Indeed, an old anteroseptal infarct is possible because there are QS complexes in leads V1–V3 with almost no R-wave progression. However, this patient was young without any history of coronary artery disease. Other causes of poor R-wave progression (for example, left ventricular hypertrophy, dextrocardia or emphysema) do not seem likely. As noted earlier, one other common explanation for "poor R-wave progression" is an error in precordial lead placement, where the recording electrodes are placed too high on the chest, so that they fail to record depolarization of the mass of the left ventricle.

### Clinical Course

This ECG was repeated 14 minutes later with the precordial leads placed one interspace lower; as shown in the follow-up tracing, the "evidence" of old anterior wall myocardial infarction has disappeared.

## Case 1.15 Same patient, now with the chest leads placed one interspace lower.

In this tracing, the normal R-wave progression has suddenly reappeared (although the lead V1 R-wave is still absent). The computer reading changed and affirmed: "Sinus tachycardia, when compared with ECG of [14 minutes ago], criteria for anterior infarct are no longer present."

## Case 1.16 A 65-year-old man with a history of severe emphysema and a recent hospitalization for pneumonia presented with worsening shortness of breath, cough and purulent sputum. At home, he used 3 liters oxygen 24 hours per day. On presentation to the ED, he had marked hypoxemia and hypercarbia.

### The Electrocardiogram

Of course, the computer algorithm is not correct. This is not normal sinus rhythm. The P-waves are inverted in the inferior leads (with a short PR interval measured at 116 msec), and the P-wave is upright in aVR. Therefore, this is a junctional rhythm. The QRS axis is also abnormally rightward for a 65-year-old patient; while this should raise the suspicion of acute right heart strain (acute pulmonary thromboembolism), it is also consistent with chronic right ventricular enlargement (cor pulmonale) in this patient with severe COPD.

### Clinical Course

In fact, right axis deviation (RAD) was seen on numerous previous ECG tracings. Another interesting finding: the amplitude of the (inverted) P-waves seems unusually large, possibly indicating right atrial enlargement. RAE was confirmed on an ECG taken 24 hours later, when his rhythm had converted to a sinus tachycardia.

## Case 1.16 Same patient, 24 hours later.

### The Electrocardiogram

The patient now has a sinus tachycardia with a short PR interval. The right axis deviation persists. The tall, steepled P-waves in leads II and III, accompanied by an inverted P-wave in lead aVL, suggest RAE (P-pulmonale). The technical criterion for diagnosing "P-pulmonale" is a P-wave in leads II and III that exceeds 2.5 mm in amplitude.

### Clinical Course

The patient's hemodynamic and respiratory status stabilized in the hospital, and he was discharged home to continue his regimen of supplemental oxygen, bronchodilators and other medications.

# References

ECGpedia.org. www.google.com/search?hl=
en&site=imghp&tbm=isch&source=hp&
biw=1280&bih=923&q=ecgpedia+limb+lea
d+reversal&oq=ecgpedia+limb+lead+rever
sal&gs_l=img.12 … 1824.9990.0.12263.27.6.
0.21.21.0.97.439.6.6.0 …. 0 … 1ac.1.64.im
g..0.10.444.DZuGwkgvWhI#imgrc=S92XY
HFxQrfueM%3A. Accessed April 11, 2016.

Gorgels A. P. M., Engelen D. J. M., Wellens
H. J. J. Lead aVR, a mostly ignored but very
valuable lead in clinical electrocardiography.
*J Am Col Cardiol.* 2001; **38**:1355–1356.

Hancock E. W., Deal B. J., Mirvis D. M. et al.
AHA/ACCF/HRS Recommendations for the
standardization and interpretation of the
electrocardiogram. Part V: Electrocardiogram
changes associated with cardiac chamber
hypertrophy. A scientific statement from the
American heart Association
Electrocardiography and Arrhythmias
Committee, Council on Clinical Cardiology;
the American College of Cardiology

Foundation; and the Heart Rhythm Society. *J
Am Coll Cardiol.* 2009; **53**:992–1002.

Harrigan R. A., Chan T. C., Brady W. J.
Electrocardiographic electrode
misplacement, misconnection and artifact. *J
Emerg Med.* 2012. **43**:1038–1044.

Kligfield P., Gettes L. S., Bailey J. J. et al.
Recommendations for the standardization
and interpretation of the electrocardiogram.
Part I: The electrocardiogram and its
technology. A scientific statement from the
American Heart Association
Electrocardiography and Arrhythmias
Committee, Council on Clinical Cardiology;
the American College of Cardiology
Foundation; and the Heart Rhythm Society. *J
Am Coll Cardiol.* 2007; 491109–491127.

Mirowski M. Left atrial rhythm. Diagnostic
criteria and differentiation from nodal
arrhythmia. *Am J Cardiol.* 1966; **17**:203–210.

Rosen A. V., Koppikar S., Shaw C.,
Baranchuk A. Common ECG lead placement
errors. Part 1: Limb lead reversals. In *J Med*

*Students.* 2014; **2**:92–98. Part 2: Precordial
misplacements. Limb lead reversals. In *J Med
Students.* 2014; 2:99–103.

Surawicz B., Knilans T. K. *Chou's
electrocardiography in clinical practice.* Sixth
edition. Philadelphia, PA: Elsevier Saunders,
2008.

Thygesen K., Alpert J. S., Jaffe A. S. et al. Third
universal definition of myocardial infarction. *J
Am Coll Cardiol.* 2012;**60**:1581–1598.

University of Minnesota. Atlas of human
cardiac anatomy. Conduction system tutorial.
2014. www.vhlab.umn.edu/atlas/conduction-s
ystem-tutorial/overview-of-cardiac-conduc
tion.shtml. Accessed May 24, 2016.

Wagner G. S., Strauss D. G. *Marriott's
Practical Electrocardiography.* Twelfth
edition. Philadelphia, PA: Lippincott,
Williams & Wilkins, 2014.

Wellens H. J. J., Conover M. *The ECG in
emergency decision-making.* Second edition.
St Louis, MO: Elsevier, Inc., 2008.

# Inferior Wall Myocardial Infarction

Inferior wall myocardial infarction (IMI) is the most common ST-elevation myocardial infarction (STEMI). The classic features of inferior STEMI are unmistakable:

- The hallmark is the presence of ST-segment elevations in the "inferior limb leads" – II, III and aVF.
- In most cases, there is reciprocal ST-segment depression in the high lateral (or "superior") leads – I and, especially, aVL. As illustrated in Chapter 1, the positive pole of lead aVL is electrically opposite to lead III.
- In the earliest hours of acute IMI, the ST-segments in II, III and aVF may be normal or near-normal, but frequently, there is ST-segment depression in aVL. Thus, ST-segment depression in AVL constitutes a critical "early warning" sign of acute inferior wall STEMI.
- In most cases of inferior wall STEMI (approximately 80 percent), the culprit event is an acute occlusion of the right coronary artery (RCA). In the remaining cases, the clotted vessel is the left circumflex artery (LCA). RCA (rather than LCA) occlusion is more likely if the ST-segment is elevated to a greater extent in lead III than in lead II, the ST-segment is markedly depressed ($\geq$ 1mm) in lead aVL, or there is electrocardiographic evidence of right ventricular myocardial infarction (RVMI). Lead III is the most sensitive lead for the diagnosis of inferior wall STEMI caused by RCA occlusion.
- ST-segment depressions in aVL are sometimes absent in acute inferior wall STEMI, if the culprit occluded artery is the LCA; in fact, the ST-segments in aVL may even be slightly elevated if occlusion of the LCA has caused not only the inferior STEMI but also a *high lateral infarction*.

- In 90 percent of patients, there is a "dominant" RCA that supplies branches to the anterior and lateral walls of the right ventricle, the AV-node and the posterior left ventricular wall. Thus, acute inferior wall STEMI is often complicated by one or more of the *big three:* right ventricular myocardial infarction (RVMI), AV nodal block or concomitant infarction of the posterior wall. ST-segment depressions in precordial leads V1–V3 are highly suggestive of extension of the STEMI to the posterior wall.
- Although inferior STEMI has a more favorable prognosis than anterior wall STEMI, the presence of RVMI, AV block or posterior wall extension helps define a high-risk subset of IMI patients; patients with one or more of these complications have a higher incidence of cardiogenic shock, ventricular and atrial arrhythmias and in-hospital and late mortality.
- The right-sided leads (V4 R and V1) should be examined carefully in every patient who presents with acute inferior wall STEMI. ST-elevations in leads V4 R or V1 signify that an RVMI is present. These ECG findings: also put the culprit lesion in the proximal RCA, before the take-off the right ventricular (acute marginal) branches; identify a subset of inferior STEMI patients at heightened risk of AV block, atrial and ventricular arrhythmias, shock and death; and help avoid complications during treatment.

## Inferior Wall ST-Elevation Myocardial Infarction

ECGs 2.1 and 2.2 are typical 12-lead electrocardiograms from patients with acute inferior wall STEMIs.

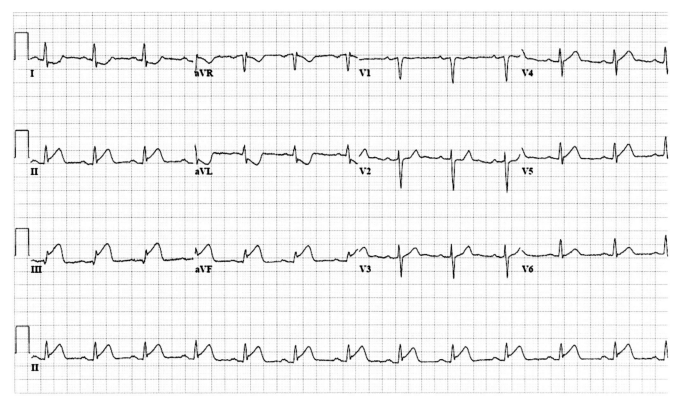

**ECG 2.1** A 37-year-old man presented with chest pain and diaphoresis.

## The Electrocardiogram

The ECG shows classic features of an inferior STEMI. ST-segment elevations are present in II, III and aVF. There is obvious reciprocal ST-segment depression in the high lateral leads (I and aVL). The ST-segment elevations are much greater in III than in II; as discussed in more detail later, this helps identify the right coronary artery (RCA) as the likely infarct-related vessel. ST-segment elevation in lead III > lead II also increases the probability that a right ventricular infarction is present.

The elevated ST-segments, often called epicardial "currents of injury," reflect transmural ischemia that extends from the endocardial to the epicardial surface (Birnbaum, Nikus et al., 2014; Wagner et al., 2009). Most importantly, ST-segment elevations announce the onset of a "STEMI" and the need for emergent reperfusion therapy. Like other acute coronary syndromes, a STEMI is usually caused by "an occlusive blood clot that is formed on a ruptured atherosclerotic plaque in an epicardial coronary artery" (Birnbaum, Wilson et al. 2014).

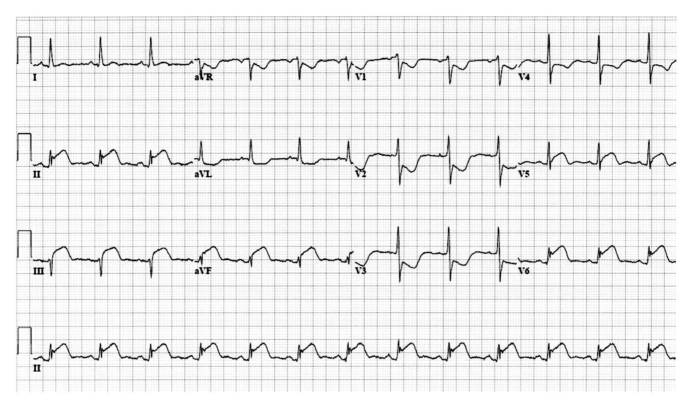

**ECG 2.2** A 56-year-old man presented at 3:45 A.M. with nausea and epigastric pain.

## The Electrocardiogram

The ECG demonstrates an acute inferior wall STEMI. Reciprocal ST-segment depression is present in lead aVL. The ST-segments are also elevated in the lateral precordial leads (V5–V6), indicating extension of the infarct to the lateral wall. As discussed later in this chapter, involvement of the lateral leads (V5–V6) in addition to the inferior leads is a marker of a larger infarct territory.

Importantly, there are marked ST-segment depressions in the right precordial leads (V1–V3); this indicates extension of the infarction to the posterior wall (also a marker of a larger infarct territory). Right-sided leads were negative for right ventricular infarction. The proper reading of this 12-lead ECG is "acute inferior, posterior and lateral STEMI."

## Identifying the Infarct Artery

Acute inferior wall STEMI is usually caused by occlusion of the right coronary artery (RCA, 80 percent) or left circumflex artery (LCA, 20 percent). Identifying the infarct-related artery may be of clinical importance, as RVMI and heart block are more likely in RCA occlusions.

Although the 12-lead ECG is an imperfect tool to identify the infarct-related artery, there are some helpful clues (Kontos et al., 1997; Chia et al., 2000; Zimetbaum et al., 1998; Zimetbaum and Josephson, 2003; Surawicz and Knilans, 2008; Wang et al., 2009; Wagner et al., 2009).

## RCA Occlusion More Likely

The RCA perfuses the inferior and posteromedial portions of the left ventricle along with the right ventricle (see Figure 2.1; Wellens and Conover, 2006). This is the territory of limb lead III. Therefore:

- If the ST-segment elevation is higher in lead III than in lead II, a proximal RCA clot is more likely. This is expected, as the positive pole of lead III is oriented to the *right inferior* segment of the heart (see Figure 2.1 and also Chapter 1). In contrast, lead II monitors the *left inferior* segment and is more influenced by LCA occlusions.
- If the ST-segment depression in lead aVL is ≥ 1.0 mm, a proximal RCA clot is more likely. This is also understandable: in a RCA occlusion, the electrical vector of the injury current is directed toward the right side of the heart – that is, toward lead III and away from lead aVL. Leads III and aVL are near-electrical opposites.

These same ECG findings (ST-segment elevations in III > II and marked ST-segment depressions in aVL) are also strong predictors of a concomitant RVMI.

## LCA Occlusion More Likely

The LCA primarily perfuses the posterior and left lateral walls of the left ventricle, which is the segment directly monitored by inferior limb lead II (see Figure 2.1; Wellens and Conover, 2006). There are three ECG clues that suggest LCA occlusion in patients presenting with an acute inferior wall STEMI:

- LCA occlusion is more likely if the ST-segment elevations are equal or greater in lead II than in lead III (since the injury current is directed in a more leftward and posterior direction).
- LCA occlusion is more likely if the ST-segment is isoelectric, or even elevated, in lead aVL. In the setting of IMI, this suggests an occlusion of the LCA because the injury current is directed more leftward and posterior (toward, not away from, aVL). The LCA supplies the high lateral region, typically via one or more obtuse marginal (OM) branches. Elevation of the ST-segment in aVL usually signifies an acute inferior and high lateral STEMI. Here, the ST-segment elevation in lead aVL may cancel out the expected ST-segment depression in this lead.
- In some studies, the presence of concomitant ST-segment elevations in leads V5–V6 (signifying lateral wall involvement) or ST-segment depressions in leads V1–V4 (signifying posterior wall involvement) moderately increases the likelihood that the LCA is the culprit vessel (Surawicz and Knilans, 2008; Assali et al., 1998). Similarly, ST-segment depressions (> 1 mm) in lead aVR may be more common in inferior STEMIs caused by obstruction of the LCA (Tamura, 2014; Vales et al., 2011). Lead aVR is electrically opposite to lead II (see Chapter 1).

**Figure 2.1** Predicting the infarct-related artery in patients with acute inferior wall STEMI.

Right coronary a. (RCA)
Left circumflex a. (LCX)
Posterior descending a. (PDA)
Left anterior descending a. (LAD)

III     II     aVF

The following ECGs demonstrate acute inferior wall STEMIs caused by RCA occlusion (ECG 2.3) or LCA occlusion (ECG 2.4).

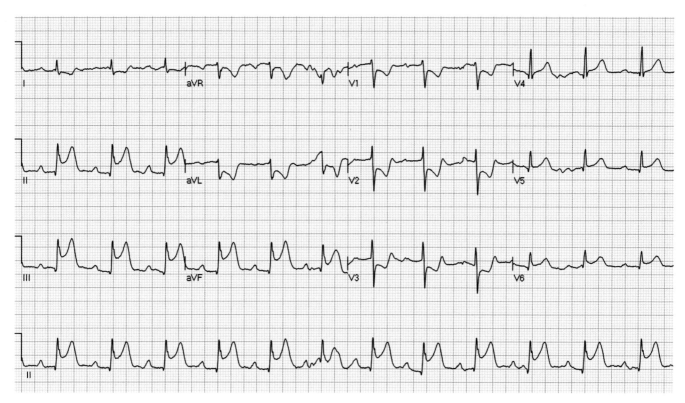

**ECG 2.3**   A 49-year-old female collapsed in her bathroom. On arrival in the emergency department, she was lethargic and mildly hypotensive.

## The Electrocardiogram

The ECG demonstrates an acute inferior wall STEMI, with extension to the posterior and lateral left ventricular wall. First-degree AV block is present. The ST-segment elevations are larger in lead III than in lead II. There is also marked ST-segment depression in aVL. Thus, the culprit infarct-related artery is almost certainly the RCA, based only on this 12-lead ECG. Right-sided leads were obtained (see next ECG).

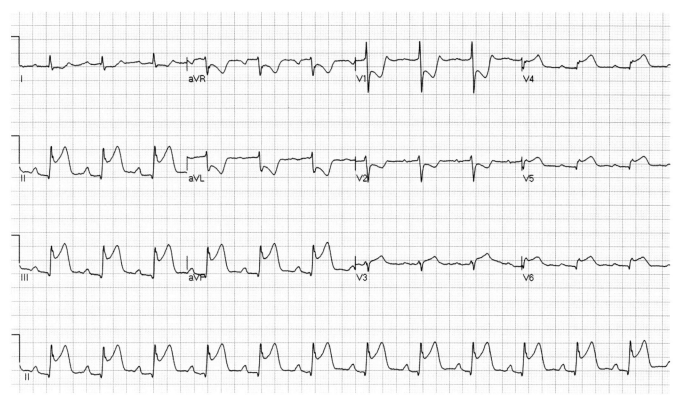

**ECG 2.3** Same patient (right-sided leads).

## The Electrocardiogram

Although not marked by the computer, these are the right-sided leads. The lack of normal R-wave progression identifies this as a right-sided tracing.

The right-sided leads are positive for right ventricular infarction: V4 R demonstrates marked ST-segment elevation. This ECG finding alone puts the culprit lesion in the RCA, before the take-off the right ventricular (acute marginal) branches. ST-segment elevation in V4 R also identifies a subset of inferior STEMI patients at heightened risk of AV block, atrial and ventricular arrhythmias, shock and death. In fact, each of the *big three* complications of IMI (RVMI, posterior wall extension and AV block) is present in this patient.

## Clinical Course

Her initial troponin was normal (0.01) but later peaked at 45.5. She underwent emergency coronary angiography, which revealed a large, dominant RCA. According to the cath report, "There was a 99 percent eccentric, thrombotic stenosis in the proximal RCA that was the culprit vessel for the patient's acute presentation." Not surprisingly, an echocardiogram in this patient demonstrated inferior and lateral wall hypokinesis and hypokinesis of the right ventricle.

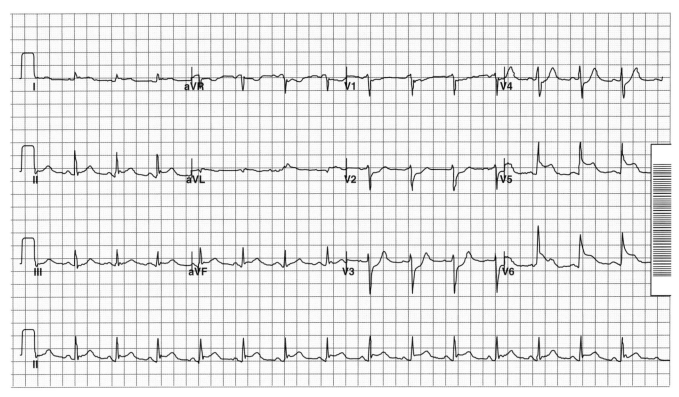

**ECG 2.4** A 59-year-old female, previously healthy except for hypercholesterolemia, presented after a single episode of chest pain accompanied by dyspnea and slight discomfort in both arms. After calling 911, she had a syncopal episode. In the presence of paramedics, she had a VF arrest. After defibrillation, she was hemodynamically stable and alert.

## The Electrocardiogram

The ECG demonstrates an acute inferior and lateral wall STEMI. The ST-segment depressions in V1–V4 indicate extension of the STEMI to the posterior wall. There are several clues that suggest a left circumflex artery (LCA) occlusion. First, the ST-segments are more elevated in lead II than in lead III. In addition, the ST-segments are not depressed in the high lateral leads (I and aVL) – in fact, the ST-segments are slightly elevated in these leads. In the setting of an acute inferior wall STEMI, ST-segment elevation in leads I and aVL often indicates that the LCA or one of its branches is obstructed. Pronounced ST-segment elevations are also present in the lateral precordial leads (V5–V6), which is sometimes a marker of LCA occlusion.

## Clinical Course

On angiography, she had a 99 percent occlusion of the proximal obtuse marginal (OM), a large branch of the LCA. The LAD and RCA were not obstructed. She recovered uneventfully after placement of an LCA stent. Her initial troponin level was 0.06; later, the troponin peaked at 114.

# Early Warning Signs: Subtle Presentations of Inferior STEMI

Sometimes, in the earliest hours of acute inferior STEMI, the ST-segments in the inferior leads are normal or almost normal. There are no "tombstone" ST-segment elevations. Traditional "cath lab activation criteria" are not met. The computer algorithm reassures us that the ECG is normal. And we are left to wonder: Is the ECG abnormal? Are the minor ST-elevations or ST-segment straightening in lead III important? Should we activate the cath lab?

Even in the face of ambiguity, the astute clinician will recognize two important early warning signs of impending inferior wall STEMI:

## 1. The ST-segments in II, III or aVF may be straightened, even if they are not noticeably elevated.

One of the earliest changes in the evolution of acute STEMI is a simple straightening of the ST-segment. That is, the ST-segment loses its normal upward concavity. See Figure 2.2.

## 2. There is often ST-segment depression in lead aVL.

ST-segment depression in aVL and lead I may occur early in the evolution of inferior wall STEMI, even hours before there is any noticeable ST-elevation in leads II, III or aVF (Hassen et al., 2014; Birnbaum et al., 1993; Turhan et al., 2003; Bischof et al., 2016).

In 1993, Birnbaum and colleagues published an important review of 107 consecutive patients with evolving inferior wall myocardial infarctions (Birnbaum et al., 1993). They concluded:

> ST depression in aVL . . . is found in the majority of patients with evolving inferior wall myocardial infarction and . . . may be the sole electrocardiographic sign of the inferior infarction . . . Transient ST depression in aVL is a sensitive, early electrocardiographic sign of acute inferior wall myocardial infarction.

Marriott made a similar point (Marriott, 1997):

> Whenever a change resembling this is found in aVL in a patient under suspicion of angina pain, that patient should be kept under wraps until the diagnosis is clarified.

To summarize: leads III and aVL, which are electrical near-opposites, are the most critical leads for the diagnosis of early or subtle inferior wall STEMIs.

- Often, in the early phases of inferior STEMI, the only abnormality may be ST-segment straightening or minimal ST-elevation in lead III.
- ST-segment depression in aVL (and sometimes in lead I) is the other critical "early warning" sign of acute inferior wall STEMI.

Therefore, carefully examine lead aVL in all patients where STEMI is a possibility. Lead aVL can help us notice and interpret subtle and ambiguous ST-segment abnormalities in the inferior leads. And importantly, when there are ST-elevations involving the inferior or the anterior leads (or both), the finding of ST-segment depressions in lead aVL eliminates any consideration that these ST-elevations are the result of pericarditis or benign early repolarization (Bischof et al., 2016).

Examine ECGs 2.5 and 2.6 for clear examples of Birnbaum's and Marriott's lesson. Each of these tracings is diagnostic of acute inferior wall STEMI. However, the ST-segment elevations in the inferior leads are subtle. In each case, the diagnosis of acute inferior wall STEMI was missed or delayed. But each case also demonstrates clear ST-segment depression in aVL, which should have alerted the clinicians to the correct diagnosis.

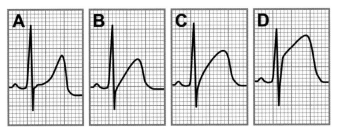

**Figure 2.2** ST-segment straightening in the early evolution of a STEMI. In Panel A, the ST-segment has a normal configuration. Panel B shows straightening of the ST-segment; even without noticeable elevation of the ST-segment, an acute STEMI may be present. Often, in the earliest stages of an acute STEMI, there is little ST-segment elevation. The only clues to an evolving STEMI may be ST-segment straightening, along with reciprocal ST-segment depressions in one or more opposite-facing leads. These are "don't-miss" clues; we can't wait for "tombstone" ST-segment elevations to appear (Panels C and D).

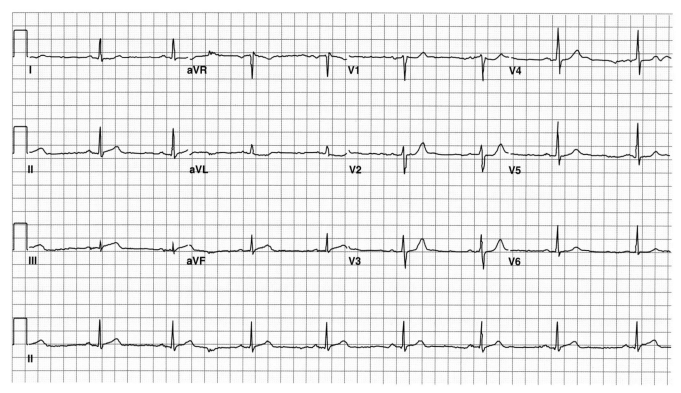

**ECG 2.5** A 55-year-old man presented with intermittent chest pain and mild dyspnea. The computer reading was "Sinus bradycardia, otherwise normal ECG." He was admitted for "Possible Acute Coronary Syndrome, Rule-out M.I."

## The Electrocardiogram

The clinicians did not immediately recognize the early inferior wall STEMI, probably because the ST-segment in lead III is barely elevated. The computer reading was also reassuring. However, upon careful inspection, there is straightening of the ST-segments in leads III (and also in leads II and aVF); the normal, upward concavity in these leads is gone. There is also subtle ST-segment elevation in III and aVF. If, at the bedside, there was any doubt about these abnormalities, lead aVL provides a telltale clue: the ST-segment is depressed. While at first glance the sagging ST-segment in aVL may seem minor, it is actually quite pronounced when considered in light of the very small R-wave in the same lead. *The disproportionate ST-depression in aVL provides proof that the subtle ST-segment abnormalities in the inferior leads represent a true, "actionable" STEMI.*

The computer cannot make this diagnosis, but we have to. At the very least, the patient needs a repeat ECG within 10–15 minutes. In the words of Marriott, he must be "kept under wraps." Note: sinus bradycardia is also present. Sinus bradycardia is common in acute inferior STEMI, since the SA node is supplied by the RCA in 60 percent of individuals (and by the LCA in the remaining 40 percent). Inferior wall STEMIs are also frequently accompanied by increased parasympathetic tone.

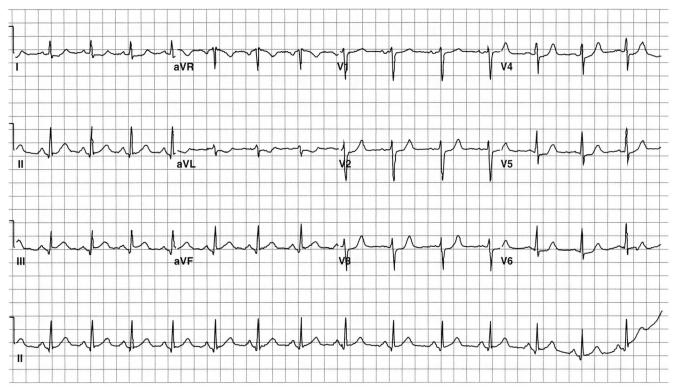

**ECG 2.6** A 41-year-old female presented with 3 days of chest pain and cough, which she attributed to "sitting in front of the computer all day." She reported mild chest discomfort and was slightly anxious.

## The Electrocardiogram

Initially, this healthy young female was felt to have atypical chest wall pain. The clinicians interpreted her ECG as either "benign early repolarization or pericarditis." But it cannot be either one of these. Reciprocal changes are present: the ST-segment depressions in the high lateral leads (I and aVL) are incompatible with early repolarization or pericarditis. ST-seg-ment depression is also present in the anterior and lateral precordial leads.

Most importantly, there is ST-segment elevation in lead III. Sure, the ST-segment in lead III is only 1 mm elevated, and it has a reassuring, "smiley face," upward concavity. But don't be fooled. This ECG demonstrates an early, subtle inferior wall STEMI. Her initial troponin was 4.25. The next figure shows her repeat ECG, taken 17 minutes later.

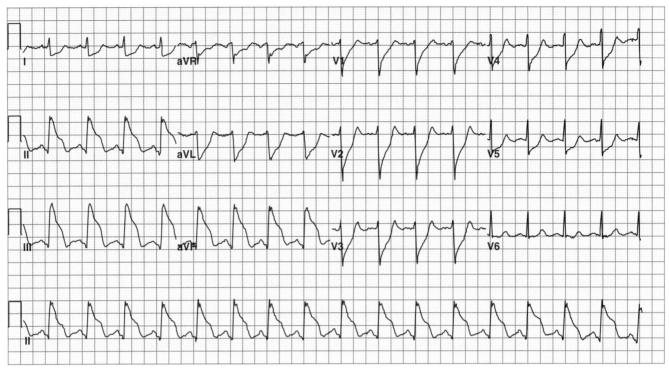

**ECG 2.6** Same patient (follow-up ECG, taken 17 minutes later).

This follow-up ECG demonstrates a more obvious acute inferior and posterior wall STEMI along with sinus tachycardia.

## The Shape of the ST-Segment: About Upward Concavity and Smiley Faces

This would be an appropriate time to consider whether "upward concavity" or "downward concavity" is a helpful clue in distinguishing between STEMI and other, more benign causes of ST-segment elevation (for example, early repolarization pattern, pericarditis or the ST-segment elevations associated with left ventricular hypertrophy). In general, ST-segments that are straightened, concave downward, "dome-shaped" or "tombstone" in appearance are much more common in STEMI. And smooth, upwardly concave ST-segments (with "J-point elevation") are more characteristic of benign conditions. But the shape of the ST-segment is simply not a reliable ECG sign in differentiating between the two. A smoothly contoured, concave-upward, "smiley face" ST-segment does not exclude acute ST-elevation myocardial infarction, as illustrated in this case (Brady et al., 2001; Birnbaum, Nikus et al., 2014).

To detect subtle STEMIs, focus on whether the ST-segment elevations are *regional* (in an anatomic territory, such as the inferior, lateral or anterior wall) and focus on the presence of *reciprocal* ST-segment depressions (here, in leads I and aVL). This topic is considered in more detail in Chapter 7, Confusing Conditions: ST-Segment Elevations and Tall T-Waves (Coronary Mimics).

The lesson from the preceding cases is clear: do not wait for the ST-segments to exceed "2 mm in elevation in at least 2 contiguous leads." Do not wait until the ST-segments look like "tombstones." Do not wait until the 12-lead ECG meets "cath lab activation criteria." And do not wait for the computer to get it right. We must make the diagnosis of acute inferior wall infarction early. Learn to detect subtle straightening and minor elevations of the ST-segments in II, III and aVF. And always check for ST-segment depressions in leads I and aVL, which can serve as a trusted ally.

## STEMI Equivalents: ST-Segment Elevations "Below the Required Threshold"

This atlas is filled with examples of acute ST-elevation myocardial infarctions in their early stages, where the ST-segment elevations are barely noticeable. Remember, there should not be a strict "minimum threshold" for the ST-segment elevation to make a diagnosis of acute STEMI (Chan et al., 2005; Birnbaum, Wilson et al., 2014; Birnbaum, Nikus et al., 2014; Nikus et al., 2014; Nikus et al., 2010). The often-repeated standard of "ST-segment elevation of at least 1 mm in at least two contiguous leads" (with various age, gender and lead variations) was derived from population-based studies and also served as the criteria for entry into the original, large randomized trials of thrombolytic therapy. It remains a cornerstone of the American Heart Association/American College of Cardiology/European Society of Cardiology criteria for the diagnosis of STEMI (Chan et al., 2005; American College of Cardiology Foundation, 2013; Thygesen et al., 2012; Birnbaum, Wilson et al., 2014).

But virtually all current consensus statements regarding the definition of STEMI include the caveat that "lesser degrees of ST-

[elevation] … do not exclude acute myocardial ischemia or evolving MI" (Thygesen et al., 2012). In clinical practice, any ST-segment elevation may be sufficient, especially when the ST-segment elevations are regional and are accompanied by reciprocal changes in the electrically opposite leads. In addition, even minimal ST-segment elevations may be significant, when they are found in leads where the QRS amplitude is very low (for example, lead aVL) (Birnbaum, Wilson et al., 2014). Straightened or minimally elevated ST-segments, when accompanied by reciprocal ST-segment depressions, are often a "STEMI equivalent." See Chapter 3 for additional discussion and examples of these and other "STEMI equivalents."

## Inferior Wall STEMI *without* ST-Segment Depressions in aVL

Even as we stress the importance of ST-segment depression in lead aVL as an early warning sign of inferior STEMI, we should not overstate our case. There is an important electrocardiographic caveat: occasionally, patients with early inferior wall STEMIs will present without any reciprocal ST-segment depressions in aVL. This is an uncommon exception, but it is important. As noted earlier, these patients often have ST-segment elevations that are more pronounced in lead II than in lead III, and the culprit coronary artery occlusion is usually the LCA rather than the RCA. Typically, the LCA is occluded proximal to the takeoff of the first obtuse marginal (OM) branch. In this circumstance, a concurrent high lateral STEMI is often present along with the inferior wall STEMI. The expected ST-segment depressions in aVL that are reciprocal to the inferior wall STEMI are "canceled out" by the ST-segment elevations in the high lateral leads (I and aVL) (Birnbaum, Wilson et al., 2014). ST-segment elevations are also frequently present in the lateral precordial leads (V5 and V6).

Refer again to ECG 2.4, presented earlier, for an example of an inferior and lateral wall STEMI without ST-segment depression in aVL (due to an LCA occlusion). Additional examples are included in the self-study ECGs in this chapter.

## Complications of Inferior Infarction: The *Big Three*

In caring for patients with acute inferior wall STEMI, it is not enough to simply identify the inferior ST-segment elevations. In every case, the clinician must examine the tracing carefully for the following *big three* complications:

- ST-elevations in lead V1 or V4 R, signifying right ventricular myocardial infarction (RVMI);
- ST-segment depressions in the right precordial leads (V1–V3), indicating extension of the STEMI to the posterior wall; and
- The presence of first-degree, second-degree or third-degree AV nodal block.

These three complications are common in patients with inferior STEMI, and they are readily apparent from the surface ECG. Importantly, each of these complications is also an independent marker of a larger infarction, and each is associated with a heightened risk of pump failure, post-infarct angina, heart block, atrial and ventricular arrhythmias and in-hospital and 1-year mortality.

## Anatomic Correlations

The electrocardiographic features and the complications of IMI (the *big three*) are completely predictable, based on the anatomy of the right coronary artery (Figure 2.3).

In 90 percent of individuals, there is a dominant RCA[1] that supplies:

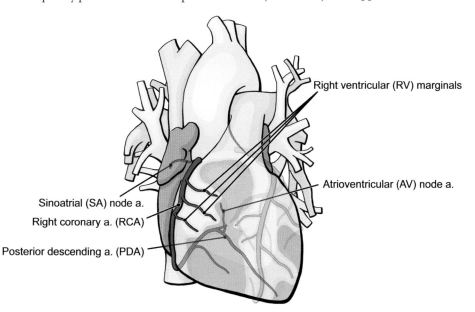

Right ventricular (RV) marginals

Atrioventricular (AV) node a.

Sinoatrial (SA) node a.

Right coronary a. (RCA)

Posterior descending a. (PDA)

**Figure 2.3** Anatomy of the right coronary artery.
The anatomy of the RCA helps to explain the frequent occurrence of RVMI, AV nodal block and posterior wall extension (the *big three* complications) in patients with acute inferior wall STEMI.

---

[1] Clinicians often refer to a patient's coronary anatomy as "right dominant" or "left dominant." Ninety percent of individuals are "right dominant," which means that the large posterior descending artery (PDA) arises from the RCA. About 10 percent of individuals are "left dominant"; in these cases, the PDA is a branch of the left circumflex artery. "Dominance" has nothing to do with the total territory subserved or with the artery's overall importance. Though the vast majority of individuals have right dominant coronary anatomy, it is still the left anterior descending artery that provides the main blood supply to the large anterior wall of the left ventricle.

- The inferior wall of the left ventricle;
- The anterior and lateral walls of the right ventricle, via the acute marginal (right ventricular) branches, which exit from the proximal to mid-portion of the RCA;
- Large portions of the posterior wall of the left ventricle and the posterior interventricular septum, via the large posterior descending artery (PDA); and
- The AV nodal artery, which is a tiny branch of the PDA (explaining the common association between inferior STEMI and AV nodal block).

One last clinical-anatomic correlation: the PDA usually supplies blood to the posteromedial papillary muscle of the mitral valve. (The anterolateral papillary muscle is involved less often in patients with ST-elevation myocardial infarction because it usually has a dual blood supply, from the left anterior descending and the left circumflex arteries.) Therefore, acute inferior wall myocardial infarction is often accompanied by papillary muscle dysfunction. It is routine to hear a soft, apical, holosystolic murmur of mitral insufficiency in patients with acute inferior wall STEMI. A loud holosystolic murmur, in a patient with an inferior STEMI and pulmonary edema, signifies acute papillary muscle rupture, a rare but potentially devastating complication. A case of inferior wall STEMI, complicated by papillary muscle rupture, is included in the self-study ECGs later in this chapter.

## Right Ventricular Myocardial Infarction

RVMI occurs in 25–50 percent of patients with acute inferior STEMI (Goldstein, 2012; Wellens, 1993; Tsuka et al., 2001; Del'Itallia, 1998; Moye et al., 2005; Kakouros and Cokkinos, 2010; O'Rourke and Dell'Italia, 2004; Zehnder et al., 1993). Almost always, RVMI results from occlusion of the RCA proximal to the acute marginal (right ventricular) branches (see Figure 2.2). Thus, RVMI is usually recognized in the context of, and as a complication of, an acute inferior wall STEMI.

The most important complication of RVMI is hypotension due to low cardiac output. Impaired cardiac output results primarily from progressive hypokinesis and dilatation of the right ventricle. Dilatation of the RV also causes bowing of the interventricular septum, which then intrudes into the left ventricular chamber, further impairing LV filling and systolic function (Goldstein, 2012; Inohara et al., 2013).

Less frequently, RVMI may result in other complications, including atrial fibrillation (due to right atrial dilatation), ventricular tachycardia or fibrillation, RV thrombus formation with subsequent pulmonary thromboembolism, ventricular septal rupture, tricuspid valve regurgitation, pericarditis or hypoxemia (caused by high RV pressures and right-to-left shunting through a patent foramen ovale).

Even though the right ventricular dysfunction is often transient (and the term right ventricular *infarction* may be a misnomer), the occurrence of RVMI is associated with an increased risk of early mortality, cardiogenic shock, ventricular tachyarrhythmia and advanced heart block compared with IMI alone (Goldstein, 2012; Zehnder et al., 1993; Inohara et al., 2013; Hamon et al., 2008).

Once RVMI is recognized on the ECG, clinicians know to avoid drugs that will reduce right ventricular preload, such as nitroglycerin, morphine and diuretics. Intravenous fluids are typically administered in order to optimize right ventricular filling and improve cardiac output (Goldstein, 2012). Inotropic agents (for example, dobutamine or dopamine) are often used for hypotension that is refractory to moderate volume resuscitation. Overzealous fluid administration in patients with RVMI can cause further bowing of the septum into the left ventricular cavity and, paradoxically, impair left ventricular function. Correction of bradycardia and heart block, which often coexist in patients with RVMI, is also critical. Emergent reperfusion speeds recovery of right ventricular function.

## Electrocardiographic Signs of RVMI

### ST-Segment Elevation in Lead V4 R

The most sensitive and specific sign of RVMI is ST-segment elevation in the right-sided precordial lead V4 R (Moye et al., 2005; Zehnder et al., 1993; Inohara et al., 2013). Indeed, ST-segment elevation in V4 R is a more sensitive and specific test for RVMI than bedside physical findings, including the classic triad of hypotension, jugular venous pressure elevation and clear lungs. The ST-segment elevation in V4 R may be quite transient (Wagner et al., 2009). Also, the ST-segment elevation in V4 R may be quite small – sometimes no more than 0.1mV. This is understandable, given that the right ventricle has only one-sixth the muscle mass of the left ventricle (Kakouros and Cokkinos, 2010).

ST-segment elevation in V4 R is strongly predictive of a mid- or proximal RCA occlusion. In addition, this ECG finding alone – ST-segment elevation in V4 R – is a strong, independent predictor of complications and early mortality. In Zehnder's classic review of 200 consecutive patients with acute IMI, the finding of ST-segment elevation in V4 R of ≥ 1 mm increased the in-hospital mortality rate five-fold, from 6 to 31 percent (Zehnder et al., 1993). Patients with ST-elevation in V4 R had a higher incidence of major in-hospital complications, including ventricular tachycardia and fibrillation, high-grade AV block that required pacing, atrial fibrillation, hemodynamic instability, pump failure and cardiogenic shock.

### Larger ST-Segment Elevations in Lead III Compared with Lead II

Disproportionate ST-elevation in lead III (> II) and pronounced (≥ 1 mm) ST-segment depression in lead aVL are also valuable markers of accompanying RVMI (Turhan et al., 2003; Moye et al., 2005). As summarized earlier in this chapter, these are the same ECG clues that are used to predict the proximal RCA as the infarct-related artery.

### ST-Segment Elevation in Lead V1

Every standard 12-lead ECG comes with one right-sided lead – for free. Precordial lead V1 is located in the fourth intercostal space, just to the right of the sternum (see Chapter 1). Thus, it is a right-sided lead, and it routinely monitors the right ventricle as well as the interventricular septum. In the setting of inferior wall STEMI, the presence of ST-segment elevation in lead V1 is highly suggestive of concomitant RVMI, accompanied by acute right ventricular dilatation (rather than, by chance, a second, anteroseptal STEMI) (Zimetbaum and Josephson, 2003; Tsuka et al., 2001; Moye et al., 2005; Wagner et al., 2009). Patients with acute inferior wall STEMI and ST-segment elevation in V1 almost always have a proximal RCA occlusion. Sometimes, in these patients, reciprocal ST-segment depressions appear in leads V5 and V6.

Keep in mind that, in patients with acute inferior STEMI, two opposing forces may be tugging on the right precordial lead ST-segments (including V1). Right ventricular infarction causes ST-segment *elevation* in V1. At the same time, posterior wall extension is a common complication of IMI and causes right precordial ST-segment *depression*. Ultimately, the position of the ST-segments results from a summing of these forces; RVMI can hide the signs of posterior wall involvement, and vice versa.

A final caveat: there is another circumstance where patients may present with simultaneous ST-segment elevations in the inferior leads and in the anteroseptal leads (including V1). This occurs in the setting of anterior wall STEMI and, specifically, when the occluded artery – the left anterior descending – includes a long, terminal branch that "wraps around" the apex of the heart to perfuse the inferior left ventricular wall. However, occlusion of a "wrap-around" LAD is likely to cause more extensive ST-segment elevations involving the anterior and lateral precordial leads, including V6. In the setting of inferior wall STEMI, accompanying ST-segment elevation limited to precordial lead V1 usually signals RV infarction (Alzand and Gorgels, 2011). Examples of concurrent anterior and inferior STEMI caused by occlusion of a "wrap-around LAD" are included in Chapter 3, Anterior Wall Myocardial Infarction.

The next two cases illustrate the electrocardiographic features of inferior wall STEMI complicated by acute RVMI.

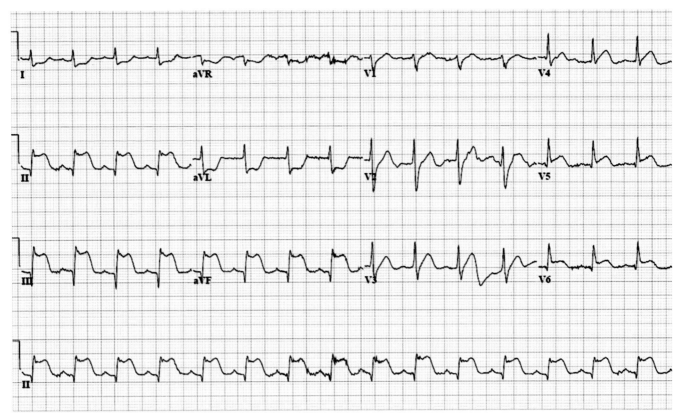

**ECG 2.7** A 35-year-old man presented with severe chest pain radiating to the jaw, accompanied by nausea, vomiting and shortness of breath. He was noted to have a soft mitral insufficiency murmur.

## The Electrocardiogram

The ECG demonstrates an acute inferior wall STEMI. There is extension to the lateral wall (V5–V6), suggesting a large infarct territory. Given the ST-segment elevations in lead III (> II) and the marked ST-segment depressions in aVL, a proximal RCA clot can be predicted; these ECG findings are also highly suggestive of concomitant RVMI. In this setting, the soft, apical holosystolic murmur usually represents papillary muscle dysfunction. Right-sided leads were obtained (see the next ECG).

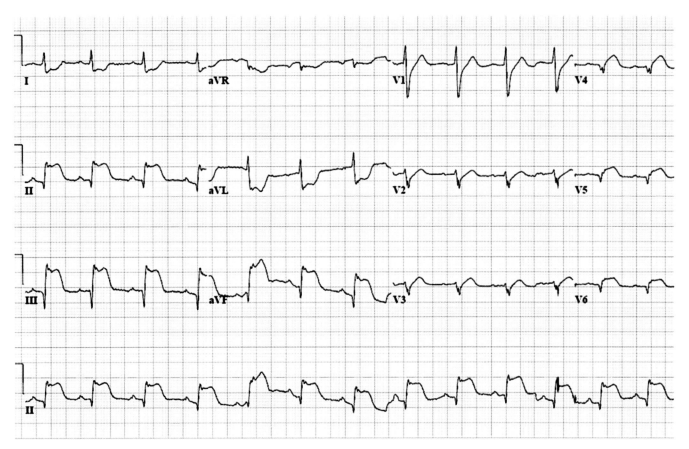

**ECG 2.7** Same patient (right-sided leads).

This is the right-sided ECG (note the decreasing R-waves across the precordial leads). There is marked ST-segment elevation in lead V4 R, consistent with acute RVMI. The ST-segment elevations in V4 R are often transient, sometimes lasting only a few hours.

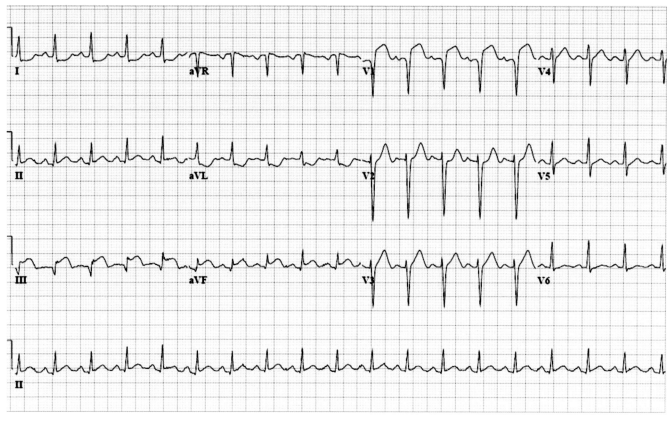

**ECG 2.8** A 52-year-old man presented with bilateral arm pain, fullness in his throat, nausea and diaphoresis.

## The Electrocardiogram

In this tracing, there is an obvious inferior wall STEMI, with reciprocal ST-segment depressions in leads I and aVL. Sinus tachycardia is also present. In the setting of acute myocardial infarction, sinus tachycardia is often an "arrhythmia of pump failure" and may presage later development of overt congestive heart failure.

There is also dramatic ST-segment elevation in lead V1. As noted previously, lead V1 is a right-sided precordial lead; therefore, ST-segment elevation in this lead, in a patient with inferior wall STEMI, provides evidence of RVMI and is typically a marker of acute RV dilatation. The ST-segment elevations in V1 do not usually imply a second, anterior wall STEMI.

## Clinical Course

Coronary angiography confirmed a tight, proximal RCA occlusion; this was predictable given the ST-segment elevations in lead III (much greater than lead II), the marked (> 1 mm) ST-segment depressions in aVL and the electrocardiographic evidence of RVMI.

Right-sided leads were also obtained in this patient, although strictly speaking they were not needed. The right-sided leads were positive for RVMI (see next ECG).

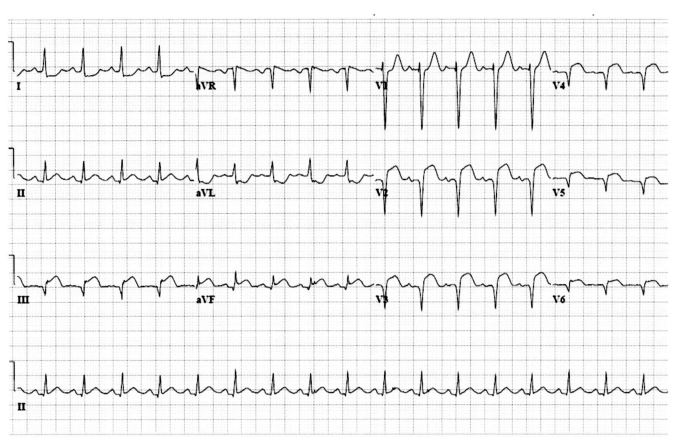

**ECG 2.8** Same patient (right-sided leads).

The right-sided leads demonstrate ST-segment elevation in V4 R, consistent with acute RVMI.

## Summary: Electrocardiographic Clues to Right Ventricular Infarction

The right-sided leads (V4 R and V1) should be examined carefully in every patient who presents with an acute inferior wall STEMI. ST-elevations in leads V4 R or V1 signify that an RVMI is present. This ECG finding also:

- Puts the culprit lesion in the proximal RCA, before the take-off the right ventricular (acute marginal) branches;
- Identifies a subset of inferior STEMI patients at heightened risk of complications during hospitalization; and
- Helps avoid complications during treatment.

## Inferior Infarction Extending into the Posterior Wall (ST-Segment Depressions in V1–V3)

About half of all patients with inferior wall STEMI also have concomitant ST-segment depressions in the right precordial leads (V1–V3). ST-segment depressions in V1–V3 are usually the reciprocal marker of a current of injury (ST-segment elevations) involving the posterior wall. Thus, they signify collateral damage (a STEMI) involving the posterior wall. Patients with IMI

accompanied by ST-segment depressions in V1–V3 have larger infarctions, greater cardiac biomarker release, more pump failure, more ventricular tachycardia, more heart block requiring pacing and higher in-hospital, 30-day and 1-year mortality rates (Zimetbaum and Josephson, 2003; Surawicz and Knilans, 2008; Birnbaum et al., 1999). When these ST-segment depressions resolve quickly (within 24 hours of presentation), the prognosis is improved.

As discussed in Chapter 4, Posterior Wall Myocardial Infarction, so-called "posterior wall STEMIs" typically involve large regions of the lateral wall and are more properly termed "posterolateral STEMIs" (Wagner et al., 2009). The diagnosis of posterior wall involvement can be confirmed by finding ST-segment elevations in the posterior leads (V7, V8 and V9).

In patients with inferior wall STEMI, ST-segment depressions can also occur in the more lateral precordial leads (V4–V6). These appear to carry a different, more ominous significance. In patients with inferior STEMI, disproportionate ST-segment depressions in leads V4–V6 may signify anterior wall ischemia and the likelihood of coronary disease involving the left anterior descending artery or one of its branches (Hasdai et al., 1997).

Refer again to ECGs 2.2, 2.3, 2.4 and 2.6, which demonstrate inferior wall STEMIs complicated by posterior wall infarction. See ECG 2.9 for another example of an acute inferior and posterior wall STEMI, misread by the computer.

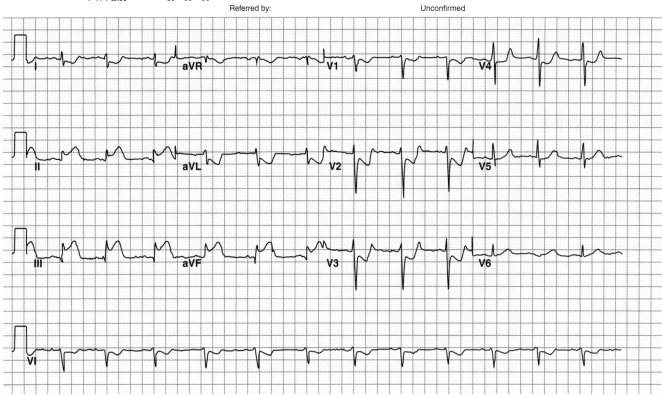

25 mm/s
10 mm/sV
40 Hz
Pgm 006B
12SLtn v74

Med:
                              Wt:
Med: M      Race:
Loc:  30     Room:
Option:        7
Vent.  rate           75 BPM
PR interval          152  ms
QRS duration        96   ms
QT/QTc         396/442  ms
P-R-T axes        59   99   96

NORMAL SINUS RHYTHM
RIGHTWARD AXIS
INFERIOR INFARCT. POSSIBLY ACUTE
T WAVE ABNORMALITY. CONSIDER ANTERIOR ISCHEMIA
ABNORMAL ECG

Referred by:                              Unconfirmed

**ECG 2.9** A 63-year-old man with 1 week of exertional chest pain and dyspnea presented with increasing chest pain at rest. The computer algorithm identified the acute inferior STEMI. The computer then added, "T-wave abnormality – consider anterior ischemia."

## The Electrocardiogram

The ECG is not subtle. There are large ST-segment elevations in leads II, III and aVF, with reciprocal ST-segment depressions in leads I and aVL. Clearly, the patient is experiencing an acute inferior wall STEMI.

There are also marked ST-segment depressions in the anterior precordial leads (V1–V3). The computer algorithm struggled with these ST-segment depressions, querying "anterior ischemia." However, we know that these right precordial ST-segment depressions do not usually represent anterior wall ischemia. Rather, they represent reciprocal changes – not reciprocal to the inferior STEMI but, rather, reciprocal to a concurrent posterior wall STEMI. Despite the marked ST-segment depressions in leads V1–V3, the T-waves remain upright; these upright T-waves may be considered the mirror image of posterior wall T-wave inversions. As highlighted in Chapter 4, Posterior Wall Myocardial Infarction, these changes – ST-segment depressions and "bolt upright" T-waves in leads V1–V3 – are highly suggestive of posterior wall STEMI rather than anterior wall ischemia.

This patient is suffering from an acute inferior and posterior STEMI. Inferior STEMIs accompanied by anterior precordial ST-segment depressions have larger infarctions, more pump failure and higher short- and long-term mortality rates. The ST-segment elevations in lead III are > II, indicating that there is a proximal RCA occlusion. This was verified at catheterization.

As stated earlier, an important distinction should be made. Patients with an inferior STEMI and *lateral, rather than right-sided, precordial ST-segment depressions* are very likely to have extensive, multivessel coronary artery disease involving the LAD or its first diagonal branch in addition to the primary infarct vessel (usually the RCA). In these patients, ST-segment depressions involving predominantly leads V4–V6 may well signify concomitant anterior wall ischemia.

## Inferior Wall STEMI Complicated by Atrioventricular (AV) Nodal Block

AV nodal block (first-degree, second-degree and third-degree) is also common in patients with acute inferior wall STEMIs. Higher grades of AV block often occur together with right ventricular myocardial infarction (RVMI); the combination

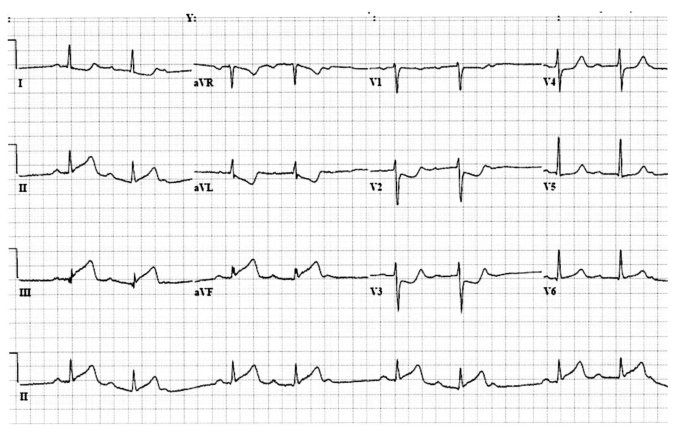

**ECG 2.10** A 54-year-old man with a history of hypertension and diabetes presented with intermittent substernal chest pain for 2 months. His pain became more frequent over 3 days and then worsened acutely over 4 hours.

of high-grade AV block and RVMI is associated with a large infarct size, congestive heart failure, cardiogenic shock and higher mortality.

The exact etiology of AV block in the setting of IMI is unclear, although ischemia of the AV node is a likely explanation. As explained earlier, the AV nodal artery is a distal branch of the PDA, which, in turn, arises from the RCA in 90 percent of patients (see Figure 2.3). Heightened vagal tone and accumulation of potassium or adenosine in the region of the AV node may also contribute to AV block during acute IMI.

Higher levels of AV block (second- or third-degree) may occur gradually or abruptly. But in most cases, the block is transient. If second-degree AV block occurs, it is usually "Mobitz Type 1" (Wenckebach) because the block resides within, not below, the AV node. Patients who are hemodynamically stable may not require pacing, and since the site of the block is within the AV node, atropine may be effective (Surawicz and Knilans, 2008).

High-grade AV block in the setting of IMI is often accompanied by acceleration of pacemaker activity in the region of the AV junction. Thus, it is common to see emergence of a narrow-complex junctional escape rhythm at a rate of 50–70 beats per minute, a rate that is often adequate to maintain the patient's blood pressure. The junctional rhythm may also accelerate to a rate of 100 or greater, a tachycardia often referred to as non-paroxysmal junctional tachycardia (NPJT) or accelerated junctional rhythm (Surawicz and Knilans, 2008).

ECG 2.10 represents an acute inferior wall STEMI complicated by *the big three.*

## The Electrocardiogram

The ECG demonstrates an inferior wall STEMI with extension into the posterior left ventricular wall. (The ST-segment depressions are most pronounced in V2–V3.) AV-nodal block (second-degree, Mobitz Type 1) is also present. (In the lead II rhythm strip, the PR interval lengthens, followed by a single dropped beat, before this pattern repeats.)

## Clinical Course

The patient's troponin level peaked at 123. Emergency coronary angiography revealed a 100 percent occlusion of the mid-RCA. The right-sided leads demonstrated an RVMI (see next tracing).

The right-sided leads demonstrate modest ST-segment elevations in V4 R, consistent with acute right ventricular infarction. The anterior precordial ST-segment depressions are absent because these are the right-sided leads. Also, in this tracing, Mobitz Type 1 second-degree heart block is no longer present; it has been replaced by first-degree AV block. (The PR interval is slightly greater than 200 msec.)

Thus, this case demonstrates all of the complications of inferior wall STEMI (the *big three*).

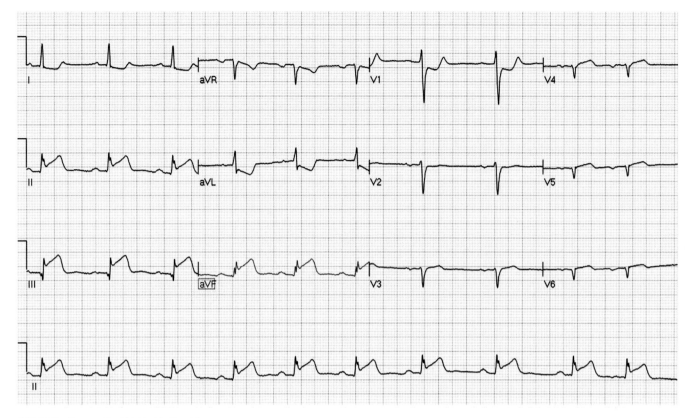

**ECG 2.10** Same patient (right-sided leads).

## Inferior Wall STEMI: Postscripts

### Recognizing Inferior Wall STEMI in Special Situations

It is important to recognize inferior wall STEMIs in several special situations: in the setting of left ventricular hypertrophy with repolarization abnormalities, when there is a right or left bundle branch block, when there are multiple premature ventricular contractions (PVCs) and in the patient who has suffered a cardiac arrest. The self-study ECGs include examples of these challenges where inferior wall STEMIs are often missed.

### "Old" Inferior Myocardial Infarctions

It is common to detect evidence of an old or "indeterminate age" myocardial infarction on the 12-lead ECG. The hallmark of an old inferior wall myocardial infarction is the presence of *pathologic Q-waves in leads II, III and aVF*. Marked diminution in the amplitude of the R-waves usually carries the same significance.

Frequently, Q-waves appear in the inferior leads (especially in lead III) in normal individuals, in the absence of coronary artery disease or prior myocardial infarction. It is usually not difficult to distinguish normal from abnormal Q-waves. As summarized in Chapter 1, the distinction depends on duration, depth and location of the Q-waves (Surawicz and Knilans, 2008; Brady et al., 2001; Thygesen et al., 2012; Goldberger, 1980).

> **Pathologic Q-Waves Signifying Old Inferior Infarction**
>
> - Q-waves are present in leads II, III and aVF.
> - The Q-waves are ≥ 0.03 seconds in duration.
> - The Q-waves are ≥ 1 mm (1 small box) deep or deeper than 25 percent of the R-wave amplitude.
> - T-wave inversions are present in the same leads.
>
> *Note:* Q-waves are often present in lead III, even in the absence of any history of myocardial infarction or other heart disease. These isolated Q-waves, which may vary with respiration or body position, are often a normal finding (Goldberger, 1980).

Development of "pathologic" Q-waves is highly variable. Sometimes, Q-waves in the infarct leads are present on the presenting ECG, even in in the first hour of symptoms; early Q-waves are especially common in anterior wall myocardial infarctions, and they do not necessarily signify old infarction or irreversible injury (Birnbaum, Wilson et al., 2014; Wellens and Conover, 2006). Conversely, not all patients who suffer a STEMI develop Q-waves. And Q-waves often disappear over days, weeks or months.

"Old" or "indeterminate age" Q-waves that are present on old, baseline ECG tracings do not represent acute disease. However, they may have great clinical significance. For example, in a patient with syncope or pre-syncope, the finding of an old infarction (pathologic Q-waves) on the presenting ECG is strongly associated with a cardiac arrhythmia, especially ventricular tachycardia, as the etiology for the patient's syncope (Bhat et al., 2014; Puppala et al., 2014). Examples of old inferior wall myocardial infarctions are included in the self-study ECGs.

# Over- and Underdiagnosis of Myocardial Infarction

The surface 12-lead ECG is not a perfect diagnostic tool for myocardial infarction. There are important limitations in both sensitivity and specificity.

### False Positives

At times, the 12-lead ECG will be falsely positive and lead to the overdiagnosis of acute STEMI. For example, ST-elevations are relatively common in patients with cardiomyopathy, pericarditis, myocarditis, left ventricular hypertrophy and the early repolarization syndrome. ST-elevations are also seen in the right precordial leads in healthy persons.

Myocarditis, in particular, can be difficult to distinguish from STEMI, since the ST-segment elevations in myocarditis are often regional (focal myocarditis) and are associated with cardiac biomarker elevations. The ECG clues to myocarditis are discussed in Chapter 5, The Electrocardiography of Shortness of Breath. The electrocardiographic features of early repolarization and pericarditis are discussed in Chapter 7, Confusing Conditions: ST-Segment Elevations and Tall T-Waves (Coronary Mimics). Left ventricular hypertrophy is discussed in Chapter 6.

### False Negatives

Clinicians are aware that patients with acute ST-elevation MI or other acute coronary syndromes may have a normal or near-normal ECG at initial presentation. Sometimes, the ECG is normal or near-normal because of collateral circulation or because there are competing vectors of ischemia (that is, ischemia or cardiac injury in remote zones may attenuate the ST-elevations in the leads facing the main infarction) (Birnbaum, Nikus et al., 2014; Birnbaum, Wilson et al., 2014; Atar and Birnbaum, 2005). ST-segment elevations may also come and go, if the obstructed coronary artery reperfuses and reoccludes. And even large infarctions may develop in electrocardiographically "silent" regions of the heart (Brady 2007).

Still, it is uncommon for a symptomatic patient to have an ECG that is normal and unchanging over a 1-hour observation period, at least when the obstructed coronary artery is the LAD or RCA (Chan et al., 2005; Smith et al., 2002). Therefore, the diagnostic sensitivity of the ECG is increased if repeated ECG tracings are obtained. According to expert panels, when patients present with chest pain or related symptoms, ECGs should be repeated at least every 15–30 minutes, for at least 1 hour, before ruling out the diagnosis of early or evolving STEMI (Thygesen et al., 2012; Birnbaum, Nikus et al., 2014). Diagnostic sensitivity can also be improved by reviewing old, baseline ECG tracings, recording posterior leads and performing echocardiography to detect regional wall motion abnormalities (Thygesen et al., 2012).

For example, consider the following case (ECG 2.11).

Room: 02
loc: 1002

Vent. rate          72 BPM          Normal sinus rhythm
PR interval         166 ms          Normal ECG
QRS duration         94 ms          No previous ECGs available
QT/QTc          360/394 ms
P-R-T axes       39  38  13

Technician: 37576
Test ind: CP

Y:                          Y:                          Referred by: SELF                          Reviewed & Interpreted by:

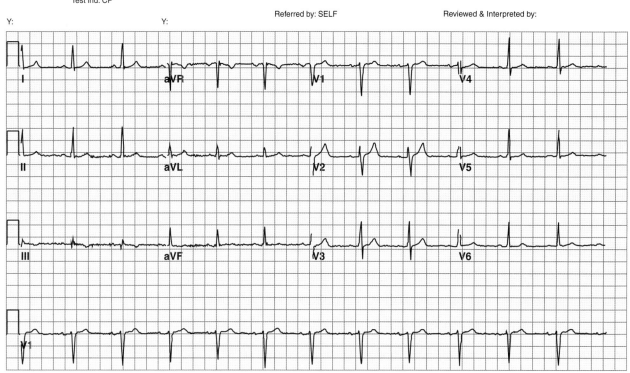

**ECG 2.11**  A 45-year-old man, a heavy smoker with a history of mild hypertension but with no known coronary artery disease, presented with intermittent, brief episodes of burning chest pain that radiated to both arms and his jaw. He was asymptomatic in the emergency department. His blood pressure was 167/114.

## The Electrocardiogram

The computer reading was technically accurate but falsely reassuring. The astute emergency clinicians interpreted this ECG correctly, noting in the electronic health record: "There is only a small amount of ST-segment straightening in lead III, with no reciprocal changes in aVL. Plan to administer Aspirin, measure troponin levels and obtain repeat ECG."

The initial troponin level was 0.22. These inferior wall ECG changes are impossibly subtle, but they prompted a repeat ECG.

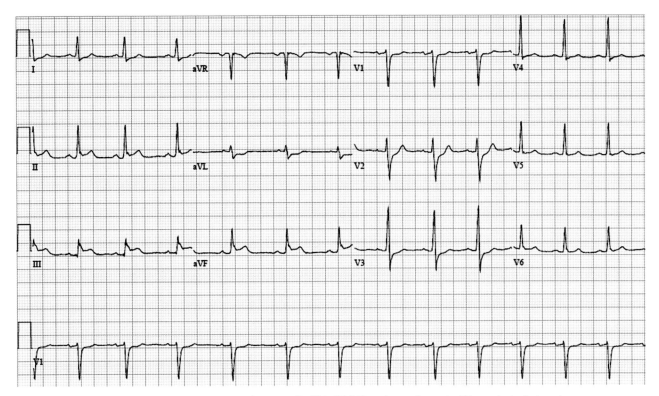

**ECG 2.11**  Same patient, now experiencing worsening chest pain. His BP is 178/102, and according to the ED note, he is diaphoretic.

## The Electrocardiogram

This ECG, obtained 1 hour and 12 minutes after the initial triage tracing shows unequivocal evidence of an acute inferior wall STEMI, with clear reciprocal ST-segment depressions in leads I and aVL. There is also evidence of extension to the posterior wall.

## Clinical Course

The patient went immediately to the catheterization laboratory, which demonstrated a 100 percent occlusion of the proximal RCA. His peak troponin level was only 11.8.

Of course, if the 12-lead ECGs are truly normal and the clinical suspicion of myocardial infarction is moderate or high, posterior leads should also be obtained; the standard 12-lead ECG is quite insensitive for the diagnosis of "true" (isolated) posterior wall ischemia or infarction. (See Chapter 4, Posterior Wall Myocardial Infarction.) Also, when patients present with chest pain and have a normal or nondiagnostic ECG, other coronary and noncoronary diagnoses should also be considered (for example, pulmonary thromboembolism, thoracic aortic dissection, myocarditis, pericarditis, pneumothorax and esophageal rupture). Point-of-care ultrasound may add immense value in the early differentiation of these conditions.

# Self-Study Electrocardiograms

**Case 2.1** A 77-year-old man with hypertension, diabetes and chronic renal insufficiency was brought by EMS with a presenting complaint of acute chest pain and dyspnea. On arrival in the ED, he had a VF arrest and was promptly defibrillated. Post-arrest, his blood pressure was 103/48.

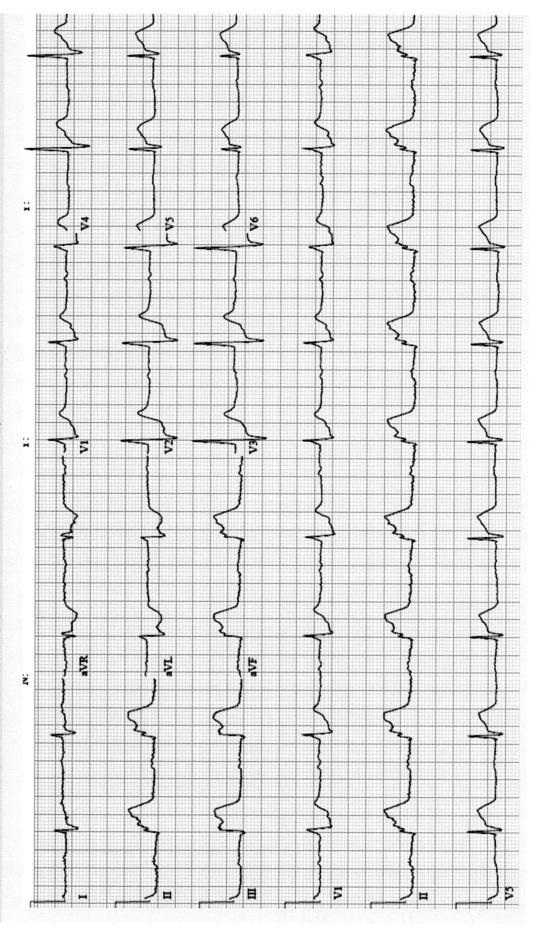

**Case 2.2** A 47-year-old man without any significant medical history presented with severe substernal chest pain, left arm pain and shortness of breath.

oom: S56
oc: 1002

| Vent. rate | 71 BPM |
| PR interval | 138 ms |
| QRS duration | 96 ms |
| QT/QTc | 364/395 ms |
| P-R-T axes | 11 50 36 |

Normal sinus rhythm
Nonspecific ST abnormality
Abnormal ECG
No previous ECGs available

Technician:
Test ind:

Referred by:

Reviewed & Interpreted by:

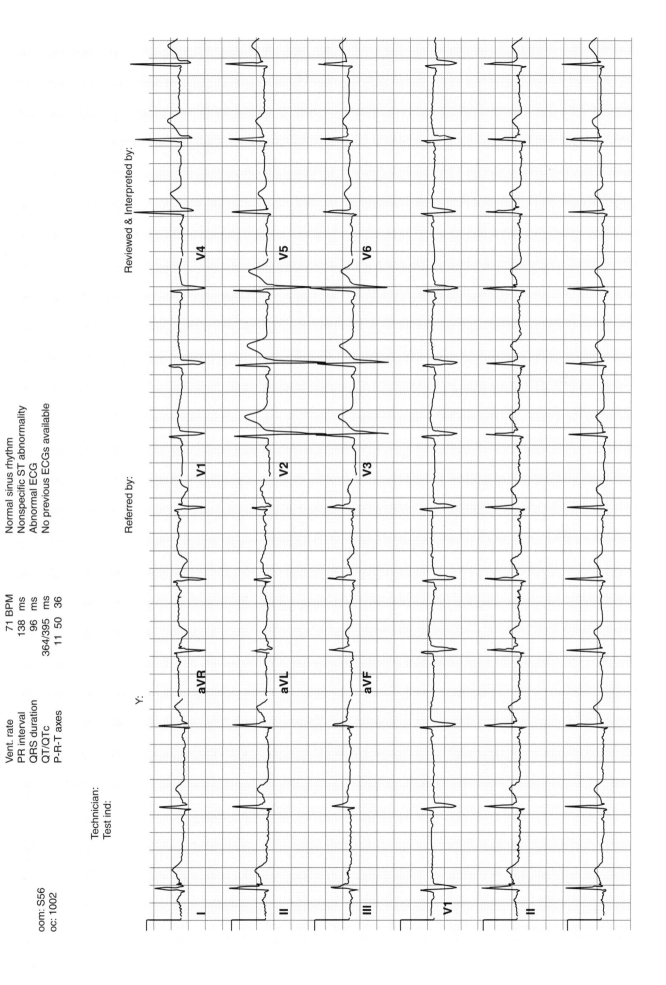

**Case 2.2 (Continued)** Same patient (18 minutes later).

**Case 2.3** A 78-year-old man presented to the emergency department in cardiac arrest. No medical history was available.

**Case 2.4** A 52-year-old female with long-standing hypertension presented to the emergency department with 1 day of stuttering chest tightness and some nausea. The emergency medicine and cardiology teams felt that her ECG was consistent with left ventricular hypertrophy with repolarization abnormalities ("strain pattern"). The computer algorithm reached the same diagnosis. Her initial troponin was 0.35, and she was admitted to the telemetry unit for "risk stratification and rule-out myocardial infarction, possible non-STEMI."

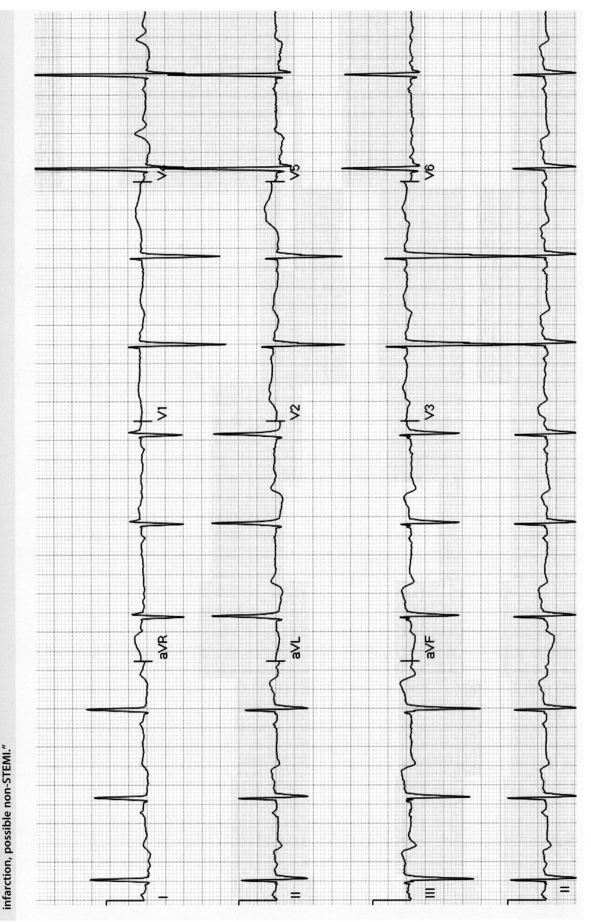

**Case 2.5** A 69-year-old female presented after a syncopal episode. She reported chest and abdominal pain over 1 hour. In the field she was initially pulseless, and the pre-hospital ECG demonstrated bradycardia and ST-elevations in the inferior leads.

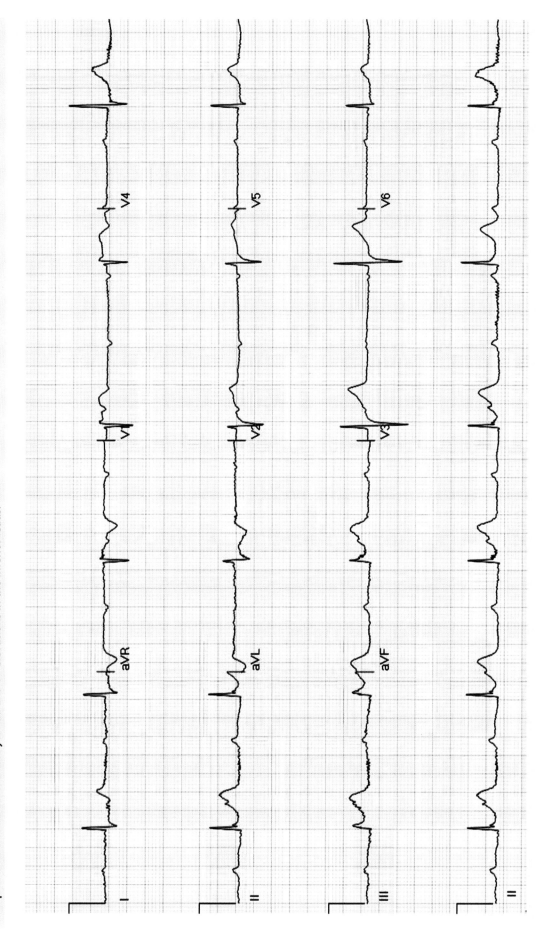

**Case 2.6** A 53-year-old man presented with dizziness and a near-syncopal episode. He had sustained an acute inferior myocardial infarction 13 days earlier.

**Case 2.7** A 53-year-old man was brought to the emergency department by paramedics after being struck by a car at very low speed. He stated that the vehicle's side mirror sideswiped the right side of his chest. His only complaint was right-sided chest pain. During his trauma evaluation, an ECG was obtained because he "didn't look good or feel good."

| | | |
|---|---|---|
| Rate 130 | - | Tachycardia with unusual P axis, rate 130..............P axis not -30 to 120, rate>= 100 |
| PR 210 | - | Multiple atrial premature complexes...................Short R-R intervals, normal QRSD |
| QRSD 189 | - | Left anterior fascicular block and..................QRS axis -45 deg., QRS > 120 mS |
| QT 471 | | nonspecific intraventricular conduction |
| QTc 471 | | delay |
| | - | Right atrial enlargement............................P > 0.25 mV |
| --Axis-- | - | ST segment elevation................................ST > .20 mV |
| P -89 | - | Lead(s) V4, V5, V6 were not used for morphology analysis |
| QRS 265 | | |
| T -80 | | — ABNORMAL ECG —        Unconfirmed diagnosis. |

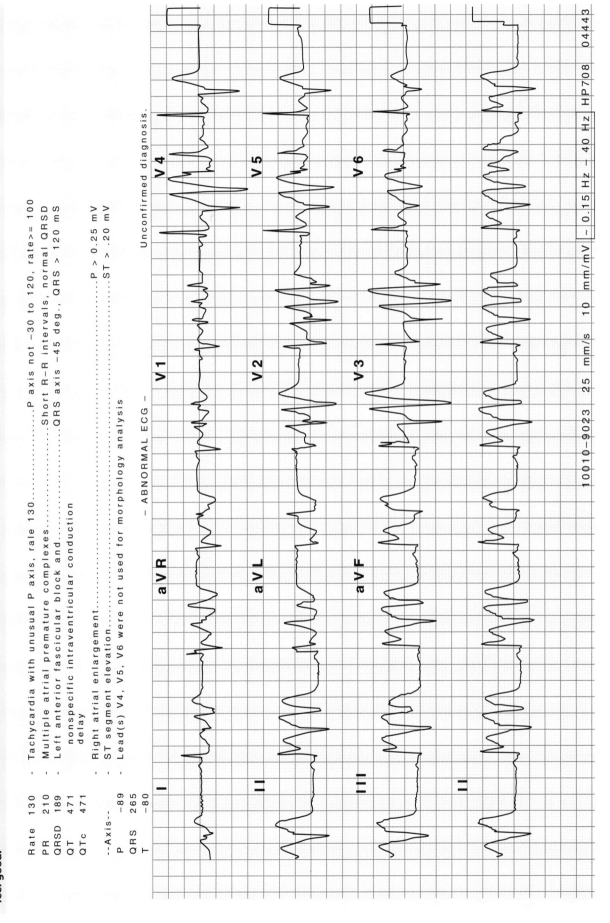

10010-9023   25 mm/s   10 mm/mV   ~ 0.15 Hz – 40 Hz HP708     04443

**Case 2.8** A 56-year-old man with a history of heavy smoking and untreated hypertension presented with acute left-sided chest pain, beginning 25 minutes prior to presentation. He had associated dyspnea, diaphoresis and nausea. The initial computer reading was "sinus tachycardia, and marked ST abnormality, possible lateral subendocardial injury." He was admitted to the hospital, where his ED note read, "Non-specific ST-T changes, not meeting STEMI criteria."

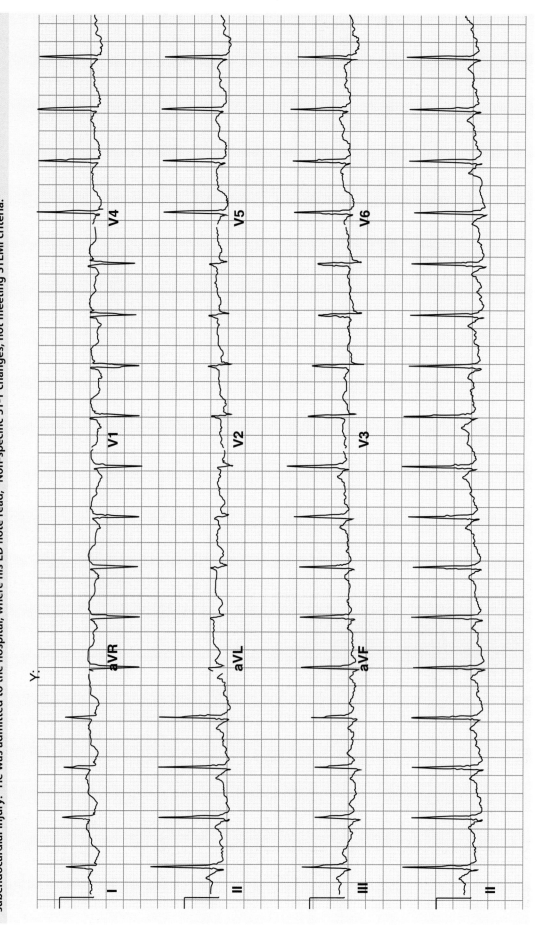

**Case 2.9** A 59-year-old woman presented with acute shortness of breath. In the emergency department, she was in pulmonary edema. Her dyspnea worsened, and she developed progressive hypoxia, requiring endotracheal intubation.

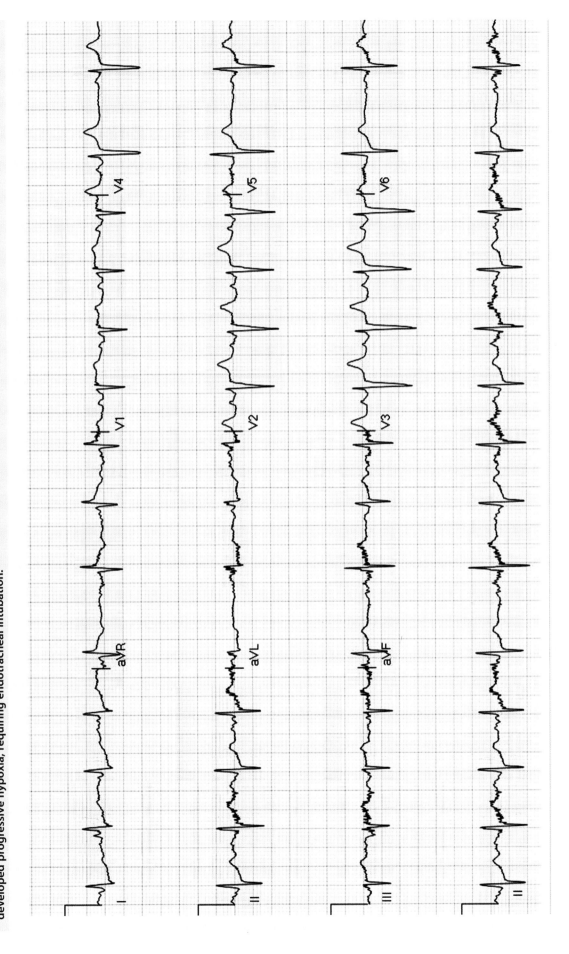

**Case 2.9 (Continued)** Same patient, follow-up ECG, 90 minutes later.

**Case 2.10** A 59-year-old man presented with chest pain, dizziness and shortness of breath.

**Case 2.11** An 80-year-old female presented with 3 hours of nausea and vomiting accompanied by light-headedness. She had a history of hypertension and hypothyroidism. She reported a normal cardiac nuclear stress test 1 year earlier. She denied chest pain and was in no distress on presentation.

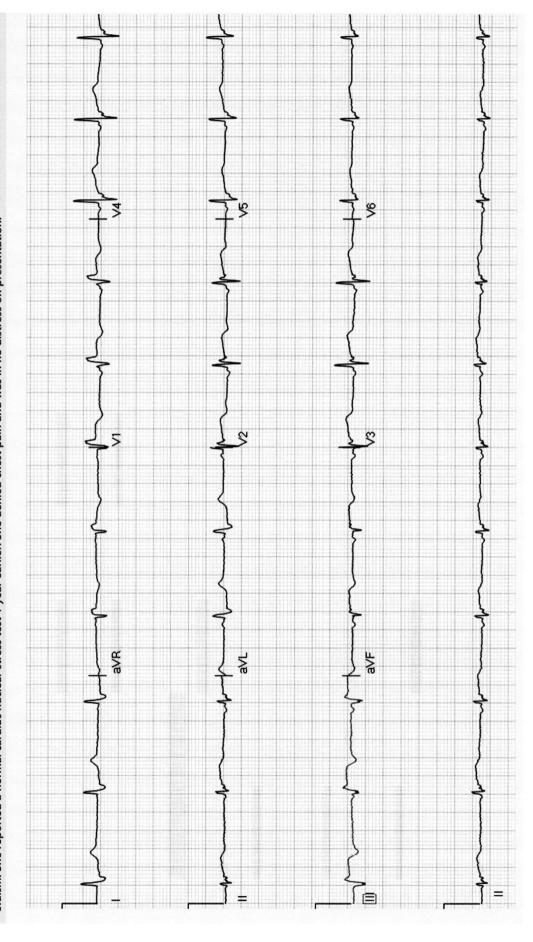

**Case 2.12** A 44-year-old man was healthy and without any known coronary artery disease or cardiovascular risk factors, except for smoking. He presented with intermittent chest pain over 8 days. On the morning of admission, he had severe chest pain, accompanied by nausea and diaphoresis.

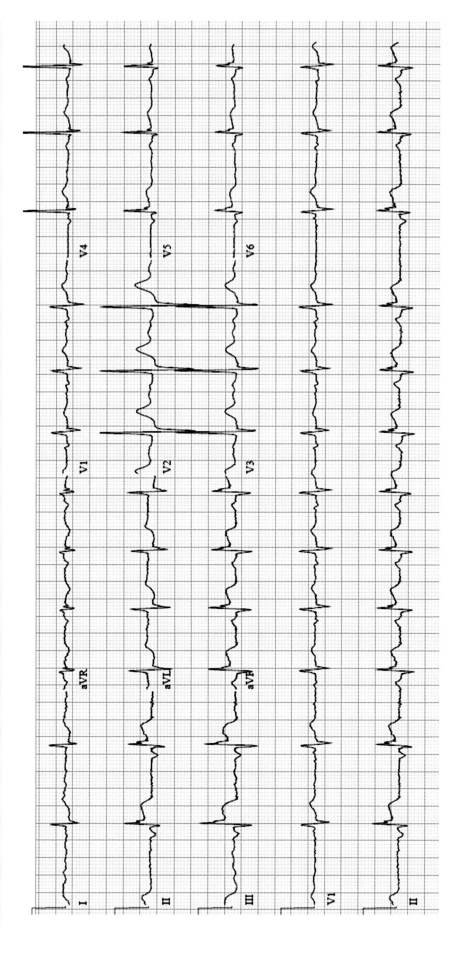

**Case 2.13** A 60-year-old man was driving. He pulled off to the side of the road and called 911. When the EMTs arrived, he was in ventricular fibrillation. A life support flight crew was also summoned. In the field, despite multiple defibrillation shocks, an epinephrine drip and other drugs, he remained in refractory VF. The resuscitation efforts continued in the emergency department. Prior to ending the resuscitation effort, a final 200 J shock was administered as shown.

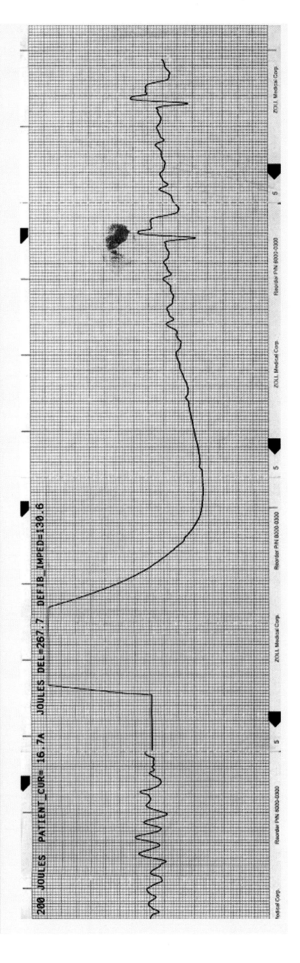

**Case 2.13 (Continued)** The same patient – 12-lead ECG after defibrillation.

| | | |
|---|---|---|
| Vent. rate | 98 | pbm |
| PR interval | * | ms |
| QRS duration | 176 | ms |
| QT/QTc | 472/602 | ms |
| P-R-T axes | * 196 | 88 |

Wide QRS rhythm
Right bundle branch block
Abnormal ECG

Opt:

Room:

Technician: 51514
Test ind:

Referred by:                    Unconfirmed

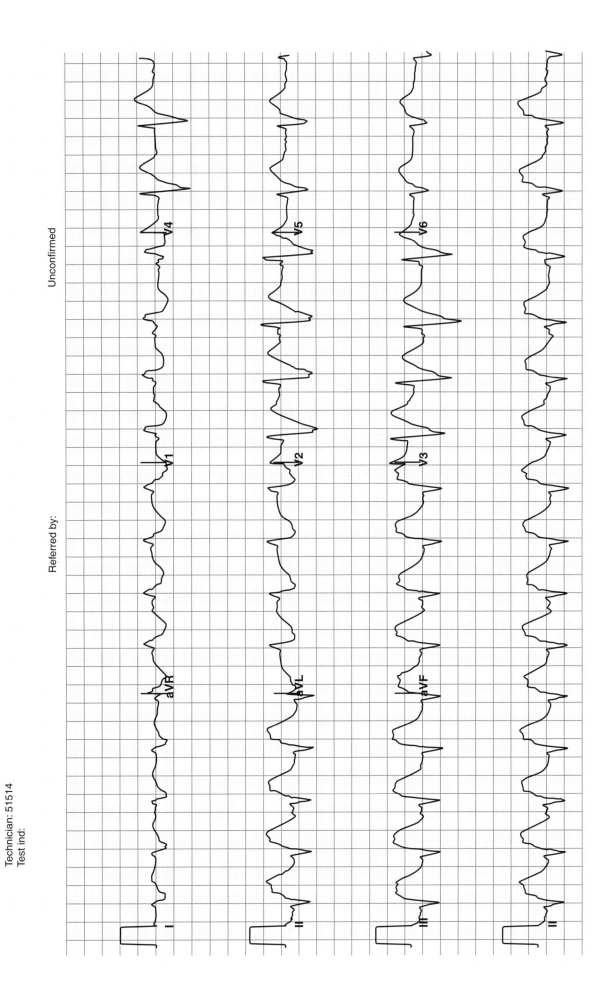

**Case 2.14** A 67-year-old female with a history of hypertension, hyperlipidemia and diabetes presented with 2 hours of left upper chest pain and mild shortness of breath. She had stable vital signs but was having chest pain in the ED. She received aspirin and sublingual nitroglycerin. Her initial troponin was 0.01.

oom: 370
c: 1002

| Vent. rate | 82 BPM |
|---|---|
| PR interval | • ms |
| QRS duration | 94 ms |
| QT/QTc | 366/427 ms |
| P-R-T axes | • 49  62 |

Atrial fibrillation with premature ventricular complexes
Low voltage QRS
Cannot rule out Anteroseptal infarct (cited on or before 30-JAN-2012)
Abnormal ECG
When compared with ECG of
Premature ventricular complexes are now present

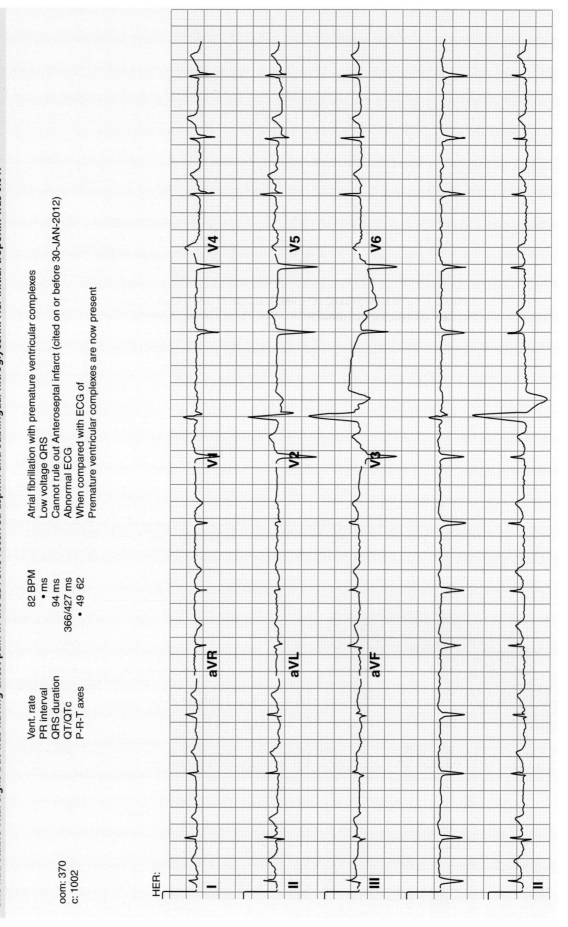

HER:

# Self-Study Notes

## Case 2.1 A 77-year-old man with hypertension, diabetes and chronic renal insufficiency was brought by EMS with a presenting complaint of acute chest pain and dyspnea. On arrival in the ED, he had a VF arrest and was promptly defibrillated. Post-arrest, his blood pressure was 103/48.

### The Electrocardiogram

The ECG demonstrates an obvious inferior and lateral wall STEMI, accompanied by two of the classic complications: posterior wall extension (ST-segment depressions in leads V1–V3) and first-degree AV block. The tall, broad R-waves in precordial leads V1 and V2 are consistent with the evolving posterior wall infarction. There is also sinus bradycardia and an abnormal right axis deviation. Lateral (V5–V6) ST-segment elevations are also present. This patient has suffered an acute inferior-lateral-posterior STEMI. Lateral wall involvement, posterior wall involvement and AV block are all markers of a larger infarct territory.

### Clinical Course

The initial troponin level was 0.24, but it later peaked at > 500. The patient underwent emergent catheterization, which revealed a heavily calcified and completely obstructed proximal RCA. Also, there was an anomalous origin of the left circumflex artery (LCA). Both the LCA and obtuse marginal (OM) arose from the proximal RCA and were obstructed by clot. The extensive STEMI, involving the inferior, lateral and posterior walls, is now easily explained. The patient was hemodynamically unstable in the catheterization laboratory, requiring pressor support with dopamine.

## Case 2.2 A 47-year-old man without any significant medical history presented with severe substernal chest pain, left arm pain and shortness of breath.

### The Electrocardiogram

The computer reading is incorrect. The ST abnormalities are not "nonspecific." The ECG shows ST-segment elevation in lead II that is more pronounced than lead III. The ST-segment is also elevated in lead III. There is no noticeable ST-segment depression in aVL. This does not exclude inferior wall STEMI; rather, it suggests that the left circumflex artery is the culprit vessel. Also, there is ST-segment elevation in the lateral precordial leads (leads V5–V6). This ECG is indicative of an acute inferior, lateral and high lateral wall STEMI in its early stages, *most likely caused by an acute occlusion of the left circumflex artery*. The ED clinicians obtained a second ECG 18 minutes later.

## Case 2.2 Same patient (18 minutes later).

### The Electrocardiogram

On the follow-up ECG, the inferior and lateral STEMI is much more obvious. It is critical to recognize an inferior wall STEMI, even if the ST-segment in lead aVL is not depressed. In this case, the ST-segment in lead aVL was normal on the initial ECG, and on this follow-up ECG, it is slightly straightened and elevated (when compared with the earlier tracing).

### Clinical Course

The initial troponin levels were 0.00 and 0.02, but later the troponin peaked at 47. Catheterization revealed an aneurysm and 100 percent obstruction of the left circumflex artery and its obtuse marginal (OM) branch.

## Case 2.3 A 78-year old man presented to the emergency department in cardiac arrest. No medical history was available.

### The Electrocardiogram

This is the patient's first post-resuscitation ECG. The emergency physicians and cardiologists interpreted the tracing as showing "wide complexes" and an "idioventricular rhythm"; this is understandable because slow, wide, pulseless and diffusely abnormal

ECGs are common after prolonged cardiopulmonary resuscitation. In fact, the patient is suffering an acute inferior wall STEMI. The "wide QRS complexes" actually represent ST-segment elevations in II, III and aVF, with ST-segment depressions in aVL – an all-too familiar regional pattern of inferior wall STEMI. The ST-segments are also elevated in V5–V6, suggesting lateral wall STEMI, and they are depressed in in V1–V2, indicating posterior wall involvement. The rhythm is likely a slow junctional bradycardia.

### Clinical Course

The clinicians felt that the QRS complexes were wide, and calcium, sodium bicarbonate, insulin and glucose were administered for possible hyperkalemia. The patient remained in arrest and expired before coronary angiography could be performed.

## Case 2.4 A 52-year-old female with long-standing hypertension presented to the emergency department with 1 day of stuttering chest tightness and some nausea. The emergency medicine and cardiology teams felt that her ECG was consistent with left ventricular hypertrophy with repolarization abnormalities ("strain pattern"). The computer algorithm reached the same diagnosis. Her initial troponin was 0.35, and she was admitted to the telemetry unit for "risk stratification and rule-out myocardial infarction, possible non-STEMI."

### The Electrocardiogram

There is little question that she has electrocardiographic findings of left ventricular hypertrophy with repolarization abnormalities. But here is what the clinicians (and the computer algorithm) missed: first, the ST-segments are straightened and elevated in the inferior leads, especially leads III and aVF. ST-segment elevation occurs commonly in the right precordial leads (V1–V3), but *not in the inferior* leads, in patients with LVH. There is also obvious ST-segment depression in leads I and aVL, consistent with acute inferior STEMI. While the ST-segment depressions in I and aVL are consistent with LVH with repolarization abnormalities (I and aVL are left-facing leads), the same cannot be said for the ST-segment depressions in the anterior precordial leads (V1–V3). In LVH with repolarization changes (the "strain pattern"), the ST-segments in the right precordial leads are typically elevated, not depressed. (See the discussion of LVH in Chapter 6.) In this patient, the anterior precordial ST-segment depressions are indicative of extension of the inferior STEMI to the posterior wall.

### Clinical Course

Two hours after admission, she sustained a VF arrest. She was successfully resuscitated. Her troponin peaked at 96. Her catheterization was performed almost 14 hours after her initial presentation. Angiography demonstrated a tight occlusion of the ostial and proximal left circumflex artery. The final ECG diagnosis: acute inferior and posterior ST-elevation myocardial infarction; also left ventricular hypertrophy with repolarization abnormalities.

## Case 2.5 A 69-year-old female presented after a syncopal episode. She reported chest and abdominal pain over 1 hour. In the field she was initially pulseless, and the pre-hospital ECG demonstrated bradycardia and ST-elevations in the inferior leads.

### The Electrocardiogram

Her ECG demonstrates an acute inferior wall STEMI and complete heart block. The ST-segment elevation in V1 is indicative of a right ventricular infarction. RVMI was confirmed with additional right-sided leads.

### Clinical Course

Upon presentation, this patient required intravenous fluids, pressors and transcutaneous pacing to stabilize her blood pressure. She was intubated because of progressive hypoxia. She was taken emergently to the catheterization laboratory, which demonstrated a "long, 90 percent stenosis of the proximal RCA and a long, 90 percent stenosis of the mid-distal RCA." She had multiple bouts of ventricular tachycardia during the procedure, but the culprit lesions were successfully treated with four bare metal stents. Her peak troponin level was 153.

## Case 2.6  A 53-year-old man presented with dizziness and a near-syncopal episode. He had sustained an acute inferior myocardial infarction 13 days earlier.

### The Electrocardiogram

The ECG demonstrates pathologic Q-waves in leads III and aVF, consistent with an old ("remote" or "indeterminate age") inferior wall myocardial infarction. Leads III and aVF meet the criteria for "pathologic Q-waves" outlined earlier in this chapter. T-wave inversions are also present in these two leads. The limb leads also suggest left ventricular hypertrophy. (The voltage in lead I is > 11 mm.)

### Clinical Course

As noted earlier in this chapter, in a patient with syncope, the mere presence of an "old" or "indeterminate age" myocardial infarction (Q-waves) on the ECG is strongly associated with ventricular tachycardia as the etiology for the patient's syncope.

## Case 2.7  A 53-year-old man was brought to the emergency department by paramedics after being struck by a car at very low speed. He stated that the vehicle's side mirror sideswiped the right side of his chest. His only complaint was right-sided chest pain. During his trauma evaluation, an ECG was obtained because he "didn't look good or feel good."

### The Electrocardiogram

The 12-lead ECG is made more challenging because of the widespread ventricular ectopy. However, the inferior wall STEMI is plainly seen in the few normally conducted beats. In the normal sinus beats, there are large ST-segment elevations in leads II, III and aVF, accompanied by ST-segment depressions in leads I and aVL, just as expected. We cannot allow the PVCs to distract us from recognizing the classic features of an inferior wall STEMI. In this case, the computer initially missed the diagnosis.

## Case 2.8  A 56-year-old man with a history of heavy smoking and untreated hypertension presented with acute left-sided chest pain, beginning 25 minutes prior to presentation. He had associated dyspnea, diaphoresis and nausea. The initial computer reading was "sinus tachycardia, and marked ST abnormality, possible lateral subendocardial injury." He was admitted to the hospital, where his ED note read, "Non-specific ST-T changes, not meeting STEMI criteria."

### The Electrocardiogram

This patient's acute inferior and posterior wall STEMI was initially missed. The ECG may not meet a hospital's "cath lab activation" criteria, but it unequivocally meets our criteria for diagnosing an acute inferior wall STEMI. There is clear ST-segment elevation in lead III; even though it is "concave upward" and may appear benign at first glance, it is accompanied by reciprocal ST-segment depression in I and aVL. There is also mild ST-segment elevation (concave downward, or "dome-shaped") in lead V1, suggesting possible accompanying RVMI.

The ST-segments are mildly elevated in aVR; aVR is a right-facing lead, and ST-elevations in aVR may increase the likelihood that the culprit occluded vessel is the RCA and even increase the likelihood that an RVMI is present. Possible posterior wall involvement is suggested by the ST-segment depressions in V2–V4. Sinus tachycardia is also present.

### Clinical Course

This patient's troponin level peaked at 13.8. Angiography demonstrated a 100 percent proximal RCA occlusion. Perfusion was restored, and a bare metal stent was placed.

## Case 2.9 A 59-year-old woman presented with acute shortness of breath. In the emergency department, she was in pulmonary edema. Her dyspnea worsened, and she developed progressive hypoxia, requiring endotracheal intubation.

### The Electrocardiogram

Her initial ECG is almost normal. The clinicians did not fully appreciate the ST-segment depressions in leads I and aVL, which should have served as an early warning sign of acute inferior STEMI (see earlier discussion of Birnbaum's warning). On this initial ECG, these ST-segment depressions in the high lateral leads are the only definitive markers of an acute inferior STEMI. A repeat ECG was obtained.

## Case 2.9 Same patient, follow-up ECG, 90 minutes later.

### The Electrocardiogram

This ECG was taken 90 minutes later, and it shows clear evolution of her inferior wall STEMI with more marked ST-segment depressions in leads I and aVL.

One likely cause of acute pulmonary edema, given her inferior wall STEMI, is acute papillary muscle rupture. The records did not comment on a mitral insufficiency murmur. As noted earlier, the RCA is a major source of blood supply to the posteromedial papillary muscle of the mitral valve. It is always important to auscultate the heart for the presence of mitral insufficiency, especially in patients with congestive heart failure or shock. Actual rupture of the papillary muscle is rare; however, when it occurs, it is catastrophic and is a "don't-miss" mechanical cause of cardiogenic shock in IMI patients.

There is another likely cause for her severe cardiac pump failure. Her ECG demonstrates extensive ST-segment depressions across the precordial leads, and the ST-segments are *disproportionately depressed in the lateral precordial leads* (V4–V6). As discussed earlier, this is often a sign of extensive LAD disease with concomitant anterior wall ischemia, even while the culprit artery is the RCA.

Other causes of pump failure and shock in acute inferior wall myocardial infarction, in addition to extensive inferior, posterior and lateral wall involvement and papillary muscle rupture, include: RV infarction (especially if the patient has received diuretics or vasodilators); interventricular septal rupture; and arrhythmias, including atrial fibrillation or high-grade AV block.

### Clinical Course

The patient developed worsening pulmonary edema and expired in the emergency department before she could be transferred to the angiography suite.

## Case 2.10 A 59-year-old man presented with chest pain, dizziness and shortness of breath.

### The Electrocardiogram

The ECG demonstrates an acute inferior wall STEMI and atrial fibrillation (AF) with a rapid ventricular response. There is also poor R-wave progression and low voltage in the limb leads. When AF occurs during the first hours of an acute inferior wall STEMI, it usually signifies one of the following: left ventricular pump failure causing left atrial distention, RVMI (with right atrial dilatation), atrial infarction, catecholamine excess or an electrolyte abnormality (hypokalemia or hypomagnesemia). An important additional point: these findings – regional ST-segment elevation, low-voltage QRS complexes and tachycardia – are also consistent with severe focal myocarditis. (See Chapter 5 for further discussion.)

## Case 2.11 An 80-year-old female presented with 3 hours of nausea and vomiting accompanied by light-headedness. She had a history of hypertension and hypothyroidism. She reported a normal cardiac nuclear stress test 1 year earlier. She denied chest pain and was in no distress on presentation.

### The Electrocardiogram

The ECG demonstrates sinus rhythm with a right bundle branch block. But the cause of her nausea and light-headedness is the inferior STEMI. The ECG shows ST-segment elevation in III (> II) and in aVF and ST-segment depression in aVL. Lead V1 shows pronounced ST-segment elevation; we know that V1 is a right-sided lead, and ST-segment elevation in V1, in the setting of an acute inferior STEMI, suggests that the inferior STEMI is complicated by RVMI. There is also diffuse low voltage in the limb and precordial leads.

RBBB, in contrast to LBBB, does not usually cause major displacements of the ST-segment; thus, RBBB should not interfere with the diagnosis of acute STEMI. (Posterior wall STEMI is sometimes an exception.) Still, the diagnosis of acute MI is often missed or delayed when RBBB is present. The prognosis of acute MI is worse in the presence of RBBB or LBBB, even if the BBB is long-standing and preceded the acute infarction.

### Clinical Course

Her initial troponin level was 8.0; later, the peak troponin was 16.2. Emergency angiography demonstrated significant three-vessel disease; the culprit lesion was a high-grade occlusion of the proximal RCA.

## Case 2.12  A 44-year-old man was healthy and without any known coronary artery disease or cardiovascular risk factors, except for smoking. He presented with intermittent chest pain over 8 days. On the morning of admission, he had severe chest pain, accompanied by nausea and diaphoresis.

### The Electrocardiogram

The ECG demonstrates an acute inferior wall STEMI. There are also ST-segment elevations in V5–V6, indicating extension of the infarction to the lateral wall. There is also ST-segment depression with upright T-waves in precordial leads V2 and V3, suggesting posterior wall involvement. Abnormally tall R-waves are present in leads V1 and V2, consistent with his posterior STEMI.

The limb leads and rhythm strip show periods of sinus bradycardia with the emergence of junctional beats. (Inverted P-waves are present in lead II.) As noted, junctional escape beats and more rapid ("accelerated") junctional rhythms are common in the setting of inferior wall STEMI.

### Clinical Course

This patient's right-sided ECG leads (not shown) were positive for RVMI. On catheterization, "the RCA was a large dominant vessel that had a total proximal thrombotic occlusion."

## Case 2.13  A 60-year-old man was driving. He pulled off to the side of the road and called 911. When the EMTs arrived, he was in ventricular fibrillation. A life support flight crew was also summoned. In the field, despite multiple defibrillation shocks, an epinephrine drip and other drugs, he remained in refractory VF. The resuscitation efforts continued in the emergency department. Prior to ending the resuscitation effort, a final 200 J shock was administered as shown.

### The Electrocardiogram

After the defibrillatory shock, there are two organized complexes that are highly suggestive of a STEMI. The catheterization laboratory was activated, and a 12-lead ECG was obtained.

## Case 2.13  The same patient – 12-lead ECG after defibrillation.

### The Electrocardiogram

The computer algorithm is fooled by the apparent "wide complex rhythm." In fact, the ECG shows an acute inferior and posterior wall STEMI. A right bundle branch block is also present.

### Clinical Course

Although this patient had not regained consciousness, he was taken emergently to the cardiac catheterization laboratory. The finding was not surprising: "The RCA is 100 percent occluded by thrombus in the proximal segment." A drug-eluting stent was inserted, and the patient underwent a cooling protocol. However, despite a prolonged period of hemodynamic and respiratory support, he showed no signs of cerebral recovery, and care was eventually withdrawn.

## Case 2.14   A 67-year-old female with a history of hypertension, hyperlipidemia and diabetes presented with 2 hours of left upper chest pain and mild shortness of breath. She had stable vital signs but was having chest pain in the ED. She received aspirin and sublingual nitroglycerin. Her initial troponin was 0.01.

### The Electrocardiogram

The ECG shows low-voltage QRS complexes in the limb and precordial leads, not changed from old tracings. Importantly, there are also changes of early, acute inferior STEMI with reciprocal ST-segment depression in aVL. The computer algorithm did not detect the acute STEMI. The ECG shows a likely "indeterminate age" anteroseptal MI, also unchanged from prior tracings. A single ventricular or aberrantly conducted premature beat is also noted. The rhythm is atrial fibrillation with a controlled ventricular response.

### Clinical Course

Given this patient's symptoms and her ECG, the correct diagnosis was reached: inferior wall STEMI. The interventional team was notified. Catheterization revealed that the LAD was occluded by a thrombus "in the very distal segment," where it wrapped around the apex. "Wraparound LAD" occlusions are discussed in Chapter 3. A "wraparound" LAD perfuses the inferior left ventricular wall; the obstructing clots are often in the middle or distal segments of the LAD and frequently carry a more benign prognosis. In this case, there was no evidence of anterior wall STEMI. Her peak troponin was only 8.13.

In this tracing, the ST-segment elevation in lead III is modest, and the ST-segment depression in lead aVL also appears "minor." But both changes are actually dramatic, in the context of these low-voltage QRS complexes. Low-voltage QRS complexes are also consistent with myocarditis, pericardial tamponade, infiltrative cardiomyopathy and other conditions. But given this patient's presentation, the diagnosis of acute inferior STEMI is clear. As we have said repeatedly, the computer did not, and cannot, make this diagnosis. But we must.

## References

Alzand B. S. N., Gorgels A. P. M. Combined anterior and inferior ST-segment elevation: Electrocardiographic differentiation between right coronary artery occlusion with predominant right ventricular infarction and distal left anterior descending branch occlusion. *J Electrocardiology*. 2011; 44:383–388.

American College of Cardiology Foundation/American Heart Association. 2013 ACCF/AHA Guideline for the management of ST-elevation myocardial infarction. *J Am Col Cardiol*. 2013; 61: e78–140. http://content.onlinejacc.org/article.aspx?articleid=1486115#tab1. Accessed April 1, 2016.

Assali A. R., Sclarovsky S., Herz I. et al. Comparison of patients with inferior wall acute myocardial infarction with versus without ST-segment elevation in leads V5 and V6. *Am J Cardiol*. 1998; 81: 81–83.

Atar S., Birnbaum Y. Ischemia-induced ST-segment elevation: Classification, prognosis and therapy. *J Electrocardio*. 2005; 38:1–7.

Bhat P. K., Pantham G., Laskey S. et al. Recognizing cardiac syncope in patients presenting to the emergency department with trauma. *J Emerg Med*. 2014; 46:1–8.

Birnbaum Y., Nikus K., Kligfield P. et al. The role of the ECG in diagnosis, risk estimation and catheterization laboratory activation in patients with acute coronary syndromes: A consensus document. *Ann Noninvasive Electrocardiol*. 2014; 19:412–425.

Birnbaum Y., Sclarovsky S., Mager A. et al. ST segment depression in aVL: a sensitive marker for acute inferior myocardial infarction. *Eur Heart J*. 1993; 14:4–7.

Birnbaum Y., Wagner G. S., Barbash G. I. et al. Correlation of angiographic findings and right (V1–V3) versus left (V4–V6) precordial ST-segment depression in inferior wall acute myocardial infarction. *Am J Cardiol*. 1999; 83:143–148.

Birnbaum Y., Wilson J. M., Fiol M. et al. ECG diagnosis and classification of acute coronary syndromes. *Ann Noninvasive Electrocardiol*. 2014; 19:4–14.

Bischof J. E., Worrall C., Thompson P. et al. ST depression in lead aVL differentiates inferior ST-elevation myocardial infarction from pericarditis. *Am J Emerg Med*. 2016; 34:149–154.

Brady W. J., The earth is flat. The electrocardiogram has 12 leads. The electrocardiogram in the patient with ACS: Looking beyond the 12-lead electrocardiogram. *Am J Emerg Med*. 2007; 25:1073–1076.

Brady W. J., Syverud S. A., Beagle C. et al. Electrocardiographic ST-segment elevation: The diagnosis of acute myocardial infarction by morphologic analysis of the ST segment. *Acad Emerg Med*. 2001; 8:961–9672001.

Chan T. C., Brady W. J., Harrigan R. A. et al. *ECG in emergency medicine and acute care*. Philadelphia, PA: Elsevier Mosby, 2005.

Chia B. L., Yip J. W., Tan H. C., Lim Y. T. Usefulness of ST elevation II/III ratio and ST deviation in lead I for identifying the culprit artery in inferior wall acute myocardial infarction. *Am J Cardiol*. 2000; 86:341–1433.

Del'Itallia L. J. Reperfusion for right ventricular infarction. *N Engl J Med*. 1998; 338:978–980.

Goldberger A. L. Recognition of ECG psuedo-infarct patterns. *Mod Concepts Cardiovasc. Dis*. 1980; XLIX (3): 13–18.

Goldstein J. A. Acute right ventricular infarction. *Cardiol Clin*. 2012; 30:219–232.

Hamon M., Agostini D., Le Page O. et al. Prognostic impact of right ventricular involvement in patients with acute myocardial infarction: Meta-analysis. *Crit Care Med.* 2008; **36**:2023–2033.

Hasdai D., Birnbaum Y., Porter A., Sclarovsky S. Maximal precordial ST-segment depression in leads V4–V6 in patients with inferior wall acute myocardial infarction indicates coronary artery disease involving the left anterior descending coronary artery system. *Inter J Cardiology.* 1997; **58**:273–278.

Hassen G. W., Talebi S., Fernaine G., Kalantari H. Lead aVL on electrocardiogram: emerging as important lead in early detection of myocardial infarction? *Am J Emerg Med.* 2014; **32**:785–788.

Inohara T., Kohsaka S., Fukuda K., Menon V. The challenges in the management of right ventricular infarction. *Eur Heart J: Acute Cardiovascular Care.* 2013; **2** (3):226–234.

Kakouros N., Cokkinos D. V. Right ventricular myocardial infarction: Pathophysiology, diagnosis and management. *Postgrad Med J.* 2010; **86**:719–728.

Kontos M. C., Desai P. V., Jesse R. L., Ornato J. P. Usefulness of the admission electrocardiogram for identifying the infarct-related artery in inferior wall acute myocardial infarction. *Am J Cardiol.* 1997; **79**:182–184.

Marriott H. J. L. *Emergency electrocardiography*. Naples, FL: Trinity Press, 1997.

Moye S., Carney M. F., Hostege C. et al. The electrocardiogram in right ventricular infarction. *Am J Emerg Med.* 2005; **23**:793–799.

Nikus K., Birnbaum Y., Eskola M. et al. Updated electrocardiographic classification of acute coronary syndromes. *Current Cardiol Rev.* 2014; **10**:229–236.

Nikus K., Pahlm O., Wagner G. et al. Electrocardiographic classification of acute coronary syndromes: A review by a committee of the International Society for Holter and Non-invasive Cardiology. *J Electrocardio.* 2010; **43**:91–103.

O'Rourke R. A., Dell'Italia L. J. Diagnosis and management of right ventricular myocardial infarction. *Curr Probl Cardiol.* 2004; **29**:1–47.

Puppala V. K., Dickinson O., Benditt D. G. Syncope: Classification and risk stratification. *J Cardiol.* 2014; **63**: 171–177.

Smith S. W., Zvosec D. L., Sharkey S. W., Henry T. D. *The ECG in acute MI. An evidence-based manual of reperfusion therapy*. Philadelphia, PA: Lippincott Williams & Wilkins, 2002.

Surawicz B., Knilans T. K. *Chou's electrocardiography in clinical practice*. Sixth edition. Chapters 7, 8. Philadelphia, PA: Elsevier Saunders, 2008.

Tamura A. Significance of lead aVR in acute coronary syndrome. *World J Cardiol.* 2014; **26**:630–637.

Thygesen K., Alpert J. S., Jaffe A. S. et al. Third universal definition of myocardial infarction. *J Am Coll Cardiol.* 2012; **60**:1581–1598.

Tsuka Y., Sugiura T., Hatada K. et al. Clinical significance of ST-segment elevation in lead V1 in patients with acute inferior wall Q-wave myocardial infarction. *Am Heart J.* 2001; **141**:615–620.

Turhan H., Yilmaz M. B., Yetkin E. et al. Diagnostic value of aVL derivation for right ventricular involvement in patients with acute inferior myocardial infarction. *A.N.E.* 2003; **8**:185–188.

Vales L., Kanei Y., Schweitzer P. Electrocardiographic predictors of culprit artery in acute inferior ST elevation myocardial infarction. *J Electrocardiol.* 2011; **44**:31–35.

Wagner G. S., Macfarlane P., Wellens H. et al. AHA/ACCF/HRS recommendations for the standardization and interpretation of the electrocardiogram. Part VI: Acute ischemia/infarction. A scientific statement from the American Heart Association, Electrocardiography and Arrhythmias Committee; Council on Clinical Cardiology; the American College of Cardiology Foundation; and the Heart Rhythm Society. *J Amer Col Cardiol.* 2009; **53**:1003–1011.

Wang S. S., Paynter L., Kelly R. V. et al. Electrocardiographic determination of culprit lesion site in patients with acute coronary events. *J Electrocardiol.* 2009; **42**:46–51.

Wellens H. J. J. Right ventricular infarction. *N Engl J Med.* 1993; **328**: 1036–1038.

Wellens H. J. J., Conover M. *The ECG in emergency decision-making*. Second edition. St Louis, MO: Elsevier, Inc., 2006.

Zehnder M., Kasper W., Kauder E. et al. Right ventricular infarction as an independent predictor of prognosis after acute inferior myocardial infarction. *N Engl J Med.* 1993; **328**:981–988.

Zimetbaum P. J., Josephson M. E. Use of the electrocardiogram in acute myocardial infarction. *N Engl J Med.* 2003; **348**:933–940.

Zimetbaum P. J., Krushnan S., Gold A. et al. Usefulness of ST-segment elevation in lead III exceeding that of lead II for identifying the location of the totally occluded coronary artery in inferior wall myocardial infarction. *Am J Cardiol.* 1998; **81**:918–919.

# Anterior Wall Myocardial Infarction

## Key Points

- Acute anterior wall ST-elevation myocardial infarction (STEMI) classically presents with ST-segment elevations in one or more precordial leads. Usually, ST-elevation in lead V1 signifies infarction of the interventricular septum. ST-elevation in leads V2–V4 indicates infarction of the anterior (or anteroapical) wall. ST-elevation in V5–V6 signals infarction of the lateral left ventricular wall.
- Anterior wall STEMI is a high-risk event, frequently complicated by cardiogenic shock, bundle branch block and ventricular arrhythmias.
- In the vast majority of cases of anterior, anteroseptal and anterolateral wall STEMIs, the culprit event is an acute occlusion of the left anterior descending (LAD) artery. The presence of concomitant ST-segment elevations in aVR may signify acute occlusion of the left main coronary artery (LCMA).
- Proximal LAD occlusions may also cause ST-elevations in the high lateral limb leads (I and aVL), signifying occlusion of the LAD before the first diagonal branch (D1). Not surprisingly, high lateral infarction is usually accompanied by reciprocal ST-segment depressions in the inferior leads. Isolated, high lateral STEMIs are often missed.
- Clinicians should also recognize the pattern of acute anterior wall STEMI accompanied by ST-segment elevations in leads II, III and aVF (concomitant inferior wall STEMI). Often, this signifies occlusion of the mid- or distal portion of a long LAD that wraps around the apex of the heart to perfuse the inferior wall. ST-segment elevations in the anterior and inferior leads may also be a sign of pericarditis, myocarditis, early repolarization or another "coronary mimic."
- Anterior STEMI is often complicated by development of bundle branch block; the most common pattern is right bundle branch, often with left anterior fascicular block, which may develop acutely and progress to complete heart block and life-threatening bradycardia. Bundle branch and bifascicular blocks develop when the LAD is occluded before the septal perforator branches.
- Clinicians must recognize several early warning signs of a critical LAD occlusion: tall or abnormally broad

("hyperacute") T-waves" in the anterior precordial leads; a biphasic T-wave in lead V2 or V3 ("Wellens' sign" Type A); and deep, symmetric T-wave inversions ("coronary T-waves") in the anterior precordial leads (Wellens' sign Type B). These early warning signs may occur while the patient is pain-free and hemodynamically stable and in the presence of little or no cardiac enzyme elevation. They may represent a critically obstructed LAD that has undergone spontaneous reperfusion but that remains at risk for rethrombosis.
- Limb lead aVR may provide critical diagnostic information. In the presence of an anterior STEMI, ST-segment elevation in aVR suggests occlusion of the left main coronary artery (LMCA) or "its equivalent." ST-segment elevation in lead aVR is also significant in patients who have ST-segment depressions in multiple inferior and lateral leads (typically, limb leads I, II and aVL and precordial leads V4, V5 and V6). In this situation ("global" or "concentric" ischemia), ST-segment elevation in aVR is often a "STEMI equivalent," indicating an obstructive thrombus of the LMCA or proximal LAD and the need for emergent reperfusion.
- The presence of a LBBB makes the recognition of acute anterior wall STEMI difficult. The weighted Sgarbossa criteria are specific, but not sensitive, for the diagnosis of acute anterior wall STEMI.
- Anterior wall STEMI must be differentiated from early repolarization pattern, left ventricular hypertrophy with repolarization abnormalities, pericarditis, takotusbo cardiomyopathy, hypothermia and other "coronary mimics."
- Clinicians must also recognize several "STEMI equivalents." These are ECG patterns that may not meet classic "threshold" definitions of "STEMI" nor standard "cath lab activation" criteria. But they often signal acute thrombotic occlusion of a major coronary artery and the need for emergent reperfusion. STEMI equivalents include ST-elevations in aVR, acute coronary syndromes with only minimal ("subthreshold") ST-elevations, ST-elevations in fewer than "two contiguous leads," ST-segment depressions in V1–V3 (signifying posterolateral STEMI) and other patterns reviewed in this atlas.

## Anterior Wall ST-Elevation Myocardial Infarction

Anterior wall ST-elevation myocardial infarction (STEMI) is a high-risk event. Compared with inferior wall STEMIs, anterior wall STEMIs have larger infarct sizes and a higher rate of left ventricular dysfunction, congestive heart failure, ventricular arrhythmias and in-hospital and overall mortality (Stone et al., 1988).

Classically, acute anterior wall STEMI presents with ST-segment elevation in one or more precordial leads. As illustrated in

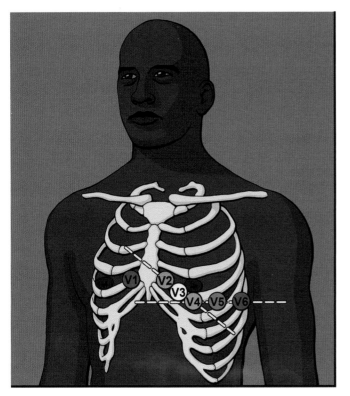

**Figure 3.1**  Standard placement of the six precordial leads.

Figure 3.1, ST-elevation in lead V1 signifies infarction of the interventricular septum. ST-elevation in leads V2–V4 indicates infarction of the anterior (or anteroapical) wall. And ST-elevation in V5–V6 signals infarction of the lateral left ventricular wall.

## Anterior Wall ST-Elevation Myocardial Infarction: A Review of the Coronary Anatomy

In the vast majority of cases of anterior, septal and anterolateral wall STEMIs, the culprit event is an acute occlusion of the left anterior descending (LAD) artery. The anatomy of the LAD is illustrated in Figure 3.2.

The most common coronary artery anatomy is illustrated in this figure. The left main coronary artery bifurcates quickly into two main branches:

- The left circumflex artery (LCA) primarily perfuses the posterior and posterolateral wall of the heart.
- The large left anterior descending (LAD) artery supplies blood to the anterior wall of the left ventricle. Note two critical branches of the LAD:
  - The large first diagonal branch ("D-1") supplies blood to the upper left (high lateral) left ventricular wall; an occlusive clot within D-1 or in the LAD proximal to D1 is likely to cause a STEMI involving the high lateral leads (I and aVL), also resulting in reciprocal ST-segment depressions in the inferior leads, especially lead III.
  - The small septal perforator branches are also critically important because they nourish the interventricular septum. Since the left and right bundle branches travel within the septum, an LAD occlusion proximal to the septal perforators often causes anteroseptal infarction (ST-segment elevation in V1–V4) and development of right or left bundle branch block. The most common pattern is right bundle branch and left anterior fascicular block, which often portends the rapid development of complete heart block and life-threatening bradycardia.

**Figure 3.2**  Anatomy of the left anterior descending coronary artery.

Left circumflex a. (LCX)

Left anterior descending (LAD) a.

1st diagonal branch

Septal perforating branches (SPs)

See ECG 3.1, which illustrates a classic anteroseptal STEMI.

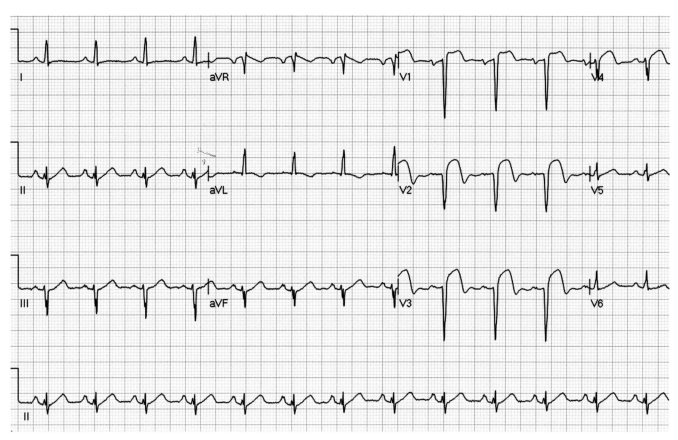

**ECG 3.1** A 46-year-old man without any significant medical history presented with 2 hours of substernal chest pain.

## The Electrocardiogram

The ECG demonstrates marked ST-segment elevations in lead V2–V4, as well as V1, indicating an acute anteroseptal STEMI. Left axis deviation is also present along with possible left atrial enlargement.

Deep "QS" complexes (Q-waves) are present in the anteroseptal leads. However, as emphasized later in this chapter, this does not mean that the evolving anterior STEMI is old, that there is irreversible myocardial necrosis or that myocardial salvage by reperfusion is not indicated.

## Clinical Course

He was taken emergently to the catheterization laboratory, which revealed a 95 percent LAD occlusion. His peak troponin was 292. On hospital day 2, an echocardiogram demonstrated hypokinesis of the mid and distal septum and apex, but the overall left ventricular ejection fraction was normal.

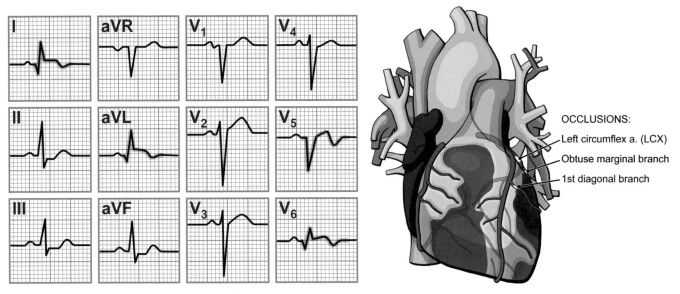

**Figure 3.3** Perfusion of the high lateral wall of the left ventricle.
A STEMI involving leads I and aVL likely signifies either an obstructive occlusion of the LAD, prior to or within the first diagonal branch; or occlusion of the left circumflex artery (LCX) or its first major branch (the obtuse marginal artery). Logically, and as illustrated in this figure, the reciprocal inferior leads, especially lead III, will show ST-segment depressions.

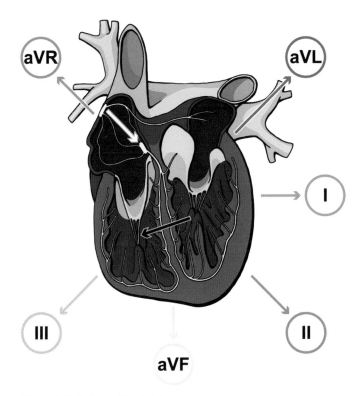

**Figure 3.4** Position of the limb leads.
Leads I and aVL monitor the high lateral portions of the left ventricle. As illustrated in Figure 3.3, the high lateral myocardium is usually supplied by the first diagonal artery (the first large, proximal branch of the LAD) or the left circumflex artery (or an obtuse marginal branch).

## STEMIs Involving the "High Lateral" Wall

Proximal LAD occlusions may cause ST-elevations not only in the anterior, septal and lateral precordial leads but also in the high lateral limb leads (I and aVL). When concomitant ST-segment elevation is present in leads I or aVL, it usually signifies occlusion of the LAD before the first diagonal branch (D1) (see Figures 3.2 and 3.3). Not surprisingly, high lateral infarction is usually accompanied by reciprocal ST-segment depressions in the inferior leads. Even if there are no noticeable ST-elevations in I or aVL, the presence of ST-segment depressions in the inferior leads, in a patient with an acute anterior wall STEMI, carries the same significance: one can predict that a high lateral STEMI is evolving and that the LAD is occluded proximal to the takeoff of D-1 (Yip et al., 2003; Arbane and Gay, 2000; Engelen, 1999; Birnbaum et al., 1994; Eskola et al., 2009; Birnbaum, Wilson et al., 2014; Wagner et al., 2009; Wang et al., 2009).

ST-segment elevations in the high lateral leads, without ST-elevations in V1–V4, may also be caused by occlusion of the left circumflex artery (LCA) or one of its major branches, especially the obtuse marginal (OM). See Figure 3.3.

See the following ECG tracing (ECG 3.2) for a typical example.

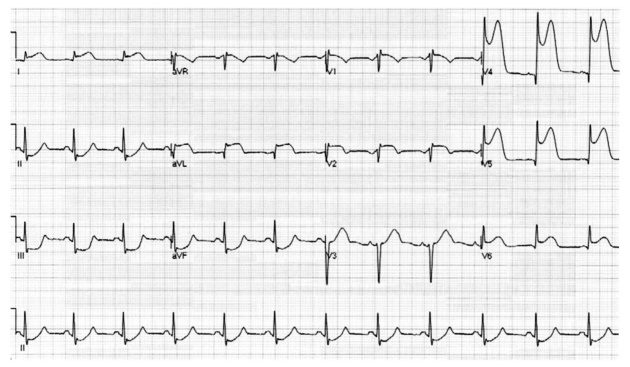

**ECG 3.2** A 61-year-old man with chest pain reported "not feeling well" for 10 hours.

## The Electrocardiogram

The ECG demonstrates an extensive STEMI involving the anteroseptal, lateral and high lateral regions of the heart. The inferior ST-depressions are reciprocal changes associated with acute injury to the high lateral wall (I and aVL).

## Clinical Course

The angiogram findings were predictable: "The left anterior descending coronary artery was totally occluded proximal to the origin of the first diagonal branch."

## Early Warnings of LAD Occlusion and Impending Anteroseptal STEMI

When patients present with chest pain, shortness of breath or related symptoms, one critical goal is to identify patients likely to have a critical LAD obstruction. Even without clear ST-segment elevations that meet standard "cath lab activation" criteria, a critical LAD occlusion may be present. Hyperacute T-waves, Wellens' syndrome and ST-segment elevations in lead aVR are among the "don't-miss" clues.

### Hyperacute T-Waves

When a major epicardial coronary artery is suddenly occluded, the first change on the electrocardiogram is a sudden increase in the amplitude of the T waves. Although these "hyperacute T-waves" may be transient, they represent a critical warning sign of coronary artery (especially LAD) occlusion (Birnbaum, 2014;

Sommers, 2002; Ayer and Terkelsen, 2014; Rokos et al., 2010; Nikus et al., 2010; Nikus et al., 2014; Thygesen et al., 2012).

In the anterior precordial leads (V1–V4), hyperacute T-waves appear abnormally tall, and often they are broad-based or "bulky" (Marriott, 1997). They can be symmetric or asymmetric. One useful clue to abnormal, hyperacute T-waves is found in precordial lead V1. The T-wave in V1 is usually small or even inverted. If the T-wave in V1 is taller than the T-wave in V6, it is usually abnormal and may be "hyperacute."

Hyperacute T-waves signify severe transmural ischemia and an impending STEMI due to a critical LAD occlusion. Although immediate reperfusion may not be indicated for hyperacute T-waves alone, repeat electrocardiograms at short intervals are required (Birnbaum, 2014).

Hyperacute T-waves signifying occlusion of the LAD and impending STEMI must be differentiated from other causes of prominent T-waves, including hyperkalemia, left ventricular hypertrophy, early repolarization, bundle branch block (or a ventricular paced rhythm), hypertrophic cardiomyopathy and stroke. For examples of some of these confusing conditions, see Chapter 7, Confusing Conditions: ST-Segment Elevations and Tall T-Waves (Coronary Mimics).

Figure 3.5 illustrates hyperacute T-waves in the precordial leads. The T-waves are tall and wide; Marriott has described these hyperacute T-waves as "broad-based" and "bulky" (Marriott, 1997). His term "wishbone effect" is also apt, as the arms of the T-wave appear to be widely splayed apart. Note that the T-wave in V1 is much taller than the T-wave in V6. This is almost never normal and serves as a clue to acute coronary insufficiency.

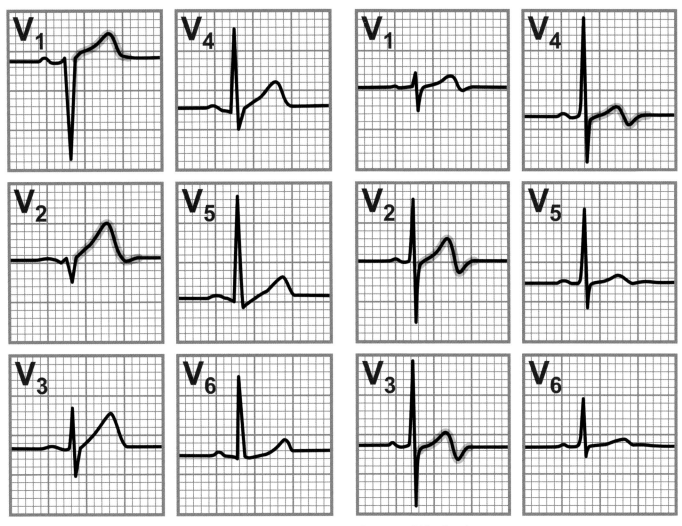

**Figure 3.5** Hyperacute T-waves.

**Figure 3.6** Wellens' syndrome.
This figure illustrates Wellens' syndrome (Type A), which is an early warning sign of a critical LAD occlusion. In leads V2, V3 and V4, the ST-segment is essentially normal. However, the T-wave is biphasic, becoming negative in its terminal portion.

## Wellens' Syndrome

Another important early warning sign of a critical LAD occlusion is "Wellens' syndrome" ("Wellens' warning"). Two patterns are recognized.

- First, precordial leads V2, V3 or V4 may show a biphasic T-wave. Classically, the ST-segment is normal or near-normal, but the T-wave is inverted in the terminal portion. This pattern, sometimes referred to as "Wellens' Type A," is usually a reflection of an acute or chronic proximal LAD occlusion. It may signify recent reperfusion of an obstructed LAD (but the obstructed LAD remains at risk).
- Deep, symmetric T-wave inversions ("coronary T-waves") in the anterior or lateral precordial leads may also signify LAD occlusion. This pattern is sometimes referred to as Wellen's sign, Type B (Tandy et al., 1999; Wagner et al., 2009; Ayer and Terkelsen, 2014; Birnbaum, 2014). These must be differentiated (clinically) from the T-wave inversions that accompany intracranial hemorrhage. Importantly, anterior precordial T-wave inversions are also a common ECG finding in patients with acute pulmonary embolism. (See Chapter 5, The Electrocardiography of Shortness of Breath.)

The ECG abnormalities of Wellens' syndrome – biphasic T-waves or deep T-wave inversions – may appear while the patient is pain-free and hemodynamically stable and in the presence of little or no cardiac biomarker elevation. Nonetheless, they are characteristic of an acute, tight LAD occlusion. Angiographic studies suggest that patients who are pain-free and who present with these biphasic or inverted T-waves in V2–V4 may have undergone spontaneous reperfusion of the LAD; that is, they are in a somewhat later, "evolutionary" phase of their acute coronary insufficiency syndrome (Nikus et al., 2014; Birnbaum, Wilson et al., 2014; Nikus et al., 2010). Nevertheless, it is likely that the proximal LAD has a ruptured plaque with residual clot and is still at risk for re-occlusion and development of a classic anterior wall STEMI within hours or days (or, possibly, weeks). These patients should not be discharged or subjected to exercise stress testing. Admission and cardiology consultation, at the very least, are indicated (Wagner et al., 2009; Birnbaum, Wilson et al., 2014; Nikus et al., 2014; Nikus et al., 2010; Birnbaum, Nikus et al., 2014).

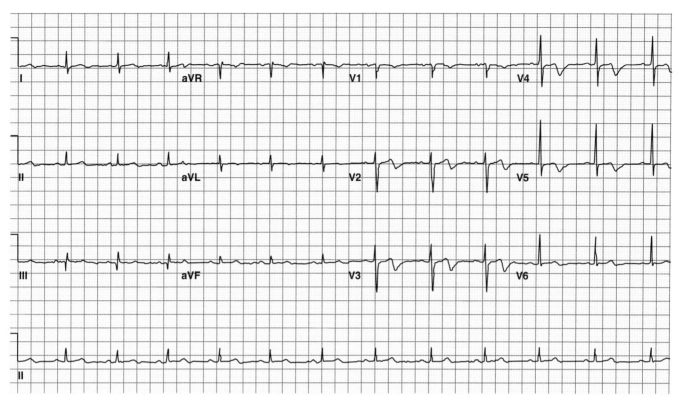

**ECG 3.3** A 75-year-old man developed chest pain while shoveling snow. He also complained of dizziness and shortness of breath. On ED arrival, he was in respiratory distress, and his initial systolic blood pressure was 80 mm Hg.

## The Electrocardiogram

The ECG shows a classic biphasic T-wave in leads V2 and V3; this is Wellens' warning. The ST-segment is essentially normal before the T-wave reverses direction and becomes inverted. The T-waves are also inverted in leads V4 and V5.

In fact, both types of Wellens' syndrome (A and B) are present on this single tracing. This pattern is strongly associated with a critical proximal LAD occlusion, even if the patient is pain-free and even if the troponin is normal. One hour later, the patient had a repeat ECG.

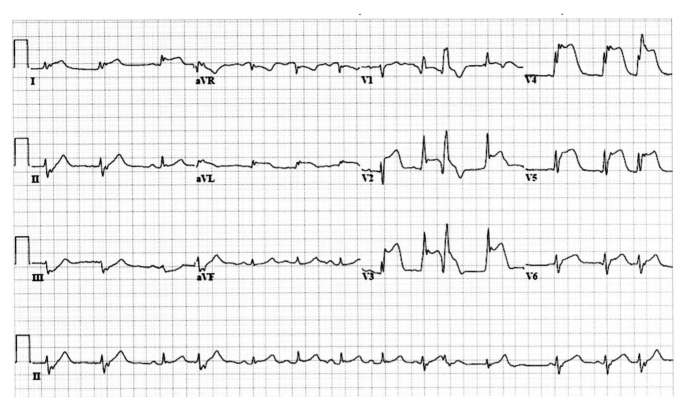

**ECG 3.3** The same patient, 1 hour later.

## The Electrocardiogram

It is usually a good idea to heed Wellens' warning. This follow-up ECG demonstrates an extensive anterior, lateral and high lateral STEMI, as evidenced by dramatic ST-segment elevations in precordial leads V2–V6 as well as leads I and aVL. As expected, there are reciprocal ST-segment depressions in lead III. There is ventricular ectopy as well.

## Clinical Course

The peak troponin was, fortunately, only 42. The ECG (with a combined anterior, septal and high lateral STEMI) is virtually diagnostic of an obstructing clot in the proximal LAD, before the first diagonal. Indeed, angiography demonstrated a *100 percent LAD occlusion proximal to D-1.*

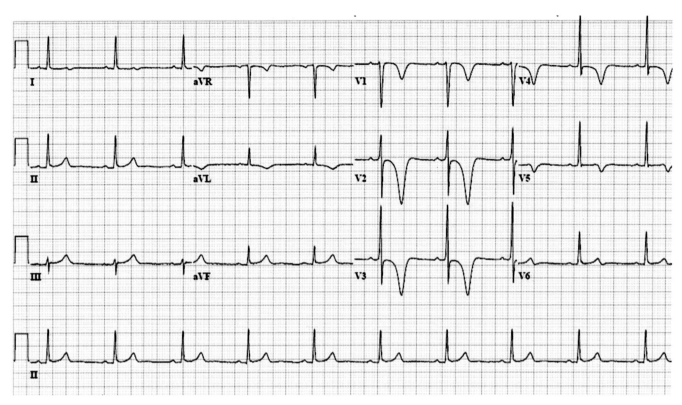

**ECG 3.4** A 46-year-old man with untreated hypertension and tobacco use reported intermittent chest pain for 2 months. The pain became suddenly worse, and he awoke on the morning of his ED visit with substernal burning. The initial troponin level was 0.7.

## The Electrocardiogram

The ECG demonstrates T-wave inversions in the anterior precordial leads (as well as T-wave abnormalities in the high lateral leads I and aVL). The precordial T-wave inversions are deep and symmetric, very suggestive of ischemia and an acute, high grade LAD occlusion. These symmetrically inverted, anterior precordial T-waves are called "coronary T-waves" or Wellens' sign, Type B. They frequently serve as an early warning sign of a critical LAD occlusion and an impending STEMI. The differential diagnosis of these deep anterior precordial T-wave inversions also includes subarachnoid hemorrhage, acute pulmonary embolism, stress (takotsubo) cardiomyopathy and, occasionally, a juvenile variant. Refer to Chapter 6, Confusing Conditions: ST-Segment Depressions and T-Wave Inversions, for further discussion.

## Clinical Course

In this case, the second troponin level was mildly elevated at 4.8. He was sent emergently to angiography, which revealed a 100 percent LAD occlusion. The troponin leak did not continue, and he did not experience a STEMI.

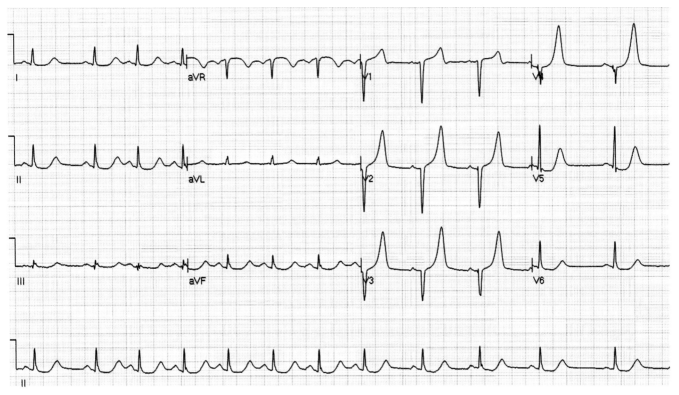

**ECG 3.5** A 49-year-old man with 4–5 hours of dull chest and interscapular pain that awoke him from sleep. He also reported several episodes of emesis and shortness of breath. He had no prior cardiac history, although he was a heavy smoker. In the emergency department, he had imaging studies to rule out pulmonary embolism or thoracic aortic dissection. His initial troponin level was normal. His serum potassium level was also normal. He was treated with nitroglycerin and morphine sulfate, and he was admitted to the intensive care unit. Catheterization was scheduled for the next morning.

## The Electrocardiogram

Hyperacute T-waves are present in precordial leads V1–V4. The T-wave in V1 is much taller than the T-wave in V6, an additional signal that the T-waves are abnormal. There are also formed Q-waves in the anterior and septal precordial leads, along with QT prolongation. There is one other important abnormality: the ST-segments are depressed in the inferior leads; as discussed earlier, this is highly predictive of a high lateral STEMI, caused by a critical LAD occlusion in the proximal segment, before the take-off of the first diagonal branch (and before the septal perforators). The ST-segments are also depressed in the lateral precordial leads, and there is mild ST-segment elevation in aVR. All of these changes are suggestive of a critical LAD or left main coronary artery occlusion or their "equivalent" (severe three-vessel disease).

## Clinical Course

Several hours after the preceding ECG was obtained, he had a witnessed episode of ventricular fibrillation that was managed successfully with a single defibrillatory shock. The following ECG was obtained.

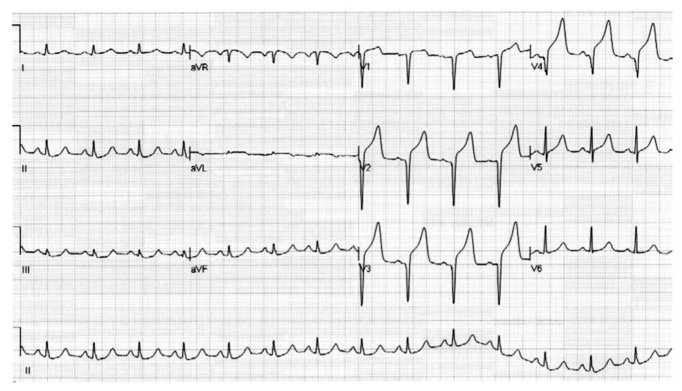

**ECG 3.5**  The same patient – 15 hours later, after an episode of ventricular fibrillation as an inpatient.

## The Electrocardiogram

As predicted by the initial hyper-acute T-waves, he has developed ECG evidence of an extensive anteroseptal myocardial infarction, with probable involvement of the high lateral leads. As noted previously, in the presence of an anterior wall STEMI, the mere presence of ST-segment depressions in the inferior leads suggests that the culprit occlusion is in the LAD proximal to D-1. This tracing indicates loss of R-wave voltage in lead aVL; and despite the low voltage in aVL, there is slight ST-segment straightening and elevation, along with the depressed ST-segments in II, III and aVF. The ST-segment depressions in V5–V6 are no longer apparent.

## Clinical Course

Catheterization revealed severe three-vessel coronary artery disease, including complete occlusions of the RCA and LCA and subtotal occlusion of the proximal LAD. His peak troponin was 242. He underwent coronary artery bypass grafting 3 days later.

# The Importance of Lead aVR

Limb lead aVR, although often ignored, may provide critical diagnostic information in patients suspected of having an acute STEMI (Tamura, 2014; Yamaji et al., 2001; Zhong-qun et al., 2008; Eskola et al., 2009; Nikus and Eskola, 2008; Gorgels et al., 2001; Rokos et al., 2010; Lawner et al., 2012; Aygul et al., 2008; Wagner et al., 2009; Williamson et al., 2006; Wang et al., 2009; Nikus et al., 2014; Birnbaum, Wilson et al., 2014).

ST-segment elevation in lead aVR may indicate an acute obstruction of the left main coronary artery (LCMA) or, alternatively, severe three-vessel disease. As explained beautifully by Wellens, "When the left main coronary artery is occluded acutely, ischemia will occur both in the territory supplied by the LAD and CX, resulting in an ST-deviation vector pointing *toward lead aVR*" (Wellens and Conover, 2006).

A more detailed discussion follows. The days of ignoring lead aVR have come to an end.

- In patients with electrocardiographic evidence of an anterior wall STEMI (ST-segment elevations in leads V1–V4), ST-segment elevation in aVR may signify acute occlusion of the left main coronary artery (LMCA). LMCA occlusion is especially likely if the ST-segment elevation is greater in aVR than in V1. In patients with acute anterior wall STEMI, the higher the ST-segment elevation in aVR, the higher the mortality rate. Complete occlusion of the LMCA is a rare occurrence; however, the LMCA perfuses at least 75 percent of the left ventricular mass, and critical LMCA occlusion is often followed by hemodynamic collapse and malignant ventricular arrhythmias (Nikus and Eskola, 2008; Yamaji et al., 2001; Tamura, 2014);

- ST-segment elevation in aVR may also be present in association with ST-segment depressions in multiple (sometimes six or more) inferior and lateral leads. Lead aVR examines the heart "from the right shoulder"; it is also reciprocal to leads I, II and aVF and leads V4, V5 and V6. Therefore, when the ST-segments are depressed in these lateral and inferior leads, it could signify "only" inferior and lateral wall ischemia. But if the ST-segment is also elevated in aVR – and especially if the widespread inferior and lateral ST-segment depressions are accompanied by inverted T-waves – the pattern is highly suggestive of an acute thrombotic occlusion of the LAD or LMCA (left main "equivalent" disease). Stated differently, this pattern is a "STEMI equivalent" (Nikus et al., 2014). According to Nikus et al., "if this ECG pattern of circumferential subendocardial ischemia also encompasses ST-elevation in lead aVR . . . and especially when associated with inverted T-waves . . . [these patients] should have high priority for urgent invasive evaluation because of high probability of severe angiographic coronary artery disease" (Nikus et al., 2014; Birnbaum, Wilson et al., 2014).

- ST-segment elevation in aVR has also been observed in patients with posterior wall STEMI, in patients with severe multivessel coronary artery disease and in patients with right heart strain due to acute pulmonary embolism.

In 2006, Williamson et al. published a review of the utility of lead aVR in emergency medicine and critical care (Williamson et al., 2006). The authors listed each of the following as a proven or potential application of lead aVR: (a) ST-segment elevations in lead aVR, suggesting left main coronary artery or proximal LAD obstruction in patients with suspected acute coronary syndromes; (b) detection of incorrect placement of the limb leads (reversal of the normal P-wave, QRS and T-wave patterns in leads I and aVR); (c) recognition of a tall, terminal R-wave in aVR, suggesting sodium channel blocker (especially tricyclic anti-depressant) poisoning; (d) supporting the diagnosis of acute pericarditis, where the PR-segment in lead aVR is commonly elevated; (e) helping to differentiate atrioventricular nodal re-entrant tachycardia (AVNRT) from atrioventricular reciprocating tachycardia (AVRT); (f) detecting inverted P-waves and AV-dissociation in aVR, confirming the diagnosis of ventricular tachycardia; and, possibly, (g) suggesting acute right heart strain and pulmonary embolus by finding ST-segment elevation in aVR.

# Understanding "STEMI Equivalents"

One of the key decision points in the emergency care of patients with chest pain, dyspnea or similar symptoms is recognition of regional ST-segment elevations (STEMIs). This ECG finding is critical because it identifies a subset of patients with acute coronary syndromes (ACS) who are highly likely to have an acute occlusion of one of the main epicardial coronary arteries. Emergent percutaneous coronary intervention (PCI), or, in many settings, thrombolytic therapy, is indicated in these patients. ACS patients who have ECG changes limited to ST-segment depressions or T-wave inversions are, for the most part, excluded from these reperfusion recommendations. So, among all the chest pain and ACS patients who present to emergency departments, finding a STEMI changes everything.

National guidelines have established "findings consistent with ST-elevation myocardial infarction (STEMI)," and these have been translated into hospital-based and prehospital "catheterization laboratory activation criteria." For the most part, these standard definitions have been derived from population-based epidemiologic studies and several large thrombolysis clinical trials. According to the 2012 Joint European Society of Cardiology/American College of Cardiology Foundation/American Heart Association/World Health Federation Task Force, a STEMI exists if the following criteria are met (Thygesen et al., 2012): new ST-segment elevation at the J-point in two anatomically contiguous leads, with the following threshold criteria: ≥ 1 mm (0.1 mV) in all leads other than leads V2–V3; and in precordial leads V2–V3, the following diagnostic criteria apply: ≥ 2 mm (0.2 mV) in men 40 years or older, ≥ 2.5 mm (0.25 mV) in men < 40 years, and ≥ 1.5 mm (0.15 mV) in women. All other ischemic changes, including regional ST-segment depressions and T-wave inversions, are, in the absence of ST-segment elevations meeting these accepted criteria, classified as "non-STEMIs or unstable angina."

Importantly, however, most experts, including the panels referenced previously, agree that the accepted definitions do not define the entirety of all ACS patients who have occluded infarct coronary arteries and who need emergent reperfusion therapy. For example, as Thygesen, Nikus and others have pointed out, "lesser degrees of ST [elevation] ... do not exclude acute myocardial ischemia or evolving MI" (Thygesen et al., 2012; Nikus et al., 2014).

In recent years, in an effort to improve ECG interpretation and emergency cardiac care, the indications for emergent reperfusion have been expanded. Some additional ECG patterns have been identified, typically called "STEMI equivalents." These ECG patterns are easily missed, and they are unlikely to be recognized by computer algorithms. Patients with these patterns do not fit the usual, "textbook" criteria for "cath lab activation;" however, these patients are highly likely to have an acute obstructing thrombus in a major coronary artery, and they are, like their counterparts with more classic ST-segment elevations, candidates for emergent reperfusion therapy.

In patients who have chest pain, dizziness, dyspnea or other symptoms compatible with an acute coronary syndrome, the following patterns are the most widely recognized "STEMI equivalents" (Rokos et al., 2010; Thygesen et al., 2012; Wagner et al., 2009; Nikus et al., 2010; Birnbaum, Nikus et al., 2014; Birnbaum, Wilson et al., 2014; Nikus and Eskola, 2008; Ayer and Terkelsen, 2014; Lawner et al., 2012).

### ST-Segment Elevations That Do Not Reach the Accepted Threshold Amplitudes

Minimal (subthreshold) ST-segment elevations may be significant, but they are easy to overlook, especially in lead aVL or other leads where the QRS voltage may be low. Even minimal ST-elevations are likely to indicate a true STEMI when there are anatomically reciprocal ST-segment depressions. As Birnbaum, Nikus and others have warned, "Not every patient with positive biomarkers and with ST-elevation lower than the threshold should be defined as having a non-STEMI, as many of them have acute occlusions of an epicardial coronary artery" (Birnbaum, Nikus et al., 2014).

### ST-Segment Elevations in Fewer Than "Two Contiguous Leads"

Early, subtle inferior wall STEMIs may present with ST-segment elevation or straightening only in lead III. Early high lateral STEMIs may present with ST-elevation limited to lead aVL. Again, the specificity for true STEMI is markedly increased when reciprocal ST-segment depressions are present.

### ST-Segment Depressions in Precordial Leads V1–V3, Indicating Posterior (or Posterolateral) Wall STEMI

As discussed in Chapter 4, these patients must not be classified as having a non-STEMI or "just anterior wall ischemia." ST-segment depressions in the right precordial leads (V1–V3), accompanied by upright T-waves, makes an acute posterior wall STEMI highly likely.

### de Winter's ST/T-Wave Complex

The de Winter complex includes upsloping ST-segment depressions in precordial leads V1–V3 that begin as sharp depressions of the J-point and then transition into an upsloping ST-segment and finally terminate in a tall, upright T-wave. Sometimes, these abnormalities are associated with ST-elevations in aVR. Although uncommon, the de Winter complex is highly suggestive of acute obstruction of the proximal LAD or, occasionally, an occlusion of the LCA (de Winter, 2015; Birnbaum, Nikus et al., 2014; Birnbaum, Wilson et al., 2014; Verouden et al., 2009). This de Winter form of hyperacute T-waves is often a persistent, rather than transient, abnormality.

### A Pattern of Inferior (Leads II and aVF) and Lateral (I, aVL, V5, V6) ST-Segment Depressions, Accompanied by ST-Segment Elevations in Lead aVR

These "global" or "concentric" or "circumferential" ST-segment depressions, when accompanied by ST-segment elevation in aVR, may indicate left main coronary artery or left anterior descending artery occlusion (discussed earlier in this chapter). These patients must not be erroneously classified as "non-STEMI" (Birnbaum, Wilson et al., 2014).

### Patients Who Have Had Return of Spontaneous Circulation (ROSC) after Out-of-Hospital Cardiac Arrest (OHCA)

Many patients with ROSC after OHCA have an occluded infarct-related vessel and are candidates for emergent reperfusion. However, ROSC after OHCA is not always a STEMI-equivalent.

One common alternative diagnosis is subarachnoid hemorrhage (SAH). Recent studies suggest that, among comatose survivors of OHCA, subarachnoid hemorrhage is more likely than an acute coronary syndrome (ACS) if: (a) the initial arrest rhythm was "unshockable (asystole or pulseless electrical activity, rather than VT or VF); (b) immediate echocardiography demonstrates a preserved (≥ 50 percent) left ventricular ejection fraction; (c) the history (if available) included pre-arrest headache rather than chest pain; and (d) if ST-segment elevations are present, they are not accompanied by reciprocal ST-depressions. None of these findings, including the history, is 100 percent discriminatory. In recent studies, T-wave inversions and QT-interval prolongation were similar in patients with ACS and SAH. The bottom line is that some patients who have ROSC after OHCA will need an emergent CT scan prior to undergoing reperfusion therapy (Lewandowski, 2014; Yamashina et al., 2015; Arnaout et al., 2015; Mitsuma et al., 2011).

### Patients with a New or Preexisting Left Bundle Branch Block and Symptoms Suggestive of an Acute Coronary Syndrome, Where the 12-Lead ECG Suggests Abnormal Concordance or Discordance (Sgarbossa Criteria)

This topic is reviewed in a later section.

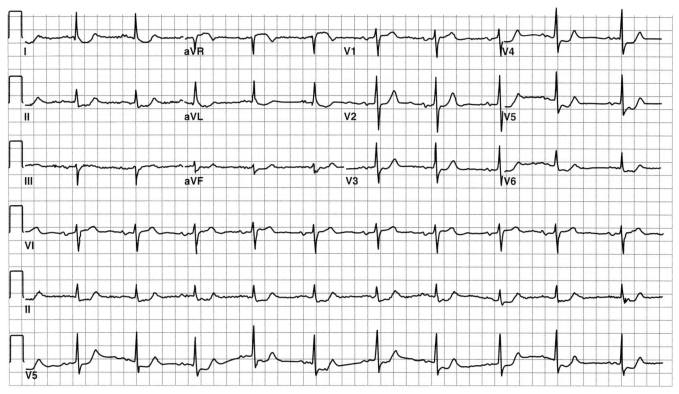

**ECG 3.6** An 86-year-old man was brought to the ED because of "itching between his shoulder blades." He also had mild chest pain. He reported a history of hyperlipidemia and glaucoma. His initial BP was 194/88. Otherwise, his physical examination was normal.

### Don't-Miss STEMI Equivalents

- Subtle, "sub-threshold" ST-segment elevations with reciprocal ST-segment depressions in the "opposite" leads
- ST-segment depressions in V1–V3, signifying posterior or posterolateral STEMI
- Hyper-acute T-waves in one or more precordial leads
- Left main coronary artery occlusion, presenting with extensive inferior and lateral ST-segment depressions, plus ≥ 1 mm ST-elevation in lead aVR
- LBBB with abnormally concordant or discordant ST-segment deviations (Sgarbossa criteria)
- de Winter ST/T-wave complex
- Wellens' syndrome
- Return of spontaneous circulation (ROSC) after resuscitation from prehospital cardiac arrest (if subarachnoid hemorrhage is unlikely)

## The Electrocardiogram

His ECG demonstrates ST-segment depression in multiple inferior and left-sided leads (I, II, aVL and V4–V6). Does this electrocardiographic pattern represent simply inferior and lateral wall ischemia? Is it enough to admit him for medical management? Or could it be something worse?

The answer lies in lead aVR. This lead, it is now recognized, provides valuable information in patients presenting with symptoms and ECG signs of an acute coronary syndrome. Lead aVR provides critical information in two situations. First, in the setting of an acute anteroseptal STEMI, if the ST-segments in aVR are elevated (≥ 0.5 mV), and, especially, if they are elevated to a greater extent than the ST-segment elevations in V1, it is highly suggestive of a left main coronary artery (LCMA) occlusion. The second situation, which applies in this case, is where there are extensive ("circumferential" or "global") lateral and inferior ST-segment depressions. As noted earlier, lead aVR explores the heart from "the right shoulder"; that is, aVR examines the heart as if it were looking at the left ventricle between leads 1 and II. Prominent ST-segment elevation in aVR may be considered "reciprocal" to the left lateral and left inferior portions of the heart (that is, reciprocal to the ST-segment depressions in leads I, II, aVL and V4–V6). If there is ST-segment depression in multiple inferior and lateral leads and if the ST-segment is elevated in aVR, this is a STEMI equivalent.

## Clinical Course

This patient had a coronary angiogram that demonstrated a 100 percent ostial left main coronary artery (LCMA) occlusion. He required hemodynamic support with an intra-aortic balloon pump. He underwent successful coronary artery bypass grafting the next day.

## Anterior Wall STEMI Complicated by Development of Bundle Branch Block

The pattern of acute anteroseptal STEMI complicated by RBBB or bifascicular block is extremely common (Nikus and Eskola, 2008; Wellens and Conover, 2006). It usually signifies an acute occlusion of the proximal LAD before the septal perforators (refer to Figure 3.2; Wellens and Conover, 2006). In these cases, there is extensive septal necrosis; and because the bundle branches course through the interventricular septum, there is a high risk of developing bundle branch block and complete heart block.

Second-degree AV block, Mobitz Type 2, may also develop. Unlike the case with heart block that develops during inferior STEMI, here the block is below the level of the AV node. There is a high mortality rate in these patients, due primarily to extensive left ventricular infarction and pump failure (Wong et al., 2006; Wellens and Conover, 2006).

The right bundle branch and the left anterior fascicle of the left bundle branch receive most of their blood supply from the LAD via the septal perforator branches (Wellens and Conover, 2006). Therefore, proximal LAD occlusion and anteroseptal STEMI are frequently complicated by development of right bundle branch block, left anterior fascicular block or both (bifascicular block) (Nikus and Eskola 2008; Wellens and Conover, 2006). The left posterior fascicle of the LBB often has a dual blood supply, from both the septal perforators of the LAD and the right coronary artery. Therefore, development of left posterior fascicular block is less common. (Neeland et al., 2012).

When BBB or bifascicular block develops during an acute anterior wall STEMI, it usually occurs within the first few hours. The BBB or bifasicular block may progress to complete heart block due to extensive necrosis of the His bundle and bundle branches.

When patients with acute STEMIs have a bundle branch block on the presenting ECG, it is not always possible to determine whether the conduction disturbance is preexisting or whether it is a complication of the acute myocardial infarction. Whether old or new, the presence of a bundle branch block is associated with delayed recognition of the STEMI, delays in administering reperfusion therapies and a higher risk of complications and in-hospital mortality. Preexisting LBBB is also a marker of chronic heart disease and elevated cardiovascular risk (Chiara, 2006; Nikus and Eskola, 2008; Wong et al., 2006; Neeland et al., 2012).

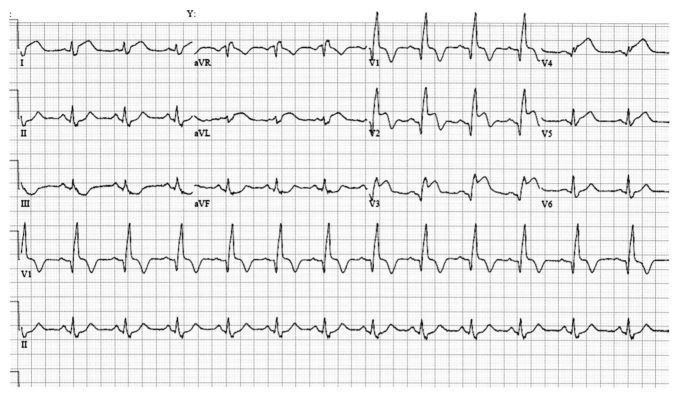

**ECG 3.7** A 49-year-old man experienced chest pain, nausea and diaphoresis. He took an aspirin, and his family drove him more than 1 hour to the emergency department. He had an episode of ventricular fibrillation immediately after triage. After defibrillation he was alert and hemodynamically stable.

## The Electrocardiogram

The ECG demonstrates a right bundle branch block (RBBB) plus an acute anteroseptal and high lateral STEMI. ST-segment elevations are widespread, involving the septal and anterior precordial leads (V1–V5) and limb leads I and aVL. The ST-segment depressions in the inferior leads are reciprocal to the high lateral STEMI.

Lead V1 has the recognizable rSR' pattern of a RBBB, except that the leading R-wave is absent. (It is now a Q-wave.) The absence of the initial R-wave indicates that the septum is infarcted. RBBB, alone or in combination with left anterior fascicular block, is a common early complication of anteroseptal STEMI, if the LAD is occluded proximal to the takeoff of the septal perforator branches.

## Clinical Course

This patient's initial troponin was 0.27. The peak troponin was 390. On catheterization, the interventional cardiologists found *a large caliber LAD that supplies multiple septal perforators and a medium caliber Diagonal 1 branch.* There was a 100 percent proximal LAD occlusion (before the septal perforators and D-1) that was treated successfully with aspiration thrombectomy and a bare metal stent.

## Recognizing Anterior Wall STEMI in the Presence of Left Bundle Branch Block

The presence of a left bundle branch block (LBBB) makes the recognition of acute anterior wall STEMI more difficult. LBBB distorts the ST-segments and T-waves in the anterior precordial leads, which may mimic or obscure the diagnosis of hyperacute T-waves, ST-segment elevation, T-wave inversion and other signs of acute or evolving STEMI.

The following ECG abnormalities, known as the "Sgarbossa criteria," suggest that an acute anterior wall STEMI is present in a patient with LBBB:

- Primary, or "concordant," ST-segment changes (that is, the ST-segment is elevated ≥1 mm in a precordial lead where the QRS complex is positive); or
- ST-segment depressions of at least 1 mm in leads V1, V2 or V3; or
- Discordant but extreme ST-segment elevation (≥ 5 mm in the anterior leads), where the QRS complexes are pointing negatively but where the ST-segments are normally elevated.

These well-studied criteria are specific but not sensitive for the diagnosis of acute anterior wall STEMI in patients with a left bundle branch block. Specificity is improved if the preceding criteria are weighted by assigning 5 points, 3 points and 2 points, respectively. Discordant ST-segment elevation is the least specific criterion, while concordant ST-segment elevation is the most specific (Sgarbossa et al., 1996; Neeland et al., 2012). According to a 2008 meta-analysis by Tabas et al., a Sgarbossa score of 3 or more (indicating at least 1 mm of concordant ST-segment elevation or 1 mm of ST-segment depression in precordial leads V1–V3) is highly specific for STEMI. However, even a Sgarbossa score of 0 has a low sensitivity and negative likelihood ratio and cannot be used to rule out myocardial infarction. A Sgarbossa score of 2 (≥ 5 mm of discordant ST-segment elevation) is neither specific nor sensitive (Tabas et al., 2008).

The vast majority of patients with chest pain and a left bundle branch block do not have an acute occlusion of a culprit infarct-related coronary artery. Therefore, the mere presence of "new or presumed new LBBB" is no longer considered a STEMI equivalent or an indication for emergent reperfusion (Neeland et al., 2012).

## "Old" Anterior Wall Myocardial Infarctions

It is common to detect evidence of an old or "indeterminate age" anterior myocardial infarction on the 12-lead ECG. The hallmark of an old anterior wall myocardial infarction is the presence of pathologic Q-waves or loss of R-waves in the anterior precordial leads. Poor R-wave progression is commonly the result of prior anterior wall STEMI.

- Q-waves are not normally present in precordial leads V1–V3, and their presence in these leads is usually indicative of a myocardial infarction (of any age) (Wagner and Strauss, 2014).
- Absence of the leading R-wave in lead V1 indicates prior infarction of the septum.
- Absent R-waves (QS complexes) or poor or reverse R-wave progression in leads V2–V4 often indicates prior anterior wall myocardial infarction. Loss of R-wave amplitude in precordial leads V5 and V6 may signify prior lateral wall infarction.
- As emphasized in Chapter 1, poor R-wave progression does not always signify that the patient has sustained a prior anterior wall infarction. Poor R-wave progression may also be caused by emphysema, a low-lying vertical heart or erroneous (high) precordial lead placement (Thygesen et al., 2012).

## Q-Waves May Appear in the *Acute Phase* of an Anterior Wall STEMI

As discussed in Chapter 2, development of Q-waves is highly variable. Sometimes, Q-waves or QS complexes in the "infarct leads" are present on the presenting ECG, even in in the first hour of symptoms. It is important to stress that *immediate Q-waves are especially common in anterior wall myocardial infarctions, and their presence does not necessarily mean that the myocardial injury is old or irreversible* (Birnbaum, Wilson et al., 2014). As Wellens emphasized, "The fact that Q-waves do not necessarily indicate [irreversible] myocardial necrosis is important knowledge ... Significant myocardial salvage by reperfusion can be accomplished in patients with new pathologic Q-waves" (Wellens and Conover, 2006).

As a separate point, not all patients who suffer a STEMI develop Q-waves. And Q-waves that do develop often disappear over days, weeks or months.

"Old" or "indeterminate" age myocardial infarctions on the ECG do not represent acute disease. However, they may have great clinical significance. For example, in a patient with syncope or pre-syncope, the finding of an old infarction (pathologic Q-waves) on the presenting ECG is strongly associated with a cardiac arrhythmia, especially ventricular tachycardia, as the etiology for the patient's syncope (Bhat et al., 2014; Puppala et al., 2014). Examples of old anterior and anteroseptal myocardial infarctions are included in the self-study ECGs.

# Self-Study Electrocardiograms

**Case 3.1** A 56-year-old man without any cardiac history presented with chest pressure. He had stable vital signs, but his lung examination showed rales bilaterally.

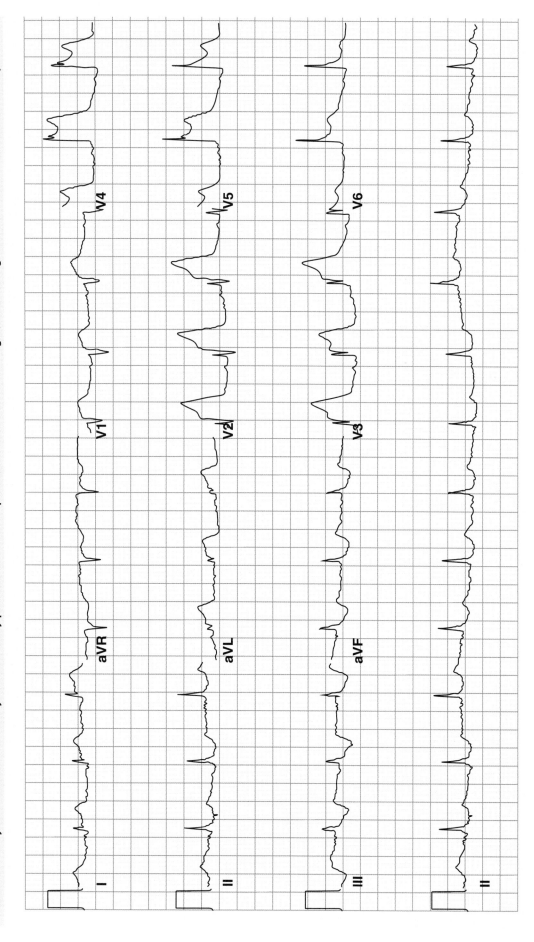

**Case 3.2** A 71-year-old female presented with acute chest pain and dizziness. The computer algorithm reading noted (in addition to atrial-paced complexes): "ST-depression, consider ischemia, anterolateral leads."

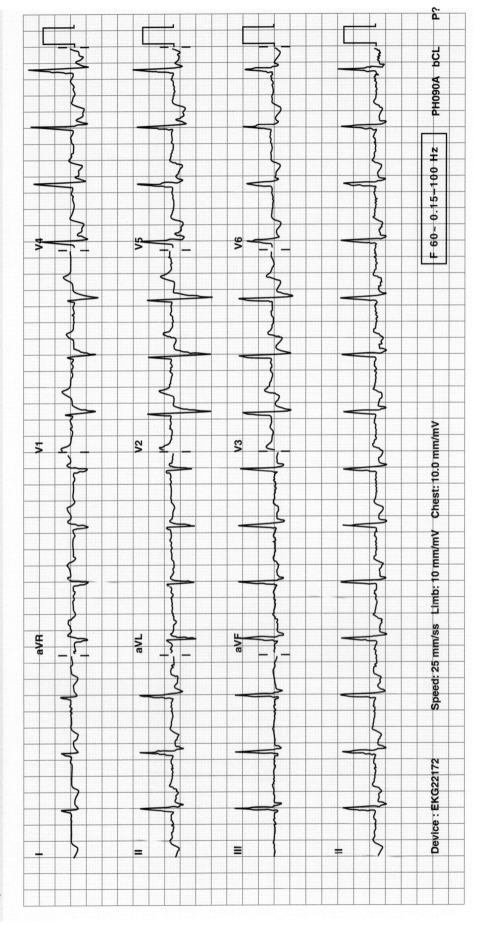

**Case 3.3** A 57-year-old man endorsed 3 hours of substernal chest pain that radiated to his jaw. His initial troponin level was 0.44.

| Vent. rate | 58 | BPM |
|---|---|---|
| PR interval | 128 | ms |
| QRS duration | 96 | ms |
| QT/QTc | 418/410 | ms |
| P-R-T axes | 36 -29 | -12 |

Room:S42
Loc:1002

Sinus bradycardia
Nonspecific ST abnormality
Abnormal ECG
When compared with ECG of 11-MAY-2013 14:23,
No significant change was found

Referred by:  SELF

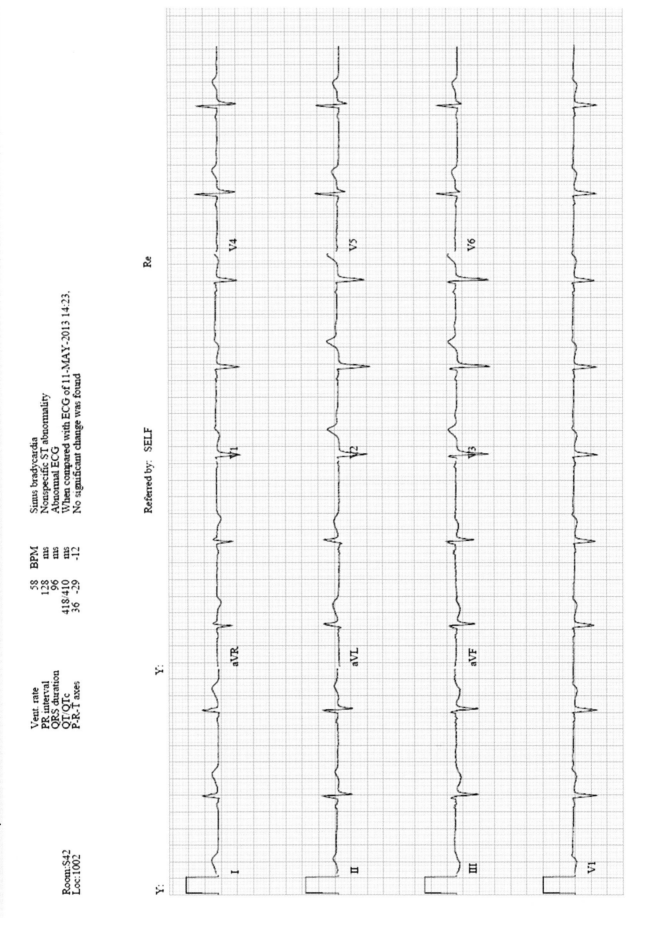

**Case 3.4** A 63-year-old man with a history of a hiatal hernia complained of intermittent "hernia pain" over several weeks. While driving his truck, he experienced severe abdominal pain, nausea and vomiting lasting 25 minutes. He called 911 from a truck stop. Initial troponin level: 0.04.

**Case 3.4 (Continued)** The same patient, 90 minutes later.

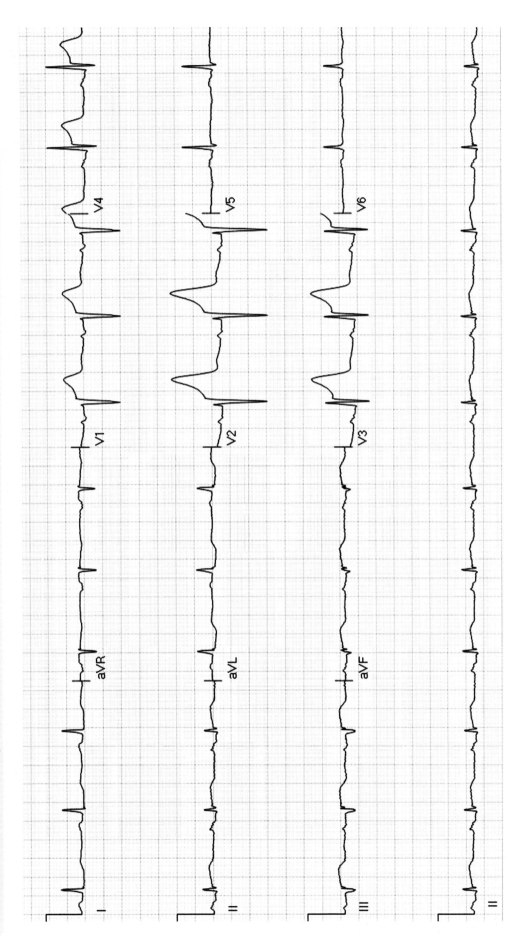

**Case 3.5** A 68-year-old man. Clinical history is unknown.

**Case 3.6** A 48-year-old man experienced chest pain while working in the yard.

**Case 3.6 (Continued)** The same patient – 12 years earlier.

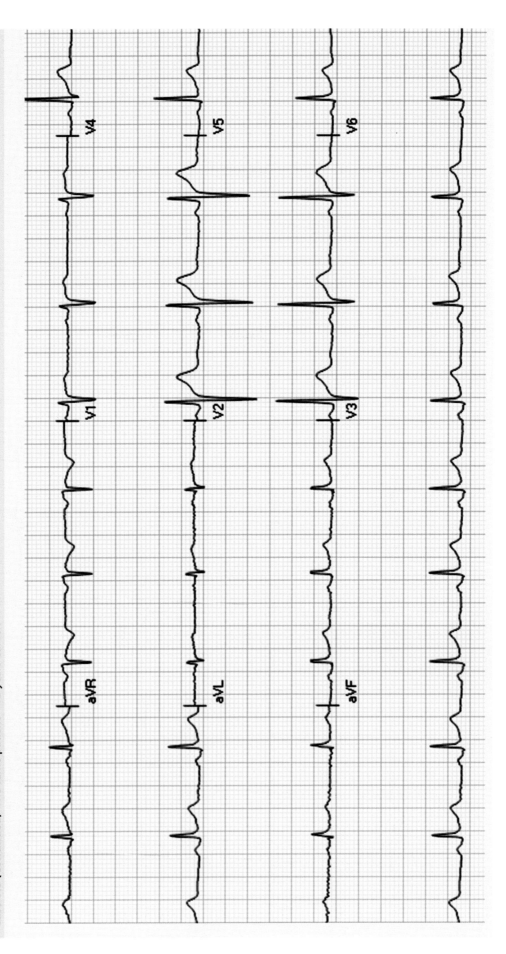

**Case 3.6 (Continued)** The same patient – 3 hours after the initial ECG.

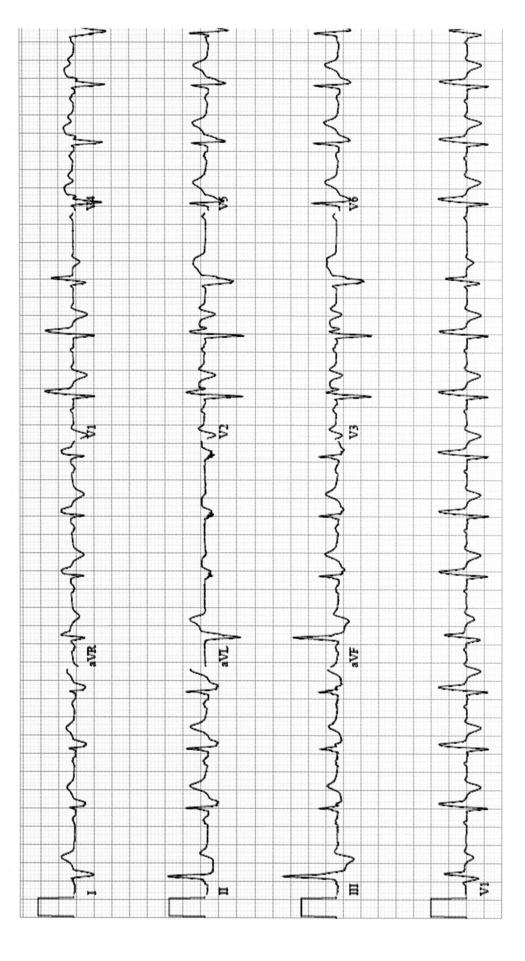

**Case 3.7** A 34-year-old man presented to the emergency department because of stuttering chest pain and shortness of breath. He was felt to have an acute coronary syndrome (ACS), and he was admitted to the intensive care unit for medical management.

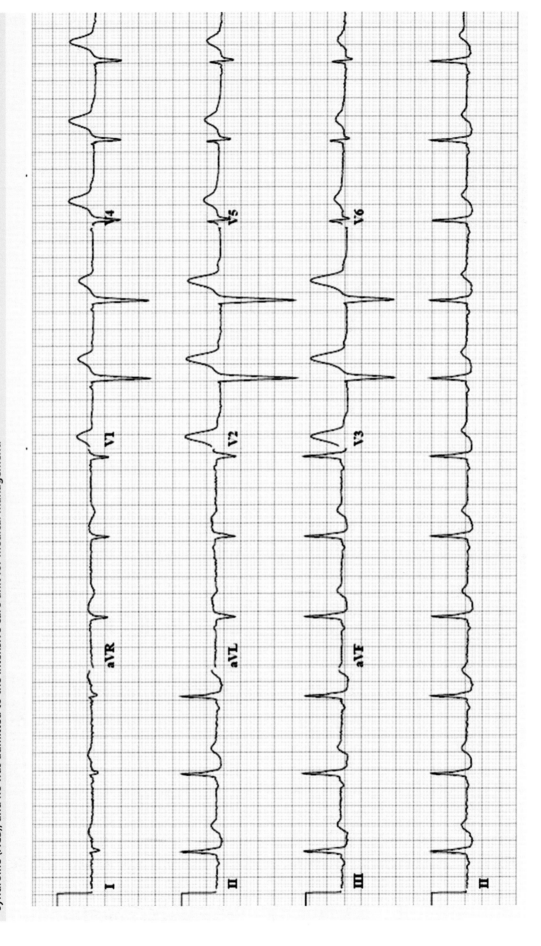

**Case 3.7 (Continued)** The same patient – 6 hours after admission (following a cardiac arrest).

**Case 3.8** A 46-year-old man presented with 1 day of chest pain with exertion and at rest.

**Case 3.8 (Continued)** The same patient – 33 minutes later.

**Case 3.9** A 44-year-old female presented with chest pain, nausea, vomiting and mild shortness of breath. She experienced three episodes of ventricular fibrillation in the emergency department. After defibrillation and treatment with amiodarone, her rhythm stabilized.

**Case 3.9 (Continued)** The same patient, follow-up ECG.

**Case 3.9 (Continued)** The same patient (an additional follow-up ECG).

**Case 3.10** A 46-year-old female called 911 because of chest pain. She had a cardiac arrest during transport and was defibrillated successfully. Her prehospital arrest and defibrillation rhythm strips are shown in the next section.

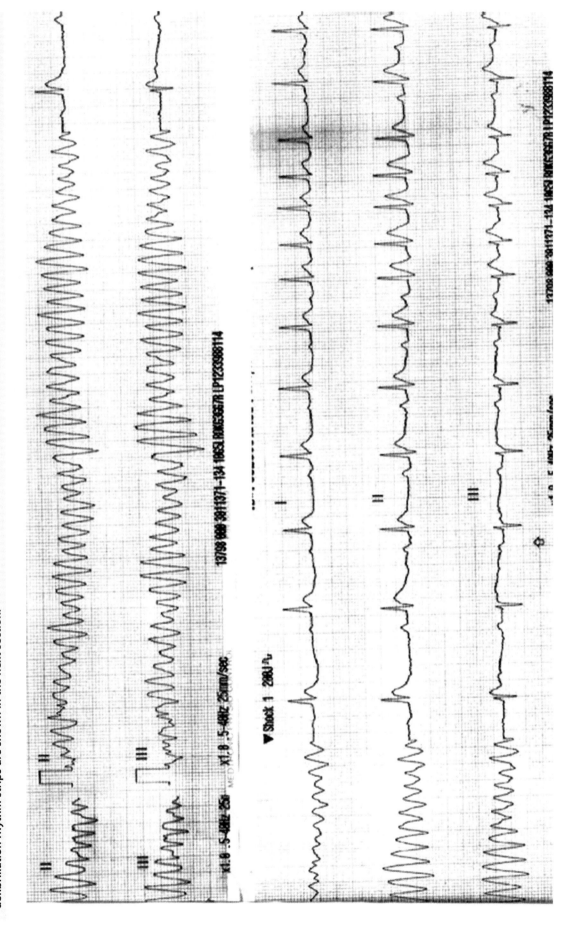

**Case 3.10 (Continued)** The same patient, after defibrillation.

**Case 3.11** A 37-year-old man with no significant past medical history presented to the emergency department with 2 weeks of intermittent chest pain. He also reported a cough productive of yellow sputum. He was admitted for "possible pneumonia and further evaluation of his chest pain, and rule out ACS." His troponin in the ED was 0.00. With respect to the ECG, the emergency department note stated, "Nonspecific T-wave changes in V5–V6 with no ST-elevation concerning to activate cath lab."

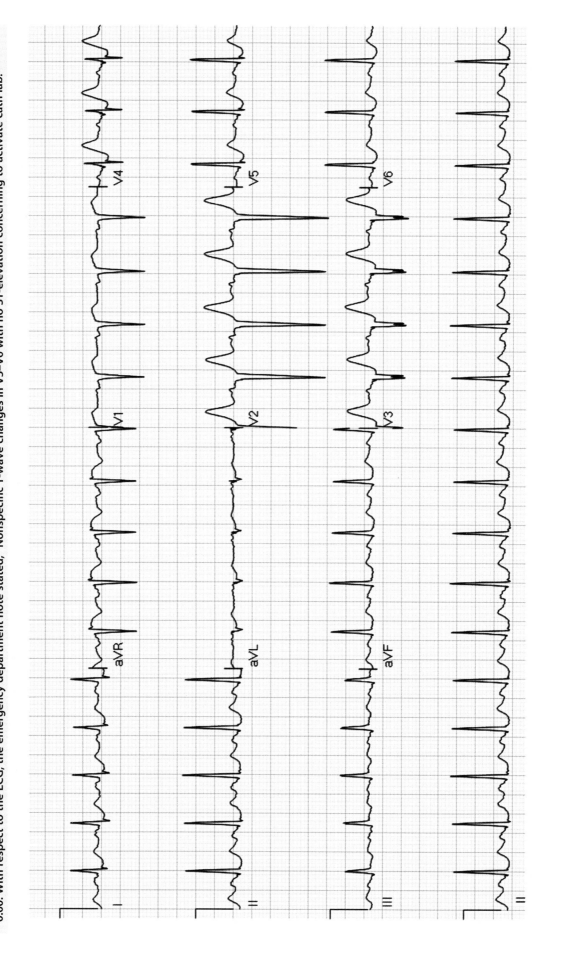

**Case 3.11 (Continued)** Same patient (follow-up ECG).

**Case 3.12** A 48-year-old man presented with diaphoresis and chest pain of sudden onset. His initial troponin level was 0.31.

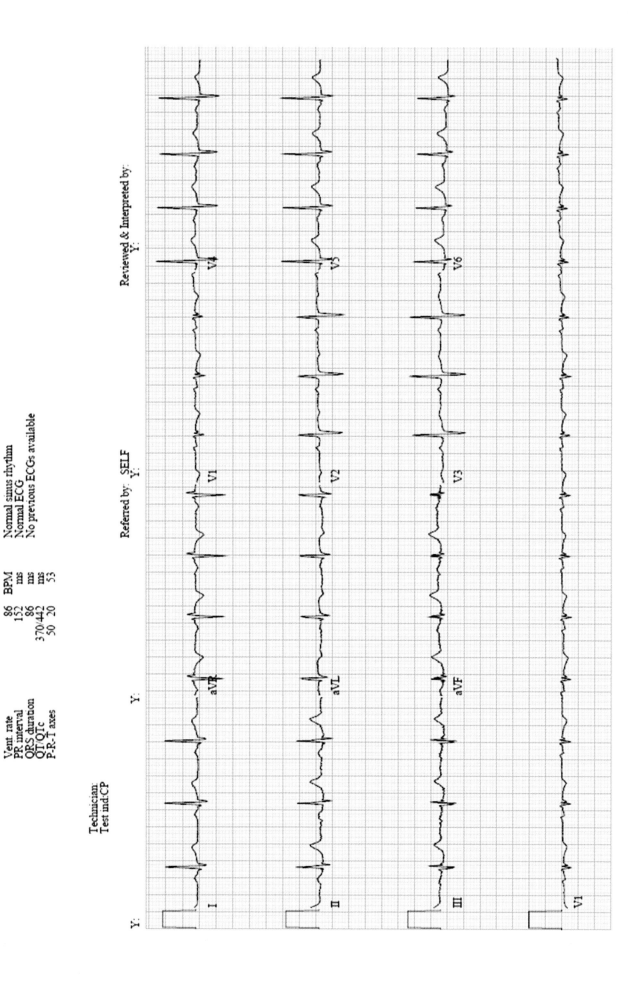

| | BPM | |
|---|---|---|
| Vent rate | 86 | |
| PR interval | 152 | ms |
| QRS duration | 86 | ms |
| QT/QTc | 370/442 | |
| P-R-T axes | 50 20 | 53 |

Normal sinus rhythm
Normal ECG
No previous ECGs available

Technician:
Test ind:CP

Referred by: SELF
Y:

Reviewed & Interpreted by:
Y:

Y:

Y:

I
II
III
V1
aVR
aVL
aVF
V1
V2
V3
V4
V5
V6

**Case 3.12 (Continued)** The same patient – 1 hour and 15 minutes later.

**Case 3.13** A 73-year-old male with a history of hypertension presented with intermittent chest pain and left arm aching for the past week. His initial troponin level was 0.16.

**Case 3.14** A 77-year-old man presented with shortness of breath. He was admitted for pneumonia. Several hours after his presentation, the following ECG was obtained.

**Case 3.15** A 61-year-old female with a history of hypertension and heavy smoking presented with intermittent chest pain over 4 days. Her chest pain became worse on the day of her emergency department visit. She also reported nausea, vomiting and shortness of breath. Her daughter convinced her to come to the hospital.

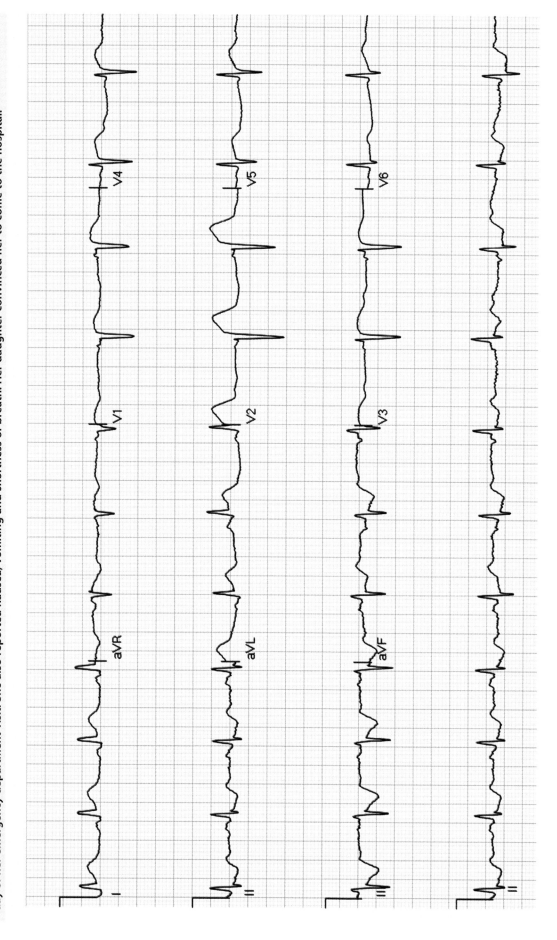

**Case 3.15 (Continued)** The same patient – 8 hours later (post-catheterization).

**Case 3.16** A 75-year-old man developed chest pain while shoveling snow. He also reported dizziness and shortness of breath. On ED arrival, he was in respiratory distress, and his initial systolic blood pressure was 80 mm Hg.

**Case 3.17** A 68-year-old female presented with 2 hours of substernal chest pain, associated with diaphoresis, nausea and vomiting.

**Case 3.18** A 66-year-old man presented with chest tightness and profuse diaphoresis. He reported no history of cardiovascular disease or risk factors. The initial troponin levels in the emergency department were normal (0.03 and 0.04).

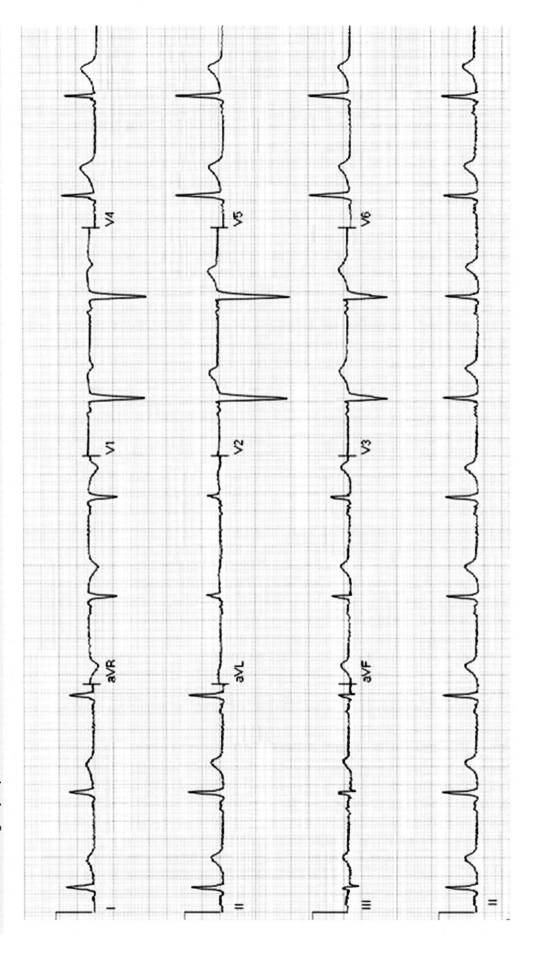

# Self-Study Notes

## Case 3.1  A 56-year-old man without any cardiac history presented with chest pressure. He had stable vital signs, but his lung examination showed rales bilaterally.

### The Electrocardiogram

The ECG demonstrates widespread ST-segment elevations in all the precordial leads (V1–V6). The STEMI also involves the high lateral leads (I and aVL), and there are reciprocal ST-segment depressions in the inferior leads. The proper reading of this ECG is "acute anterior, septal, lateral and high lateral STEMI."

### Clinical Course

On catheterization, his LAD was totally obstructed proximal to D-1. This is a classic ECG presentation among patients with acute occlusion of the LAD before the takeoff of the first diagonal branch.

## Case 3.2  A 71-year-old female presented with acute chest pain and dizziness. The computer algorithm reading noted (in addition to atrial-paced complexes): "ST-depression, consider ischemia, anterolateral leads."

### The Electrocardiogram

There are widespread ST-segment depressions and T-wave inversions, evident in multiple lateral, anterior and inferior leads. But this is not just "subendocardial ischemia." It is a STEMI-equivalent.

The clue is the marked ST-segment elevation in aVR. As discussed in earlier sections of this chapter, the combination of ST-segment depressions and T-wave inversions in multiple (6+) inferior and lateral leads (sometimes labeled "concentric" or "circumferential" ischemia), along with ST-segment elevation in aVR, is highly suggestive of a critical left main coronary artery (LMCA) occlusion.

### Clinical Course

On angiography, acute LMCA occlusion was confirmed.

## Case 3.3  A 57-year-old man endorsed 3 hours of substernal chest pain that radiated to his jaw. His initial troponin level was 0.44.

### The Electrocardiogram

Although the ECG computer algorithm suggests only a "sinus bradycardia" and "nonspecific ST abnormality," there is more. The emergency medicine team read this correctly, noting: "ECGs reviewed. Concern re: high lateral infarct with reciprocal inferior changes. Although patient does not meet activation criteria, I think this is an acute MI." Indeed, a careful inspection of the ECG reveals ST-segment elevation in aVL and reciprocal ST-segment depression in leads III and aVF. This patient has an acute high lateral STEMI.

### Clinical Course

Heparin was started, and he was transferred to the catheterization laboratory. His troponin peaked at 86.8. Predictably, catheterization revealed a 100 percent occlusion of the left circumflex artery. The patient was pain-free after placement of a stent in the mid-LCA.

High lateral STEMIs are often missed, in part because there is typically a low amplitude QRS complex in lead aVL. In this context, very small ST-segment elevations, which are disproportionate to the height of the QRS complex, may be overlooked. However, the diagnosis becomes obvious once we appreciate the ST-segment depressions in the electrically opposite lead III.

## Case 3.4   A 63-year-old man with a history of a hiatal hernia complained of intermittent "hernia pain" over several weeks. While driving his truck, he experienced severe abdominal pain, nausea and vomiting lasting 25 minutes. He called 911 from a truck stop. Initial troponin level: 0.04.

### The Electrocardiogram

Unfortunately, this patient's STEMI was overlooked, perhaps because he continued to complain of "hernia pain." An abdominal CT scan was performed, resulting in a 90-minute delay.

In this tracing, the T-waves in V1–V4 are markedly abnormal. The T-waves are tall, broad and "bulky" – that is, they are "hyperacute." The T-waves "tower" over the small R-waves. Also, the T-wave in V1 is much taller than the T-wave in V6. These hyperacute T-waves are often a marker of an impending anterior STEMI caused by complete LAD occlusion. In this case, the ST-segments in leads V1–V3 are already elevated, indicating an evolving anteroseptal STEMI.

In addition, there are subtle ST-segment elevations in leads III and aVF along with reciprocal ST-segment depressions in leads I and aVL, suggesting a concomitant STEMI involving the inferior wall. The combination of hyperacute T-waves and ST-segment elevations in V1–V3, plus an inferior STEMI, is very suggestive of an occlusion of a "wraparound LAD."

His second ECG, delayed by 90 minutes, is shown next.

## Case 3.4   The same patient, 90 minutes later.

### The Electrocardiogram

The anteroseptal and inferior ST-segment elevations are even more obvious. Leads I and aVL continue to show ST-segment depressions that are obviously reciprocal to the inferior STEMI.

### Clinical Course

The patient's troponin level peaked at 477. The catheterization results are not surprising: "There was a 100 percent mid-LAD occlusion. The LAD is a large vessel that wraps the apex and supplies the mid-inferior wall." The patient had successful placement of a stent.

In the setting of evolving anterior wall STEMI, the presence of ST-segment elevations in the inferior leads (typically accompanied by reciprocal ST-segment depressions in I and aVL) usually implies that the culprit artery is a wraparound LAD. Usually, the LAD clot is distal to the first diagonal (in the mid-LAD), and the prognosis is better (when compared with a proximal LAD occlusion).

## Case 3.5   A 68-year-old man. Clinical history is unknown.

### The Electrocardiogram

The ECG demonstrates an acute anteroseptal and lateral wall STEMI. There is also a right bundle branch block and left anterior fascicular block (bifascicular block). Normally, a RBBB is recognized by the rSR' pattern in V1 (and terminal slurring of the QRS in the lateral limb and precordial leads). In this case, there is no initial R-wave in V1, due to the septal infarction; the rSR' pattern has become only a "q-R-prime." The pattern of acute anteroseptal STEMI complicated by RBBB is common. It signifies an acute occlusion of the proximal LAD before the septal perforators. When a BBB develops acutely during an anterior wall STEMI, it represents necrosis of the septum. In this setting, it is common to develop complete heart block that is anatomically located below the level of the His bundle.

## Case 3.6   A 48-year-old man experienced chest pain while working in the yard.

### The Electrocardiogram

This ECG is trying to tell us a classic story. First, there are hyperacute T-waves in leads V1–V4. How do we know the T-waves are abnormal? First, the T-waves are abnormally tall: they tower over the small R-waves across the precordial leads. Importantly, the T-wave in V1 is abnormally prominent. (Recall that the T-wave in V1 should never be taller than the T-wave in precordial lead V6.)

If there was any question about the significance or "hyperacuity" of these T-waves, proof that they portend an LAD occlusion is evident in aVL. Already, there is ST-segment elevation in aVL, with reciprocal ST-segment depression in leads II, III and aVF.

Thus, the correct interpretation of this ECG is an acute high lateral STEMI, with hyperacute T-waves in the anterior precordial leads. This is a high-risk ECG pattern that typically evolves into a full-blown anteroseptal and high lateral STEMI. One can predict that the culprit artery is the LAD, proximal to the first diagonal branch.

### Clinical Course

In fact, catheterization revealed a 100 percent occlusion of the proximal LAD (successfully stented). His troponin peaked at 355. For comparison, the next ECG is a baseline ECG (12 years earlier), when his precordial T-waves were entirely normal. Then the next ECG shows the evolution of his acute anterior wall and high lateral STEMI.

Hyperacute T-waves are often an early sign of an acute, tight LAD occlusion, signifying transmural myocardial ischemia and impending STEMI. But tall T-waves do not always signify ischemia and infarction. Abnormally tall T-waves may represent hyperkalemia, and they are relatively common as a normal variant, especially in the early repolarization pattern. They are commonly found in patients with LBBB and, sometimes, with left ventricular hypertrophy.

## Case 3.6  The same patient – 12 years earlier.

This baseline ECG, taken 12 years earlier, is normal. The T-waves in the precordial leads are unremarkable. Note that the T-wave in lead V1 is modest and has a lower voltage than the T-wave in V6.

## Case 3.6  The same patient – 3 hours after the initial ECG.

### Clinical Course

Not surprisingly, the ECG, taken 3 hours after his initial presentation, shows evolution of the anteroseptal and high lateral STEMI. His catheterization demonstrated a 100 percent proximal LAD occlusion, so it is also not surprising that, within 3 hours, he has developed a right bundle branch block and right axis deviation (possible RBBB and left posterior fascicular block). He has already lost almost all the R-wave voltage in the affected precordial and high lateral leads.

## Case 3.7  A 34-year-old man presented to the emergency department because of stuttering chest pain and shortness of breath. He was felt to have an acute coronary syndrome (ACS), and he was admitted to the intensive care unit for medical management.

### The Electrocardiogram

The team did not immediately recognize the significance of the ECG abnormalities. First, there are hyperacute T-waves in leads V1–V4. The T-wave in lead V1 is far too tall (much taller than the T-wave in lead V6). In fact, all the T-waves are too tall for their R-waves (which are mostly absent). If there was any question about whether these hyperacute T-waves were real, there is proof in the limb leads. There are noticeable ST-segment depressions in leads II, III and aVF. This calls our attention to lead aVL, where there is subtle ST-segment straightening and elevation. Thus, this young patient is experiencing a high lateral and evolving anteroseptal STEMI.

Now we know the significance of the hyperacute T-waves: there is, more likely than not, an acute occlusion involving the proximal LAD, and given the high lateral STEMI, the obstruction is almost certainly before the first diagonal branch (D-1).

### Clinical Course

The patient was admitted and underwent emergent coronary angiography, which revealed a "90 percent occlusion of the LAD proximal to D-1 and the septal perforator branches." He sustained a ventricular fibrillation arrest about 6 hours after admission, and he was successfully resuscitated. His follow-up ECG is shown next.

## Case 3.7  The same patient – 6 hours after admission (following a cardiac arrest).

As predicted by his presenting ECG and his angiography results, he has sustained an extensive anterior, septal and high lateral STEMI, complicated by development of a new RBBB. His ejection fraction prior to discharge was 27 percent.

## Case 3.8 A 46-year-old man presented with 1 day of chest pain with exertion and at rest.

### The Electrocardiogram

The triage ECG demonstrates symmetric, deep T-wave inversions in precordial leads V4–V6 ("coronary T-waves"). Lead V3 illustrates Wellens' warning (Wellens' syndrome, Type A). In lead V3 there is a biphasic T-wave (showing terminal T-wave inversion). ST-segment elevation is already present in V3. There is also poor R-wave progression.

Given his symptoms, and based on this initial ECG, we anticipate a critical LAD stenosis and are confident that a repeat ECG and urgent reperfusion are needed. His second ECG is shown next.

## Case 3.8 The same patient – 33 minutes later.

### The Electrocardiogram

As predicted, the follow-up ECG demonstrates an extensive STEMI involving the anterior and lateral walls. We can now appreciate the time-sensitive signals that were present on the initial ECG. The patient's peak troponin level was 253. The occluded culprit artery was the mid-LAD.

## Case 3.9 A 44-year-old female presented with chest pain, nausea, vomiting and mild shortness of breath. She experienced three episodes of ventricular fibrillation in the emergency department. After defibrillation and treatment with amiodarone, her rhythm stabilized.

### The Electrocardiogram

The ECG is not diagnostic of an acute coronary syndrome. Clearly, she needs frequent repeat ECGs over the first hour while she is being observed closely. However, the presenting ECG shows broad-based, bulky T-waves in V2–V3 (along with sinus tachycardia). Follow-up ECGs (see the next ECGs) demonstrated, over a period of 90 minutes, a number of telltale early warnings of critical LAD occlusion.

## Case 3.9 The same patient, follow-up ECG.

This tracing, taken within 45 minutes of the patient's presentation to the emergency department, shows Wellens' warning: the ST-segments in V2–V3 are relatively normal (although with concerning straightening), until they are interrupted by an inverted T-wave. The biphasic T-wave in V2 and V3 is the hallmark of Wellens' syndrome, Type A. The T-waves are also inverted in leads V4 and V5. Additional ECGs were obtained.

## Case 3.9 The same patient (an additional follow-up ECG).

This ECG is remarkable for the appearance of deep, symmetric T-wave inversions in the anterior precordial leads. These "coronary T-waves" (or Wellens' syndrome, Type B) also signal that a tight proximal LAD occlusion is likely.

### Clinical Course

Serial ECGs demonstrated clear evolution of her anterior wall STEMI. Her troponin peaked at only 60. Coronary angiography revealed a "sub-total occlusion of the ostial and proximal LAD with an embolic thrombus in the downstream LAD."

## Case 3.10   A 46-year-old female called 911 because of chest pain. She had a cardiac arrest during transport and was defibrillated successfully. Her prehospital arrest and defibrillation rhythm strips are shown.

## Case 3.10   The same patient, after defibrillation.

### The Electrocardiogram

This ECG was obtained after a single defibrillation shock after her arrival to the emergency department. It demonstrates a mild sinus tachycardia and an acute injury current (STEMI) involving the high lateral wall with deep reciprocal ST-segment depressions in the inferior leads. There are also early changes of an acute anteroseptal STEMI (ST-segment elevation and loss of R-waves in precordial leads V1 and V2). This ECG is highly suggestive of a critical stenosis of the LAD, proximal to the first diagonal branch (D-1). Left main coronary artery obstruction is also a possibility given the mild ST-segment elevation in aVR.

### Clinical Course

She was taken for immediate angiography. The LMCA was not obstructed. Her catheterization report concluded that "the culprit lesion is an acute thrombotic occlusion of the ostial LAD." Her peak troponin level was 94.1. A stent was placed, and she recovered uneventfully.

## Case 3.11   A 37-year-old man with no significant past medical history presented to the emergency department with 2 weeks of intermittent chest pain. He also reported a cough productive of yellow sputum. He was admitted for "possible pneumonia and further evaluation of his chest pain, and rule out ACS." His troponin in the ED was 0.00. With respect to the ECG, the emergency department note stated, "Nonspecific T-wave changes in V5–V6 with no ST-elevation concerning to activate cath lab."

### The Electrocardiogram

The emergency physicians missed several critical electrocardiographic abnormalities. The ECG demonstrates sinus tachycardia and ST-segment depressions in leads I, II and aVF and also in the lateral precordial leads (V4–V6). Years ago, it would have been enough to interpret this ECG as showing "lateral wall ischemia" and, if the troponin was elevated, make a diagnosis of non-STEMI. Not anymore.

The ST-segment is markedly elevated in lead aVR, the no-longer-forgotten lead. The ST-segment elevation in aVR is reciprocal to the ST-segment depression in the lateral leads. Most importantly, ST-segment elevation in aVR is strongly associated with critical disease in the left main coronary artery or an "equivalent" (proximal LAD or multivessel coronary obstruction). This ECG represents a STEMI equivalent. His ECG also demonstrates abnormally tall (hyperacute) T-waves in the anterior precordial leads (V2–V4), although these could have been considered normal in the absence of the other ST-T changes.

### Clinical Course

He was admitted for antibiotics, serial troponins and ECGs and "medical management of "possible ACS." The patient's second troponin level was 37; the peak troponin level was 138. His angiography, which was delayed until the next day, revealed a 95 percent ostial LAD occlusion, and a drug-eluting stent was inserted. His echocardiogram showed hypokinesis of the anterior wall and reduced left ventricular function. His ejection fraction was 30 percent.

His follow-up ECG is shown next.

## Case 3.11   Same patient (follow-up ECG).
This ECG, taken on the second hospital day, demonstrates evolution of his acute anteroseptal STEMI.

## Case 3.12   A 48-year-old man presented with diaphoresis and chest pain of sudden onset. His initial troponin level was 0.31.

### The Electrocardiogram

The computer didn't have a chance. There is one subtle but important abnormality on the ECG tracing. There is ST-segment straightening and slight elevation in lead aVL, suggesting possible high lateral STEMI. Confirmation is provided by lead III, which demonstrates a sagging ST-segment. Given his symptoms and initial troponin, this could be enough to warrant immediate reperfusion. At the very least, he needs a repeat ECG within 15–20 minutes.

### Clinical Course

The patient continued to complain of chest tightness, and he had three ECGs over the next hour. A follow-up ECG is shown next.

## Case 3.12   The same patient – 1 hour and 15 minutes later.

### The Electrocardiogram

In this follow-up tracing, the acute high lateral STEMI is more obvious. The ST-segment elevations in I and aVL, and the reciprocal ST-segment depressions in II, III and aVF, are more dramatic. The ST-segments are also noticeably elevated in the anterior leads (V2–V5).

### Clinical Course

When angiography was performed, it revealed a 100 percent occlusion of the proximal LAD. His troponin peaked at only 15.9. Cardiac echocardiography on the second hospital day demonstrated moderate hypokinesis of anterior and anteroseptal walls with an estimated ejection fraction of 45 percent.

## Case 3.13   A 73-year-old male with a history of hypertension presented with intermittent chest pain and left arm aching for the past week. His initial troponin level was 0.16.

### The Electrocardiogram

The ECG is abnormal. The ST-segments are straightened in leads V1, V2 and V3, and they are slightly elevated in leads V1 and V2. In lead V3, there is a terminal T-wave inversion (Wellens' warning). The computer reading was simply "Cannot rule out septal infarct, age undetermined, possibly acute." Premature atrial complexes are also present.

### Clinical Course

He was taken for emergent coronary angiography, which revealed a 95 percent stenosis of the proximal LAD. He was stented successfully and never developed ECG evidence of a STEMI. The peak troponin level was only 1.7.

## Case 3.14   A 77-year-old man presented with shortness of breath. He was admitted for pneumonia. Several hours after his presentation, the following ECG was obtained.

### The Electrocardiogram

This is a challenging ECG due to the electrical artifact. Nonetheless, the ECG demonstrates lateral wall ST-segment depressions (leads I, aVL and V4–V6), accompanied by telltale ST-segment elevation in lead aVR. As discussed throughout this chapter, extensive inferior and lateral ST-segment depressions in the presence of ST-segment elevation in aVR is suggestive of left main or critical left anterior descending coronary artery occlusion (a STEMI equivalent).

### Clinical Course

His initial troponin level was 9. He underwent emergent coronary angiography, which demonstrated a 99 percent occlusion of the LMCA at the bifurcation of the LAD and LCA.

## Case 3.15 A 61-year-old female with a history of hypertension and heavy smoking presented with intermittent chest pain over 4 days. Her chest pain became worse on the day of her emergency department visit. She also reported nausea, vomiting and shortness of breath. Her daughter convinced her to come to the hospital.

### The Electrocardiogram

This patient has an obvious anterior, septal and high lateral STEMI. The ST-segment depressions in the inferior leads are reciprocal to the high lateral (I and aVL) ST-segment elevations. Patients with septal (V1) infarctions are at risk of early development of bundle branch blocks.

### Clinical Course

Her initial troponin was 0.26; the second troponin was 186.7. She underwent emergent coronary angiography, which, not surprisingly, demonstrated a 100 percent ostial and proximal LAD occlusion. Her follow-up ECG, taken 8 hours later, follows.

## Case 3.15 The same patient – 8 hours later (post-catheterization).

### The Electrocardiogram

The ECG now shows further evolution of her anteroseptal and high lateral STEMI, with development of a new RBBB.

### Clinical Course

Prior to discharge, an echocardiogram was performed, showing "apical, septal, anteroseptal and anterior wall hypokinesis to akinesis."

## Case 3.16 A 75-year-old man developed chest pain while shoveling snow. He also reported dizziness and shortness of breath. On ED arrival, he was in respiratory distress, and his initial systolic blood pressure was 80 mm Hg.

### The Electrocardiogram

The patient is suffering an extensive anterior, lateral and high lateral STEMI, as evidenced by dramatic ST-segment elevations in precordial leads V2–V6 as well as leads I and aVL. As expected, there are reciprocal ST-segment depressions in lead III. There is ventricular ectopy as well. The ECG is virtually diagnostic of a proximal LAD occlusion prior to the first diagonal branch. Ventricular ectopy is also present.

### Clinical Course

His troponin peaked at only 42. Predictably, emergency angiography revealed a 100 percent LAD occlusion proximal to the first diagonal branch.

## Case 3.17 A 68-year-old female presented with 2 hours of substernal chest pain, associated with diaphoresis, nausea and vomiting.

### The Electrocardiogram

The triage ECG shows an acute anteroseptal STEMI. PACs are also present; these are sometimes a harbinger of atrial fibrillation due to left atrial enlargement caused by left ventricular failure.

The ST-segments are depressed in lead aVL, a finding that immediately calls attention to the ST-segment straightening and mild elevation in the inferior leads. This tracing illustrates a combined anterolateral and inferior STEMI, most often explained by an obstructing thrombus in the midportion of a long LAD that "wraps around" the cardiac apex to perfuse the inferior wall.

## Case 3.18  A 66-year-old man presented with chest tightness and profuse diaphoresis. He reported no history of cardiovascular disease or risk factors. The initial troponin levels in the emergency department were normal (0.03 and 0.04).

### The Electrocardiogram

The computer interpretation was "sinus bradycardia, possible anterior wall infarction, age indeterminate, borderline ECG." However, the astute emergency physician noticed mild ST-segment depression in lead III, accompanied by super-subtle ST-segment elevation in aVL (barely noticeable but possibly significant given the low voltage QRS complex in that lead). The ECG serves as a reminder that, whenever ST-segment depressions are seen, our first obligation is to determine whether they are reciprocal to a STEMI (see Chapter 6). This ECG suggests that the patient is in the early stages of an isolated high lateral STEMI.

### Clinical Course

The catheterization laboratory was activated, and angiography revealed an isolated 100 percent occlusion of the mid-first diagonal branch (D-1). His peak troponin level was 55.5. He recovered uneventfully after placement of a stent.

## References

Arbane M., Gay J. J. Prediction of the site of total occlusion in the left anterior descending coronary artery using admission electrocardiogram in anterior wall acute myocardial infarction. *Am J Cardiol.* 2000; **85**:487–491.

Arnaout M., Mongardon N., Deye N. et al. Out-of-hospital cardiac arrest from brain cause: Epidemiology, clinical features and outcome in a multicenter cohort. *Crit Care Med.* 2015; **43**:453–460.

Ayer A., Terkelsen C. J. Difficult ECGs in STEMI: Lessons learned from serial sampling of pre- and in-hospital ECGs. *J Electrocardiol.* 2014; **47**: 448–458.

Aygul N., Ozdemir K., Tokac M. et al. Value of lead aVR in predicting acute occlusion of proximal left ananterior descending coronary artery and in-hospital outcome in ST-elevation myocardial infarction: an electrocardiographic predictor of poor prognosis. *J Electrocardiol.* 2008; **41**:335–341.

Bhat P. K., Pantham G., Laskey S. et al. Recognizing cardiac syncope in patients presenting to the emergency department with trauma. *J Emerg Med.* 2014; **46**:1–8.

Birnbaum Y., Nikus K., Kligfield P. et al. The role of the ECG in diagnosis, risk estimation and catheterization laboratory activation in patients with acute coronary syndromes: A consensus document. *Ann Noninvasive Electrocardiol.* 2014; **19**:412–425.

Birnbaum Y., Solodky A., Herz I. et al. Implications of inferior ST-segment depressions in anterior acute myocardial infarction: Electrocardiographic and angiographic correlation. *Am Heart J.* 1994; **127**: 1467–1473.

Birnbaum Y., Wilson J. M., Fiol M. et al. ECG diagnosis and classification of acute coronary syndromes. *Ann Noninvasive Electrocardiol.* 2014; **19**:4–14.

Chiara A. D. Right bundle branch block during the acute phase of myocardial infarction: modern redefinitions of old concepts. *Eur Heart J.* 2006; **27**:1–2.

de Winter R. W., Adams R., Verouden N. J. W., de Winter R. J. Precordial junctional ST-segment depression with tall symmetric T-waves signifying proximal LAD occlusion. Case reports of STEMI equivalence. *J Electrocardiol.* 2016; **49**:76–80.

Engelen D. J. Value of the ECG in localizing the occlusion site in the LAD coronary artery in acute anterior myocardial infarction. *J Am Coll Cardiol.* 1999; **34**:389.

Eskola M. J., Nikus K. C., Holmvang L. H. et al. Value of the 12-lead electrocardiogram to define the level of obstruction in acute anterior wall myocardial infarction: Correlation to coronary angiography and clinical outcome in the DANAMI-2 trial. *International J Cardiol.* 2009; **131**: 378–383.

Gorgels A. P. M., Engelen D. J. M., Wellens H. J. J. Lead aVR, a mostly ignored but very valuable lead in clinical electrocardiography. *J Am Col Cardiol.* 2001; **38**:1355–1356.

Lawner B. J., Nable J. V., Mattu A. Novel patterns of ischemia and STEMI equivalents. *Cardiol Clin.* 2012; **30**:591–599.

Lewandowski P. Subarachnoid hemorrhage imitating acute coronary syndrome as a cause of out-of-hospital cardiac arrest – case report. *Anesthesiology Intensive Therapy.* 2014; **46**:289–292.

Marriott H. J. L. *Emergency electrocardiography.* 1997; Naples, Florida: Trinity Press.

Mitsuma W., Ito M., Kodama M. Clinical and cardiac features of patients with subarachnoid hemorrhage presenting with out-of-hospital cardiac arrest. *Resuscitation.* 2011; **82**:1294–1297.

Neeland I. J., Kontos M. C., de Lemos J. A. Evolving considerations in the management of patients with left bundle branch block and suspected myocardial infarction. *J Am Coll Cardiol.* 2012; **60**:96–105.

Nikus K, Birnbaum Y, Eskola M et al. Updated electrocardiographic classification of acute coronary syndromes. *Current Cardiol Rev.* 2014; **10**: 229–236.

Nikus K., Pahlm O., Wagner G. et al. Electrocardiographic classification of acute coronary syndromes: A review by a committee of the International Society for Holter and Non-invasive Cardiology. *J Electrocardiol.* 2010; **43**:91–103.

Nikus K. C., Eskola M. J. Electrocardiogram patterns in acute left main coronary artery occlusion. *J Electrocardiol.* 2008; **41**:626–629.

Puppala V. K., Dickinson O., Benditt D. G. Syncope: Classification and risk stratification. *J Cardiol.* 2014; **63**:171–177.

Rokos I. C., French W. J., Mattu A. et al. Appropriate cardiac cath lab activation: Optimizing electrocardiogram interpretation and clinical decision-making for acute ST-elevation myocardial infarction. *Am Heart J.* 2010; **160**:995–1003.

Sgarbossa E. B., Pinski S. L., Barbagelata A. et al. Electrocardiographic diagnosis of evolving acute myocardial infarction in the presence of left bundle branch block. GUSTO-1 (Global Utilization of Streptokinase and Tissue

Plasminogen Activator for Occluded Coronary Arteries) Investigators. *N Engl J Med.* 1996; **334**:481–487.

Somers M. P., Brady W. J., Perron A. D., Mattu A. The prominent T-wave: Electrocardiographic differential diagnosis. *Am J Emerg Med.* 2002; **20**:243–251.

Stone P. H., Raabe D. S., Jaffe A. S. et al. Prognostic significance of location and type of myocardial infarction: independent adverse outcome associated with anterior location. *J Am Coll Cardiol.* 1988; **11**: 453.

Tabas J. A., Rodgriguez R. M., Seligman H. K., Goldschlager N. F. Electrocardiographic criteria for detecting acute myocardial infarction in patients with left bundle branch block: A meta-analysis. *Ann Emerg Med.* 2008; **52**:329–336.

Tamura A. Significance of lead aVR in acute coronary syndrome. *World J Cardiol.* 2014; **26**:630–637.

Tandy T. K., Bottomy D. P., Lewis J. G. Wellens' syndrome. *Ann Emerg Med.* 1999; **33**:347–351.

Thygesen K., Alpert J. S., Jaffe A. S. et al. Third universal definition of myocardial infarction. *J Am Coll Cardiol.* 2012; **60**:1581–1598.

Verouden N. J., Koch K. T., Peters R. J. et al. Persistent precordial "hyperacute" T-waves signify proximal left anterior descending artery occlusion. *Heart.* 2009; **95**:1701–1706.

Wagner G. S., Macfarlane P., Wellens H. et al. AHA/ACCF/HRS recommendations for the standardization and interpretation of the electrocardiogram. Part VI: Acute ischemia/infarction. A scientific statement from the American Heart Association, Electrocardiography and Arrhythmias Committee; Council on Clinical Cardiology; the American College of Cardiology Foundation; and the Heart Rhythm Society. *J Amer Col Cardiol.* 2009; **53**:1003–1011.

Wagner G. S., Strauss D. G. *Marriott's practical electrocardiography.* Twelfth edition. Philadelphia, PA: Lippincott Williams & Wilkins, 2014.

Wang S. S., Paynter L., Kelly R. V. et al. Electrocardiographic determination of culprit lesion site in patients with acute coronary events. *J Electrocardiol.* 2009; **42**:46–51.

Wellens H. J. J., Conover M. *The ECG in emergency decision-making.* Second edition. St. Louis, MO: Elsevier, Inc., 2006.

Williamson K., Mattu A., Plautz C. U., Binder A., Brady W. J. Electrocardiographic applications of lead aVR. *Am J Emerg Med.* 2006; **24**:864–874.

Wong C. K., Gao W., Stewart R. A. H. et al. Risk stratification of patients with acute anterior myocardial infarction and right bundle branch block: Importance of QRS duration and early ST-segment resolution after fibrinolytic therapy. *Circulation.* 2006; **114**:783–789.

Yamaji H., Iwasaki K., Kusachi S. et al. Prediction of acute left main coronary artery obstruction by 12-lead electrocardiography: ST-segment elevation in lead aVR with less ST-segment elevation in lead V1. *J Am Coll Cardiol.* 2001; **38**: 1348–1354.

Yamashina Y., Yagi T., Ishida A. et al. Differentiating between comatose patients resuscitated from acute coronary syndrome-associated and subarachnoid hemorrhage-associated out-of-hospital cardiac arrest. *J Cardiol.* 2015; **65**:508–513.

Yip H. K., Chen M. C., Wu C. J. et al. Acute myocardial infarction with simultaneous ST-segment elevation in the precordial and inferior leads. *Chest.* 2003; **123**:1170–1180.

Zhong-qun Z., Chong-quan W., Shu-yi D. et al. Acute anterior wall myocardial infarction entailing ST-segment elevation in lead V3 R, V1 or aVR: Electrocardiographic and angiographic correlations. *J Electrocardiol.* 2008; **41**: 329–334.

# Posterior Wall Myocardial Infarction

## Key Points

- Posterior wall ST-elevation myocardial infarction commonly occurs as a complication (or extension) of acute inferior wall STEMI. In this setting, ST-segment depressions appear in the right precordial leads (V1, V2 and V3) along with classic ST-segment elevations in the inferior leads. The precordial ST-segment depressions are the "mirror image" of ST-segment elevations over the posterior left ventricular wall. The culprit infarct-related artery is almost always the right coronary artery (RCA) (which perfuses the posterior wall of the heart by way of its posterior descending branch) or the left circumflex artery (LCA). Patients with inferior wall STEMIs complicated by ST-segment depressions in the right precordial leads (V1–V3) have larger infarct sizes and higher rates of pump failure, arrhythmias and early and late mortality.

- Posterior wall STEMI may also occur in combination with lateral wall or high lateral wall STEMI. ST-segment depressions are present in precordial leads V1, V2 and V3 in combination with ST-segment elevations (or simply loss of R-wave voltage) in the lateral (V5–V6) or high lateral (leads I and aVL) regions of the heart.

- Posterior wall STEMI may also occur alone. "True" or "isolated" posterior wall STEMI is not common (approximately 3–8 percent of all STEMIs) and is often missed. Usually, isolated posterior wall STEMI is caused by occlusion of the LCA or one of its branches (especially an obtuse marginal branch). The culprit artery may also be the terminal posterior descending branch of the RCA.

- Most "true" or "isolated" posterior STEMIs are not isolated at all; they actually involve the posterior and lateral left ventricular walls and can include a large at-risk territory.

- The right precordial leads (V1, V2 and V3) are critically important in diagnosing posterior wall STEMIs. Acute posterior wall STEMI should be suspected whenever the ST-segments are depressed in leads V1, V2 and V3. *Classically, the T-waves in these leads are unusually upright, despite the markedly depressed ST-segments.* ST-segment depressions and tall, upright T-waves in these right precordial leads are the electrical mirror image of ST-segment elevations and T-wave inversions over the posterior wall. Broad (≥0.04 seconds) and tall R-waves, often with a slurred upstroke, may also appear in leads V1 and V2; usually, these prominent R-waves are the reciprocal to posterior wall Q-waves, although they may reflect conduction system disturbances in some patients. The constellation of ST-segment depressions, upright T-waves and prominent R-waves in the right precordial leads (V1–V3) represents the "reciprocal sign" of true posterior wall STEMI.

- By definition, *isolated* posterior STEMIs present without any ST-segment elevations on the 12-lead ECG. These patients present with only with anterior (right precordial) ST-segment depressions and upright T-waves. They should still be considered as candidates for immediate reperfusion therapy. According to current guidelines, right precordial ST-segment depressions suggestive of posterior wall STEMI are *a STEMI equivalent.*

- ST-segment depressions in the right precordial leads (V1, V2 and V3) may also be caused by anterior wall ischemia. Not surprisingly, isolated posterior wall STEMI is often misclassified as "anterior wall ischemia or non-STEMI," leading to a delay in reperfusion therapy. *Acute posterior wall STEMI is* likely if the anterior precordial ST-segment depressions are: most marked in the right precordial leads (V1, V2 and V3); accompanied by tall, upright T-waves in these leads; accompanied by ST-segment elevations in the lateral (V5–V6) or high lateral (I and aVL) leads; or accompanied by signs of concomitant inferior wall STEMI. *Anterior wall subendocardial ischemia (or non-STEMI) is* more likely if the ST-segment depressions disproportionately involve the lateral precordial leads (V4–V6) and are accompanied by T-wave inversions.

- The standard 12-lead ECG is not a sensitive tool for diagnosing isolated posterior STEMI because it does not include any exploring leads that face the posterior left ventricular wall. The sensitivity can be increased by adding the three "posterior leads" (V7, V8 and V9). Clinicians should obtain posterior leads if a patient presents with symptoms that suggest an acute coronary syndrome (ACS) *in the absence of diagnostic ST-segment elevations in any leads.*

# Posterior Wall ST-Elevation Myocardial Infarction

Posterior wall ST-elevation myocardial infarction commonly occurs as a complication (or extension) of acute inferior wall STEMI. As discussed in Chapter 2, ST-segment depressions appear in the right precordial leads (V1, V2 and V3) along with classic ST-segment elevations in the inferior leads (Ayer and Terkelsen, 2014). The precordial ST-segment depressions are the "mirror image" of ST-segment elevations over the posterior left ventricular wall. The culprit infarct-related artery is usually the right coronary artery (RCA) or, less often, the left circumflex artery (LCA).

Posterior wall STEMI may also appear in conjunction with a lateral wall or high lateral wall STEMI. Here, the ST-segment depressions in the right precordial leads (V1, V2 and V3) are accompanied by ST-elevations in leads V5 and V6 (lateral wall STEMI) or in leads I and aVL (high lateral STEMI).

"True" or "isolated" posterior wall STEMIs are the subject of this chapter. True posterior STEMIs are not especially common (perhaps 3–8 percent of all myocardial infarctions), but they are often missed. Long delays in reperfusion therapy are almost the rule. This is not surprising because in posterior wall myocardial infarctions, the current of injury develops in an electrically "silent" region of the myocardium, where there are no exploring electrodes (Brady et al., 2001; Ayer and Terkelsen, 2014; Lawner et al., 2012; Brady 2007). Nonetheless, these are true STEMIs.

Typically, true posterior wall STEMIs present with only ST-segment depressions in one or more of the right precordial leads (V1–V3), sometimes accompanied by development of tall or broad R-waves. As befits any other STEMI, there is an occluded infarct-related artery, most often the LCA or one of its major branches. Acute posterior STEMI can also be caused by occlusion of the posterior descending artery, the terminal posterior branch of the RCA.

Recent echocardiographic and cardiac magnetic resonance imaging studies now make it clear that "true" or "isolated" posterior wall STEMI is, in fact, not isolated at all. In most patients with STEMIs characterized as "true posterior," there is extensive lateral wall ischemia and a large area of myocardium at risk (Nikus et al., 2010; Wagner et al., 2009; Ayer and Terkelsen, 2014; Rokos et al., 2010; Brady, 2007).

In some patients who present with right precordial (V1–V3) ST-segment depressions, the diagnosis is anterior wall subendocardial ischemia or non-STEMI. In other patients with right precordial lead ST-segment depressions, the correct diagnosis is posterior wall STEMI. It is our job to tell one from the other (Rokos et al., 2010; Birnbaum, Nikus et al., 2014; Birnbaum, Wilson et al., 2014).

## The Coronary Anatomy

Usually, "isolated" posterior wall STEMI is caused by a thrombotic occlusion of the left circumflex artery (LCA) or one of its major branches, most often a large obtuse marginal (OM) branch. Isolated posterior wall STEMI may also occur if the posterior descending artery (PDA), the large terminal branch of the right coronary artery, is occluded. Review Figures 3.3 and 4.1; it is no surprise that "true" posterior wall STEMIs almost invariably extend to the lateral left ventricular wall when the LCA or OM is the culprit vessel.

## Posterior Wall STEMI: The ECG "Reciprocal Sign"

Figure 4.2 illustrates the electrocardiographic hallmarks of a true posterior wall STEMI. There are dominant (tall and wide) R-wave in leads V1 and V2, which are the mirror image of posterior Q-waves. The ST-segments are depressed in the right precordial leads (V1, V2 and V3), the reciprocal to the posterior wall ST-segment elevations. And the T-waves are unusually tall, as if they are "determined" to stay upright,

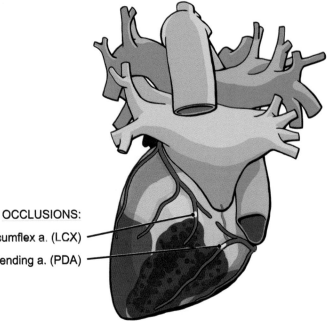

**Figure 4.1** Culprit artery occlusions in true posterior wall STEMI.

This figure shows the posterior wall of the left ventricle. True (isolated) posterior wall STEMI may be caused by occlusion of the left circumflex artery (or one of its major branches) or, occasionally, by occlusion of a terminal branch of the RCA (usually the posterior descending artery).

OCCLUSIONS:

Left circumflex a. (LCX)

Posterior descending a. (PDA)

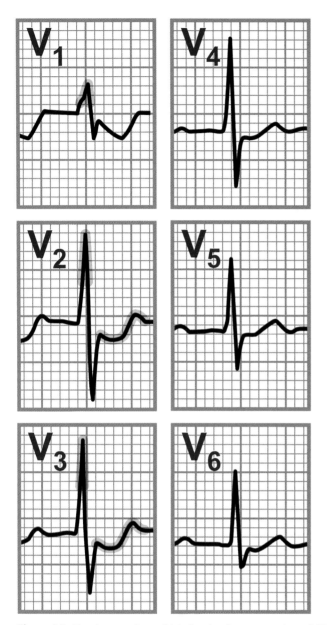

**Figure 4.2** The electrocardiographic hallmarks of a true posterior wall STEMI. From Marriott, 1997.

- *Tall or broad R-waves in precordial leads V1 and V2.* The R-wave is noticeably broad (≥0.04 seconds wide) and often has a slurred upstroke. The R:S ratio in lead V2 is ≥ 1.0. Like the mirror image Q-waves, prominent R-waves may not appear on the initial ECG[1] (Brady, 2007; Brady, 1998).

Another clue to a posterior wall STEMI is the presence of a concomitant lateral or high lateral or inferior STEMI. Therefore, whenever the ST-segments are depressed in V1–V3, raising the possibility of a posterior STEMI, check for:

- *Concomitant ST-segment elevations in the lateral (V5–V6) or high lateral (I and aVL) leads.* Lateral wall infarction may also manifest as loss of R-wave amplitude in leads V5 and V6 (the lateral wall "voltage drop-off" sign).
- *Concomitant ST-segment elevations in the inferior leads (or simply ST-segment depressions in lead aVL).*

## An Approach to Chest Pain Patients Who Have Anterior Wall ST-Segment Depressions

All too often, patients with chest pain, shortness of breath, dizziness or other related symptoms – who have ST-segment depressions in the right precordial leads (V1, V2 and V3) – are labeled as having "unstable angina" or anterior wall ischemia or a "non-STEMI." Some of these patients are experiencing acute posterior wall STEMIs, not anterior wall ischemia, and they could benefit from emergent reperfusion therapies (Pride et al., 2010; Brady et al., 2001).

ST-segment depressions in the anterior precordial leads may be caused by a posterior wall STEMI. Or they may be caused by anterior wall ischemia (unstable angina or a non-STEMI). Or anterior wall ST-segment depressions may be a sign of acute or chronic pulmonary hypertension (for example, in the setting of acute pulmonary embolism). Our objective is to discern when right precordial ST-segment depressions are a posterior wall "STEMI equivalent" (Brady et al., 2001; Wagner et al., 2009; Thygesen et al., 2012; Nikus et al., 2010; Rokos et al., 2010; Fesmire et al., 2006; Birnbaum, Nikus et al., 2014; Birnbaum, Wilson et al., 2014; Smith et al., 2002). The ECG features of acute pulmonary embolism are discussed in detail in Chapter 5, The Electrocardiography of Shortness of Breath.

One important point first: *Any ST-segment depression in V1, V2 and V3, even subtle deviations, should be taken seriously.* Remember that most normal individuals have some degree of ST-segment elevation in one or more of the right precordial leads. This means that any degree of anterior precordial ST-segment depression should raise the possibility of posterior wall STEMI or anterior wall ischemia. Also keep in mind that the anterior precordial leads are at some distance from the posterior wall of the left ventricle. Not surprisingly, even in the presence of an evolving posterior STEMI, the ST-segment

despite the sagging ST-segments. In this atlas, we refer to these as "bolt upright" T-waves. These are the mirror image of posterior wall T-wave inversions. Together, these ECG abnormalities represent the "reciprocal sign" of posterior STEMI. The reciprocal sign is usually limited to the right precordial leads (V1, V2 and V3), but they sometimes extend to V4 (Lawner et al., 2012; Brady 2007; Brady, 1998; Boden et al., 1987).

Therefore, true posterior wall STEMI should be considered whenever the following ECG abnormalities are present:

- *ST-segment depressions in the right precordial leads (V1–V3), accompanied by upright T-waves.*

---

[1] Prominent right precordial R-waves may also represent right ventricular enlargement or strain (for example, in COPD or pulmonary embolism), right bundle branch block, Type A Wolf-Parkinson-White syndrome, hypertrophic cardiomyopathy, dextroversion or other causes. Prominent right precordial R-waves may also appear in normal individuals, including children and adults ("early precordial transition" pattern) (Goldberger, 1980).

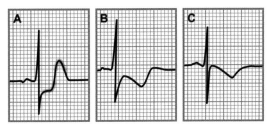

**Figure 4.3** Differentiating anterior wall ischemia from posterior wall STEMI. Posterior wall STEMI is highly likely when the right precordial ST-segments are accompanied by upright T-waves (Panel A). Panel C demonstrates symmetric T-wave inversions and is more characteristic of anterior wall ischemia (unstable angina or non-STEMI). Panel B has features of anterior ischemia and posterior STEMI; posterior leads should be obtained, along with echocardiography, whenever the diagnosis is in doubt. Remember: Panels B and C are also characteristic of acute pulmonary embolism (see Chapter 5).

depressions in V1, V2 and V3 may appear modest. Use old, baseline ECGs for comparison, if they are available.

Following are several important clues that can help to differentiate anterior wall ischemia or non-STEMI from posterior wall STEMI.

- Acute posterior wall STEMI is likely if the anterior precordial ST-segment depressions are limited to or are most prominent in the three right precordial leads (V1, V2 and V3). Anterior wall ischemia (unstable angina or a non-STEMI) is more likely if the anterolateral leads (V4–V6) are most affected by the ST-segment depressions and if the ST-T-wave changes are transient or dynamic (Smith et al., 2002).

- Acute posterior wall STEMI is also more likely if the right precordial ST-segment depressions are accompanied by tall, upright T-waves. T-wave inversions are more common in anterior wall subendocardial ischemia (and in acute pulmonary embolism). Again, the "bolt upright" T-waves in V1–V3 are the mirror image of posterior wall T-wave inversions. See Figure 4.3.

- Posterior wall STEMI is more likely if the R-waves in leads V1 or V2 are tall, are broad or have a slurred upstroke.

- Posterior STEMI is more likely if the ECG demonstrates: (a) signs of concomitant lateral wall STEMI (ST-segment elevations or loss of R-wave voltage in the lateral precordial leads V5 or V6); (b) signs of concomitant high lateral STEMI (ST-segment elevations in leads I and aVL); or (c) signs of evolving inferior wall STEMI (Nikus et al., 2010; Lawner et al., 2012).

## The Importance of ST-Segment Depressions in V1–V3 as a "STEMI Equivalent"

Patients with "only" ST-segment depressions in any of the ECG leads are often classified as "non-STEMI" or "unstable angina," conditions that may not always require emergent reperfusion therapy. However, patients felt to have a posterior wall STEMI are an exception, a position supported by published clinical guidelines. For example, while guidelines published by the American College of Emergency Physicians and the American Heart Association/American College of Cardiology

exclude patients with ST-segment depressions from the listed indications for emergent reperfusion therapies, they both single out the patient with a suspected posterior wall STEMI for special consideration. According to the 2004 AHA/ACC Guidelines (Antman et al., 2004), "In the absence of ST-elevations, there is no evidence of benefit of fibrinolytic therapy ... and there is some suggestion of harm for patients with ST-segment depression only ... Notwithstanding this, fibrinolytic therapy may be appropriate when there is marked ST-segment depression confined to leads V1 through V4 and accompanied by tall R-waves in the right precordial leads and upright T-waves indicative of a true posterior injury current and circumflex coronary artery occlusion."

The policy adds, "in circumstances where there is a suggestive clinical history and suggestive evidence of true posterior infarction, confirmatory data from posterior leads (V7 and V8) as well as 2-dimensional echocardiography may be especially helpful." Indeed, as highlighted later, posterior leads (and point-of-care echocardiography) should be obtained whenever there is doubt about the meaning of anterior precordial ST-segment depressions (Nikus et al., 2010; Lawner et al., 2012; Brady et al., 2001; Brady, 1998; Brady, 2007).

As noted earlier, even while the term "isolated posterior wall" STEMI is frequently applied, these are not necessarily small or isolated in terms of myocardial territory at risk. Often, the STEMI involves an extensive region of the lateral left ventricular wall. Not surprisingly, emergent reperfusion is associated with improved outcomes. Unfortunately, recognition of posterior wall STEMI and reperfusion interventions are often delayed (in one study, an average of 29 hours); and delay in instituting reperfusion results in adverse clinical outcomes for these patients (Brady, 2007; Pride et al., 2010; Rokos et al., 2010; Waldo et al., 2013).

In summary, when confronted with a patient with symptoms consistent with an ACS, recognition of a posterior wall STEMI may change treatment plans from routine medical management to immediate reperfusion. Just because the ST-segment elevations are "on the back," in an electrically silent area of the heart, does not make them any less important.

## Posterior Leads

The standard 12-lead ECG is not a sensitive tool for diagnosing isolated posterior STEMI because it does not include any monitoring leads that face the posterior left ventricular wall (Brady, 2007). The sensitivity can be increased by adding the three "posterior leads" (V7, V8 and V9). Clinicians should obtain posterior leads if a patient presents with symptoms that suggest an acute coronary syndrome (ACS) *in the absence of diagnostic ST-segment elevations in other leads.*

Posterior leads should be considered in patients with possible ACS if (a) the ECG appears normal, or there are only nonspecific ST- and T-wave changes; (b) there are ST-segment depressions and upright T-waves in the anterior precordial leads (V1, V2 and V3) suggesting posterior wall STEMI; or (c) there are subtle or borderline ST-segment elevations in the lateral or high lateral leads. The posterior leads are "positive" for STEMI if the ST-segment elevations are ≥ 0.5 mV.

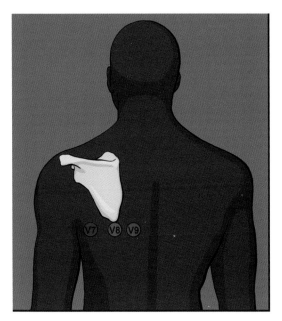

**Figure 4.4** Placement of the posterior leads.

Posterior leads may also be considered for patients with obvious inferior or lateral wall STEMIs to check for posterior wall involvement (that is, to gain additional information about the extent of the STEMI and the patient's prognosis).

Most studies indicate that using posterior leads increases the sensitivity of the ECG in the diagnosis of isolated posterior STEMI (Aqel et al., 2009; Lawner et al., 2012; Nikus et al., 2010; Brady, 2007; Brady et al., 2001; Brady, 1998). Indeed, in as many as one-third of patients with acute LCA occlusion, the maximum or only ST-segment elevations are found in leads V7, V8 or V9.

It is not known whether obtaining posterior leads adds diagnostic information if a cardiac echocardiogram is immediately available. If posterior leads are normal or equivocal, bedside echocardiography may be the most useful test in patients with anterior wall ST-segment depressions to differentiate posterior STEMI, anterior wall ischemia and pulmonary thromboembolism.

As highlighted in Figure 4.4, V8 is placed on the patient's back at the tip of the left scapula. V7 is placed at the level of V6 in the posterior axillary line. V9 is positioned halfway between V8 and left paraspinal muscles.

# Self-Study Electrocardiograms

**Case 4.1** A 56-year-old man, status-post coronary artery bypass surgery, presented with chest pain.

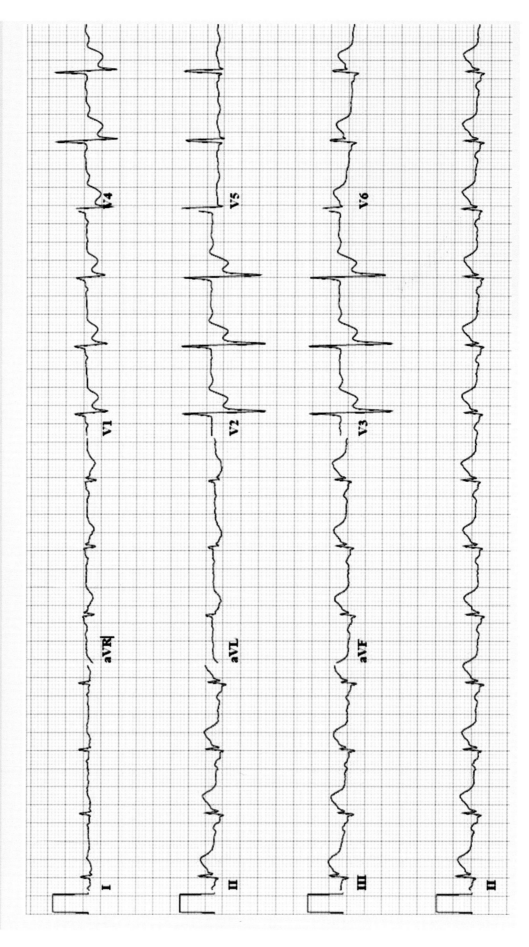

**Case 4.1 (Continued)** The same patient – 1 day later.

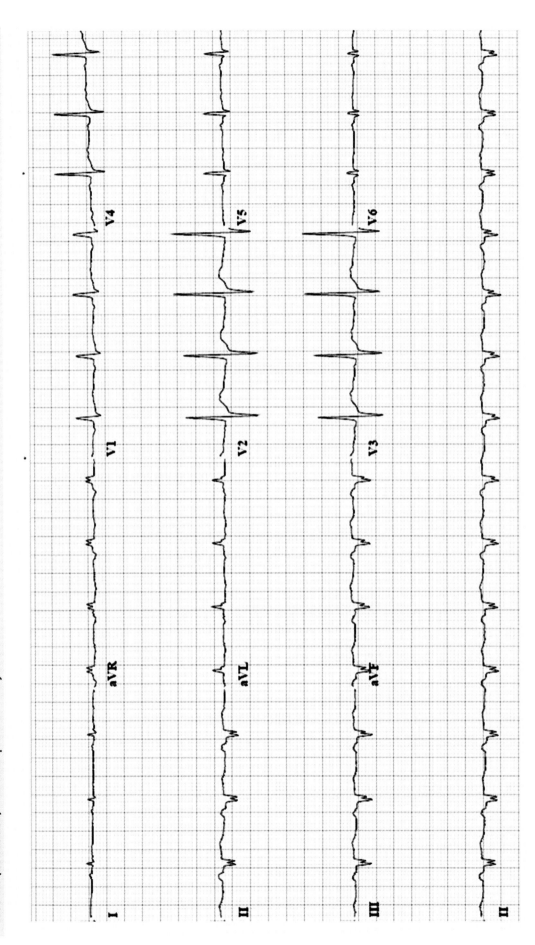

**Case 4.2** An 80-year-old female presented with confusion, diaphoresis and laboratory abnormalities of diabetic ketoacidosis.

**Case 4.3** A 71-year-old man with a history of coronary artery disease presented with intermittent chest pain (over 1 week), nausea, vomiting and shortness of breath.

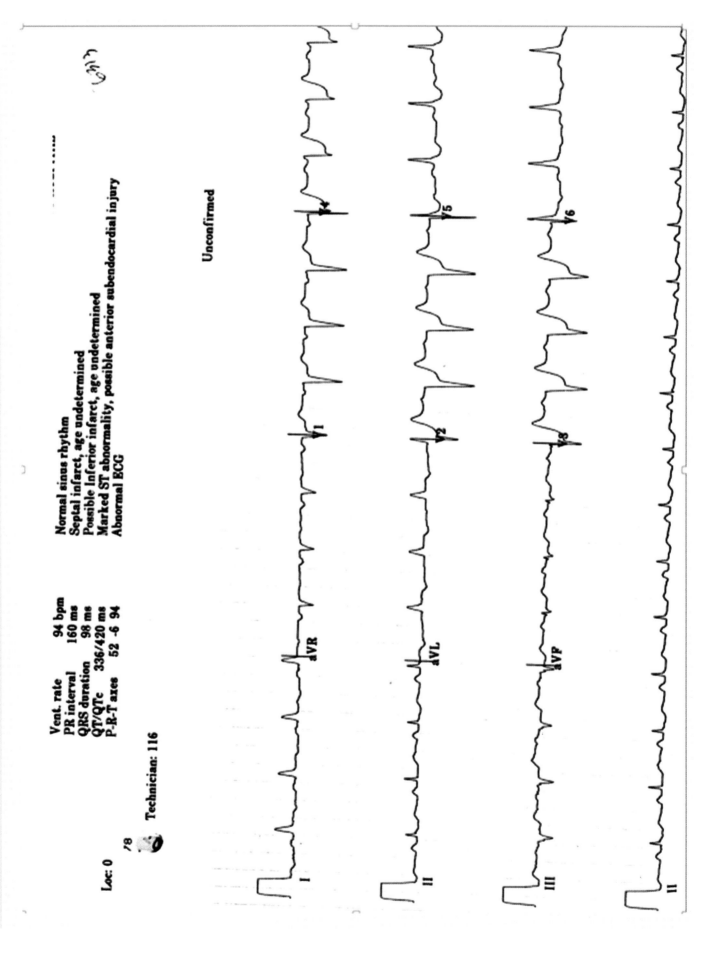

| | |
|---|---|
| Vent. rate | 94 bpm |
| PR interval | 160 ms |
| QRS duration | 98 ms |
| QT/QTc | 336/420 ms |
| P-R-T axes | 52 -6 94 |

Normal sinus rhythm
Septal infarct, age undetermined
Possible Inferior infarct, age undetermined
Marked ST abnormality, possible anterior subendocardial injury
Abnormal ECG

Unconfirmed

Loc: 0

Technician: 116

aVR · aVL · aVF · V1 · V2 · V3 · V5 · V6 · I · II · III · II

**Case 4.4** A 54-year-old man presented with the sudden onset of substernal chest pain while sitting at his desk at work. He also experienced nausea and diaphoresis. His initial troponin level was 0.04.

**Case 4.4 (Continued)** The same patient – posterior leads.

**Case 4.5** A 63-year-old man had the sudden onset of central chest pressure and severe dyspnea. His blood pressure was 100/78, and his heart rate was 123. He had a loud, holosystolic murmur, and his lung examination was consistent with pulmonary edema. His chest x-ray showed venous cephalization, bronchial cuffing and indistinct hilar vessels, also indicative of lung edema.

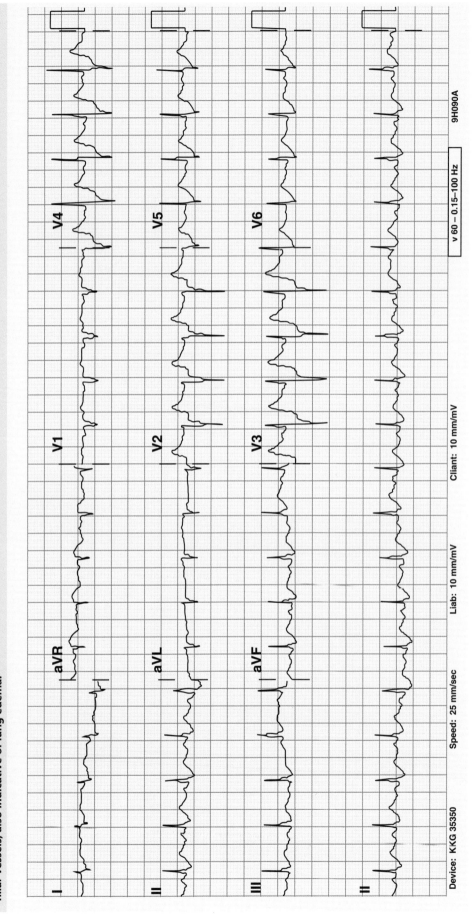

Device: KKG 35350          Speed: 25 mm/sec          Liab: 10 mm/mV          Cliant: 10 mm/mV          v 60 – 0.15–100 Hz          9H090A

**Case 4.6** A 66-year-old man with exertional dyspnea and dizziness.

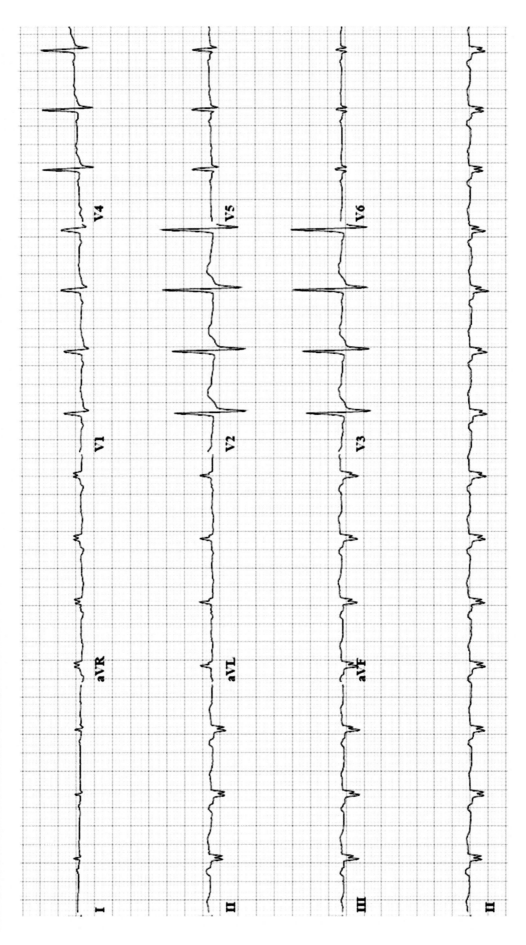

Case 4.6 (Continued) The same patient – 2 days earlier.

# Self-Study Notes

## Case 4.1 A 56-year-old man, status-post coronary artery bypass surgery, presented with chest pain.

### The Electrocardiogram

The ECG shows a typical inferior wall STEMI with extension of the STEMI to the lateral and posterior left ventricular walls. In the right precordial leads (V1, V2 and V3), the ST-segments are depressed, while the T-waves remain upright. These features are highly suggestive of posterior wall STEMI. This ECG tracing represents the most common presentation of posterior STEMI – in the setting of an inferior and lateral wall STEMI. In most cases, the occluded artery is the RCA or the LCA.

A follow-up ECG was obtained 1 day later.

## Case 4.1 The same patient – 1 day later.

On the follow-up ECG, there is an abnormally tall T-wave in precordial lead V2, where the R:S ratio is greater than 1.0. The R-wave in lead V1 is also abnormally tall and broad. These findings are highly suggestive of a posterior wall STEMI of indeterminate age. There is also loss of R-wave voltage in the lateral leads (V5 and V6); the "lateral voltage drop-off sign" is also common during and after an acute posterior wall STEMI; in fact, most posterior wall STEMIs actually involve large portions of the lateral left ventricular wall. Finally, and not surprisingly, the ECG reveals the expected changes after an inferior wall infarction; pathologic Q-waves have developed in II, III and aVF.

## Case 4.2 An 80-year-old female presented with confusion, diaphoresis and laboratory abnormalities of diabetic ketoacidosis.

### The Electrocardiogram

The most obvious abnormality is the presence of ST-segment elevations and with low R-wave voltage ("voltage drop-off") in the lateral precordial leads. These findings are diagnostic of an acute lateral wall STEMI. A high lateral STEMI may also be present (ST-segment elevation is present in lead I).

In addition, there are unmistakable signs of a posterior wall STEMI: ST-segment depressions are present in the right precordial leads (V1, V2 and V3), where there are also upright T-waves. PVCs are also present. The ECG is consistent with an acute posterior, high lateral and lateral wall STEMI. The ECG also suggests an old (indeterminate age) inferior wall infarction.

### Clinical Course

Emergent catheterization was performed, which demonstrated, as expected, a 100 percent occlusion of the left circumflex artery. Chronic LAD disease was also present. This patient expired 24 hours after her admission.

## Case 4.3 A 71-year-old man with a history of coronary artery disease presented with intermittent chest pain (over 1 week), nausea, vomiting and shortness of breath.

### The Electrocardiogram

This is a tracing from the early 1990s that was interpreted as showing "anterior subendocardial injury." He was treated initially as an acute coronary syndrome (ACS), and after a delay, he received intravenous streptokinase. His creatine phosphokinase (CPK) peaked at 1,537. While anterior wall subendocardial ischemia is in the differential, acute, true posterior wall STEMI is much more likely, given the marked right precordial (V1, V2, V3, V4) ST-segment depressions and remarkably "bolt upright" T-waves.

### Clinical Course

The posterior wall STEMI was confirmed by an echocardiogram that demonstrated basal, posterior and lateral wall hypokinesis. As noted repeatedly in this chapter, most "isolated" posterior wall STEMIs are not isolated at all; they usually involve the posterolateral myocardium. As predicted, catheterization performed later demonstrated a 100 percent proximal LCA occlusion.

## Case 4.4  A 54-year-old man presented with the sudden onset of substernal chest pain while sitting at his desk at work. He also experienced nausea and diaphoresis. His initial troponin level was 0.04.

### The Electrocardiogram

The ECG is, of course, diagnostic of an acute inferior wall and posterior wall STEMI. Lead V2 is especially classic, showing ST-segment depressions, upright T-waves and an emerging tall R-wave (the "reciprocal sign" of an acute posterior wall STEMI). First-degree AV block is also present, suggesting that the culprit occluded artery is likely to be the RCA rather than the LCA.

Although not specifically required, the ED team obtained posterior leads (next figure).

## Case 4.4  The same patient – posterior leads.

The posterior leads are labeled (*V7, V8* and *V9*). ST-segment elevations are present in these leads, signifying an acute posterior wall STEMI.

### Clinical Course

Catheterization revealed a 100 percent occlusion of the distal RCA. The culprit artery (RCA) was predictable, given the ST-segment elevations in lead III > lead II and the very deep ST-segment depressions in aVL. His troponin level peaked at only 12.40.

## Case 4.5  A 63-year-old man had the sudden onset of central chest pressure and severe dyspnea. His blood pressure was 100/78, and his heart rate was 123. He had a loud, holosystolic murmur, and his lung examination was consistent with pulmonary edema. His chest x-ray showed venous cephalization, bronchial cuffing and indistinct hilar vessels, also indicative of lung edema.

### The Electrocardiogram

An acute, "true" posterior wall STEMI is present. There are ST-segment depressions and "bolt upright" T-waves in V2 and V3. Sinus tachycardia is also present. ST-segment elevation is also present in lead aVR, which could also have suggested left main coronary artery occlusion. ST-elevations in aVR are sometimes observed in posterior wall STEMIs.

### Clinical Course

Catheterization revealed a 100 percent occlusion of the distal RCA and its posterior descending artery (PDA) terminal branch. This explains the posterior STEMI as well as holosystolic murmur and pulmonary edema, which were caused by posteromedial papillary muscle rupture.

The posteromedial papillary muscle is a part of the endocardium and, in most individuals, receives a single blood supply from the right coronary artery, usually from the PDA. In contrast, the blood supply to the anterolateral papillary muscle is supplied by both the left anterior descending and left circumflex arteries. Rupture of the posteromedial papillary muscle is more common because of the single blood supply. Echocardiography can be useful in confirming the diagnosis of papillary muscle rupture.

It is critical to auscultate the heart of the patient with pulmonary rales or shock; papillary muscle rupture is a "don't-miss" mechanical cause of pulmonary edema and cardiogenic shock in patients with acute inferior or posterior wall STEMIs.

## Case 4.6  A 66-year-old man with exertional dyspnea and dizziness.

### The Electrocardiogram

The ECG shows unmistakable evidence of an old (indeterminate age) myocardial infarction involving multiple regions of the heart. First, there are only Q-waves in the inferior leads, indicating a prior inferior wall infarction. Second, the R-wave in V1 is abnormally tall and broad and is accompanied by tall R-waves in lead V2; these changes are consistent with a prior posterior wall STEMI. Lastly, the ECG demonstrates a dramatic drop-off in R-wave voltage in precordial leads V5 and V6; thus, his prior inferior and posterior infarctions also involved the lateral wall.

In fact, as shown in the next ECG, just 2 days earlier he presented to the emergency department with an acute inferior-posterior-lateral wall STEMI.

## Case 4.6  The same patient – 2 days earlier.

### The Electrocardiogram
The ECG demonstrates an acute STEMI involving the inferior, posterior and lateral walls.

# References

Antman E. M., Anbe D. T., Armstrong P. W. et al. ACC/AHA guidelines for the management of patients with ST-elevation myocardial infarction: a report of the American College of Cardiology/American Heart Association Task Force on Practice Guidelines (Committee to Revise the 1999 Guidelines for the Management of Patients with Acute Myocardial Infarction). *Circulation.* 2004 Aug 31; 110(9):e82–292.

Aqel R. A., Fadi G. H., Ellipeddi P. et al. Usefulness of three posterior chest leads for the detection of posterior wall acute myocardial infarction. *Am J Cardiol.* 2009; 103:159–164.

Ayer A., Terkelsen C. J. Difficult ECGs in STEMI: Lessons learned from serial sampling of pre- and in-hospital ECGs. *J Electrocardiol.* 2014; 47:448–458.

Birnbaum Y., Nikus K., Kligfield P. et al. The role of the ECG in diagnosis, risk estimation and catheterization laboratory activation in patients with acute coronary syndromes: A consensus document. *Ann Noninvasive Electrocardiol.* 2014; 19:412–425.

Birnbaum Y., Wilson J. M., Fiol M. et al. ECG diagnosis and classification of acute coronary syndromes. *Ann Noninvasive Electrocardiol.* 2014; 19:4–14.

Boden W. E., Kleiger R. E., Gibson R. S. et al. Electrocardiographic evolution of posterior acute myocardial infarction: importance of early precordial ST-segment depression. *Am J Cardiol.* 1987; 59:782–787.

Brady W. J. Acute posterior wall myocardial infarction. *Am J Emerg Med.* 1998; 16:409–413.

The earth is flat. The electrocardiogram has 12 leads. The electrocardiogram in the patient with ACS: Looking beyond the 12-lead electrocardiogram. *Am J Emerg Med.* 2007; 25:1073–1076.

Brady W. J., Erling B., Pollack M., Chan T. C. Electrocardiographic manifestations: Acute posterior wall myocardial infarction. *J Emerg Med.* 2001; 20:391–401.

Fesmire F. M., Brady W. J., Hahn S., Decker W. W. et al. Clinical policy: Indications for reperfusion therapy in emergency department patients with suspected acute myocardial infarction. American College of Emergency Physicians Clinical Policies Subcommittee (Writing Committee) on Reperfusion Therapy in Emergency Department Patients with Suspected Acute Myocardial Infarction. *Ann Emerg Med.* 2006 Oct; 48 (4):358–383.

Goldberger A. L. Recognition of ECG pseudo-infarct patterns. *Mod Concepts Cardiovasc. Dis.* 1980; 49(3):13–18.

Lawner B. J., Nable J. V., Mattu A. Novel patterns of ischemia and STEMI equivalents. *Cardiol Clin.* 2012; 30:591–599.

Marriott H. J. L. *Emergency electrocardiography.* Naples, FL: Trinity Press, 1997.

Nikus K., Birnbaum Y., Eskola M. et al. Updated electrocardiographic classification of acute coronary syndromes. *Current Cardiol Rev.* 2014; 10:229–236.

Nikus K., Pahlm O., Wagner G. et al. Electrocardiographic classification of acute coronary syndromes: A review by a committee of the International Society for

Holter and Non-invasive Cardiology. *J Electrocardio.* 2010; 43:91–103.

Pride Y. B., Tung P., Mohanavelu S. et al. Angiographic and clinical outcomes among patients with acute coronary syndromes presenting with isolated anterior ST-segment depression. *J Amer Coll Cardiol Intv.* 2010; 3:806–811.

Rokos I. C., French W. J., Mattu A. et al. Appropriate cardiac cath lab activation: Optimizing electrocardiogram interpretation and clinical decision-making for acute ST-elevation myocardial infarction. *Am Heart J.* 2010; 160:995–1003.

Smith S. W., Zvosec D. L., Sharkey S. W., Hentry T. D. *The ECG in acute MI. An evidence-based manual of reperfusion therapy.* Philadelphia, PA: Lippincott Williams & Wilkins, 2002.

Thygesen K., Alpert J. S., Jaffe A. S. et al. Third universal definition of myocardial infarction. *J Am Coll Cardiol.* 2012; 60:1581–1598.

Wagner G. S., Macfarlane P., Wellens H. et al. AHA/ACCF/HRS recommendations for the standardization and interpretation of the electrocardiogram. Part VI: Acute ischemia/infarction. A scientific statement from the American Heart Association, Electrocardiography and Arrhythmias Committee; Council on Clinical Cardiology; the American College of Cardiology Foundation; and the Heart Rhythm Society. *J Amer Col Cardiol.* 2009; 53:1003–1011.

Waldo S. W., Armstrong E. J., Kulkarni A. et al. Clinical characteristics and reperfusion times among patients with an isolated posterior myocardial infarction. *J Invasive Cardiol.* 2013; 25:371–375.

# The Electrocardiography of Shortness of Breath

**Chapter**

**5**

## Key Points

- There are at least three common "shortness of breath emergencies" – pulmonary thromboembolism, pericardial effusion and myocarditis – where the ECG often provides the first diagnostic information. While the ECG is not the definitive test for any of these conditions, the ECG is often the first test performed. In many cases, the ECG provides unmistakable clues that can guide initial treatment and further diagnostic testing.

- Pulmonary embolism (PE) is a common cause of dyspnea. The most common ECG abnormalities are sinus tachycardia; T-wave inversions in leads V1, V2 and V3; a rightward QRS axis (or an axis that is more rightward than normal for the patient's age); the S1-Q3-T3 pattern; and an rSR' pattern in lead V1. Atrial flutter and atrial fibrillation occur less commonly.

- Concurrent T-wave inversions in the anterior and inferior leads are a vital clue to the presence of acute PE; however, these T-wave inversions are often misinterpreted by clinicians and computer algorithms as "possible anterior ischemia, possible inferior ischemia."

- In patients with acute PE, anterior T-wave inversions, an rSR' complex in V1 and acute right axis deviation are markers of acute pulmonary hypertension and right heart strain. They are associated with more severe pulmonary hypertension, right ventricular dysfunction, extensive pulmonary vascular obstruction (clot burden) and mortality.

- Myocarditis often presents with dyspnea as well as chest pain, palpitations and, frequently, signs of congestive heart failure. Classically, a viral prodrome is present. The combination of low voltage in the limb or precordial leads and sinus tachycardia should raise the suspicion of acute myocarditis. The ECG may also demonstrate diffuse ST- and T-wave changes, including ST-segment elevations, ST-segment depressions, T-wave inversions, premature atrial or ventricular beats and conduction abnormalities. Echocardiography is frequently the key test that defines the global wall motion abnormalities that are characteristic of diffuse myocarditis.

- Some patients develop a focal myocarditis; here, the ECG may show ST-segment elevations in a regional pattern (for example, suggesting inferior wall STEMI). Acute myocarditis is a "don't-miss" diagnosis because patients may develop fulminant congestive heart failure or malignant ventricular arrhythmias.

- Shortness of breath is the most common symptom in patients with cardiac tamponade. The characteristic ECG findings include sinus tachycardia, low-voltage QRS complexes and, frequently, electrical alternans.

- Chronic emphysema also presents characteristic ECG changes. The most common are abnormal right axis deviation and other features of right ventricular enlargement, right atrial enlargement (p-pulmonale), low QRS voltage in the limb or precordial leads, the "Lead I sign," and poor R-wave progression. Tachycardias, including multifocal atrial tachycardia, also occur commonly in patients with severe emphysema, especially during hypoxic respiratory emergencies.

## The Electrocardiography of Shortness of Breath

There are dozens of causes of shortness of breath; in most cases, the diagnosis does not depend on the electrocardiogram. Pneumonia, asthma, emphysema, congestive heart failure, upper airway obstruction and other common conditions are usually evident after performing a careful history and physical examination.

At the same time, there are at least three common "shortness of breath emergencies" – pulmonary thromboembolism, pericardial effusion and myocarditis – where the ECG often provides the first diagnostic information. The ECG is not the definitive test for any of these conditions; in terms of "diagnostic test characteristics" (sensitivity and specificity), the ECG may perform poorly. However, the ECG is often the first test performed. In many cases, the ECG provides unmistakable clues to these critical conditions.

## The ECG in Pulmonary Embolism

Pulmonary embolism (PE) is a common cause of dyspnea. Even though the ECG is not a sensitive or specific test for acute pulmonary embolism and even though the exact contribution of the ECG to other clinical decision tools (for example, Wells, Geneva, PERC, the d-dimer or other cardiac biomarkers) is unknown, the ECG often presents early clues to this diagnosis (Digby et al., 2015). In addition, PE typically presents with chest pain, dyspnea, dizziness or syncope. Since virtually every patient with one of these symptoms receives an ECG, it will always be important to recognize the telltale electrocardiographic features of PE (Digby et al., 2015).

If sinus tachycardia and "nonspecific ST-T-wave changes" are included, the ECG is abnormal in most patients with an acute PE (Geibel et al., 2005; Pollack, 2006; Petrov, 2001; Ferrari et al., 1997; Wagner and Strauss, 2014; Surawicz and Knilans, 2008; Chan et al., 2005; Chan et al., 2001). The most common and helpful ECG findings are listed in the table and are described later.

Increasingly, the ECG is recognized for providing valuable prognostic, as well as diagnostic, information in patients with suspected PE (Digby et al., 2015). Many of the ECG abnormalities (for example, right axis deviation, S1Q3T3, right bundle branch block and, especially, right precordial T-wave inversions) are reflections of elevated pulmonary artery pressures and right heart strain. They are associated with more severe pulmonary hypertension and right ventricular dysfunction; they are also associated with more extensive pulmonary vascular obstruction (clot burden) and in-hospital complications, such as cardiogenic shock and mortality (Ferrari et al., 1997; Geibel et al., 2005; Petrov, 2001; Digby et al., 2015). The ECG findings in patients with acute PE are often transient, and they may lessen or disappear after successful lytic therapy (Surawicz and Knilans, 2008; Chan et al., 2001).

In 2015, Digby et al. published a comprehensive review of the prognostic value of the ECG in patients presenting with acute PE (Digby et al., 2015). They summarized decades of evidence regarding sinus tachycardia, right axis deviation, S1Q3T3, right bundle branch block and T-wave inversions in the right precordial and other leads. The review also highlighted several more recently recognized ECG manifestations of PE, including ST-segment elevations in V1, ST-segment elevations in aVR, QT prolongation and low QRS voltage.

## Right Axis Deviation

One critical ECG clue to pulmonary embolism is the finding of right axis deviation. The QRS axis must be interpreted in light of the patient's age. ECG textbooks and computer algorithms often assert that the QRS axis is abnormally rightward only if the measured QRS axis is outside the range between −30 and +105 degrees. However, the clinician has to be more flexible (and more astute). The axis in newborns and children is rightward, reflecting the dominance of the right ventricle and right ventricular outflow tract. However, the axis shifts leftward as people age (Stephen, 1990; Wagner and Strauss, 2014; Surawicz and Knilans, 2008; Rijnbeek et al., 2014). Therefore, any degree of rightward axis – that is, *any visible S-wave in lead I* – may be abnormal in patients older than age 45–50 years. In older patients with chest pain, dyspnea, syncope or other cardiovascular symptoms, the presence of an S-wave in lead I, signifying a QRS axis that is abnormally rightward for the patient's age,

**Box 5.1 ECG Clues to Pulmonary Embolism**

- Sinus tachycardia
- Right axis deviation (including S1-Q3-T3)
- T-wave inversions in right precordial leads
- T-wave inversions in *both anterior precordial and inferior limb leads*
- Complete or incomplete right bundle branch block (rSR′ in V1)
- Atrial fibrillation or atrial flutter
- Right atrial enlargement (P-pulmonale)

may be the only clue to acute right heart strain and PE. Examples are provided later in this chapter.

## S1-Q3-T3

While sinus tachycardia is the most common ECG abnormality in patients with acute PE, the S1-Q3-T3 pattern is often considered a "classic" or even "pathognomonic" finding (Pollack, 2006). However, the S1-Q3-T3 pattern is uncommon, and it is neither sensitive nor specific for acute PE.

The most important component of the S1-Q3-T3 is probably the right axis deviation (S-wave in lead I), indicating acute right heart strain. The Q3-T3 is harder to explain; it may reflect acute clockwise rotation of the heart due to right ventricular dilatation. This would result in an abnormal direction of septal and ventricular depolarization in a posterior and leftward direction (away from lead III) (Chan et al., 2005).

## T-Wave Inversions

T-wave inversions in the right precordial leads (V1–V3) are, in some series, the most common ECG abnormality in patients with acute PE, occurring more frequently than sinus tachycardia or the S1Q3T3 pattern (Ferrari et al., 1997). In patients who present with symptoms suggestive of an acute coronary syndrome and T-wave inversions in the right precordial leads, acute PE, as well as anterior wall ischemia, should be considered in the differential diagnosis.

Even more diagnostic, *if there are concurrent T-wave inversions in the anterior and inferior leads, PE should be strongly considered* (Marriott, 1997). All too often, when the T-waves are inverted in the anterior and inferior leads, clinicians and computer algorithms misinterpret this finding. It is common for the computer to suggest, "T-wave abnormality, consider anterior ischemia; T-wave abnormality, consider inferior ischemia." Of course, simultaneous inferior and anterior ischemia is quite uncommon. Thus, in a patient with dyspnea, chest pain, dizziness, syncope or other cardiovascular symptoms, acute PE should rise to the top of the differential list. T-wave inversions are a critical finding that suggests a greater clot burden and a higher risk of hemodynamic collapse and mortality. T-wave inversions also tend to persist longer on the ECG, even after successful lytic therapy or spontaneous lysis (Surawicz and Knilans, 2008; Ferrari et al., 1997).

Consider the ECG, which is nearly diagnostic of acute PE.

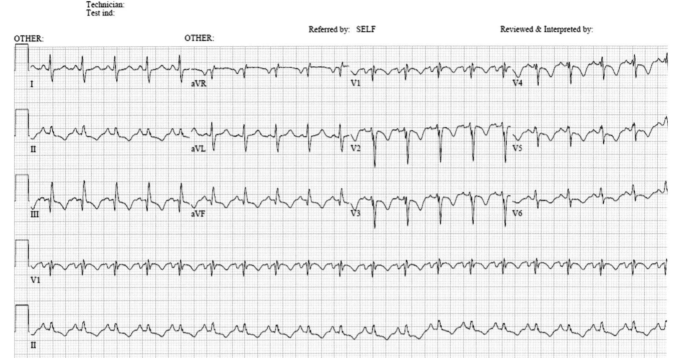

| Male | Black | Vent. rate | 119 | BPM | Sinus tachycardia |
|---|---|---|---|---|---|
| | | PR interval | 116 | ms | Possible Left atrial enlargement |
| | | QRS duration | 102 | ms | Non-specific intra-ventricular conduction delay |
| Room:1024 | | QT/QTc | 356/500 | ms | Cannot rule out Anterior infarct , age undetermined |
| Loc:1002 | | P-R-T axes | 43  82  -71 | | ST & T wave abnormality, consider anterolateral ischemia |
| | | | | | Abnormal ECG |
| | | | | | No previous ECGs available |

**ECG 5.1** A 62-year-old man, with a history of hypertension, presented with a sore throat, cough, fatigue, bilateral lower extremity swelling and periodic bouts of hemoptysis. On presentation, he had severe hypoxemia (pulse oximetry reading of 68 percent on room air).

## The Electrocardiogram

This ECG demonstrates an array of features that are nearly diagnostic of acute pulmonary embolism. The computer algorithm did not detect any of them, with the exception of sinus tachycardia. All of the following are present: sinus tachycardia; a marked right axis deviation, especially for this patient's age (including the well-known S1-Q3-T3 pattern); an abnormal rSR' in lead V1 (an "incomplete RBBB"); and T-wave inversions in both the anterior and inferior leads. These features correlate strongly with ultrasonographic and CT-scan evidence of pulmonary hypertension, right ventricular dysfunction and an extensive clot burden. Obviously, the computer algorithm is completely befuddled, and we must overrule it.

## Clinical Course

He underwent an emergent CT–pulmonary embolism (CTPE) study, which revealed the following: "Extensive bilateral pulmonary emboli, more extensive on the right, with left lung base pulmonary infarction. Bowing of the intraventricular septum is noted, suggestive of right heart strain."

He had a markedly elevated BNP (1,484). Point-of-care ultrasound demonstrated severe right heart strain with right ventricular dilatation and reduced RV systolic function. His lower extremity ultrasound studies were positive for extensive, bilateral deep venous thrombosis. He was treated with intravenous heparin, and an IVC filter was placed.

## Myocarditis

Patients with acute myocarditis often present with shortness of breath, chest pain, palpitations, syncope or other cardiovascular symptoms. Often, signs of congestive heart failure are present.

The *combination of low QRS voltage in the limb or precordial leads plus sinus tachycardia* should raise the suspicion of acute myocarditis. The ECG may also demonstrate ST-segment elevations, which may be diffuse or regional (Sarda et al., 2001). ST-segment depressions, T-wave inversions, premature atrial and ventricular ectopic beats and conduction abnormalities, including bundle branch blocks, are also common. Q-waves may also develop in patients who have fulminant myocarditis that has resulted in significant myocyte necrosis (Demangone, 2006). Cardiac biomarker elevation is almost always present.

Echocardiography is the most important test in defining the global wall motion abnormalities that are characteristic of diffuse myocarditis. But some patients will present with a *focal myocarditis*; here, the ECG may show ST-segment elevations in a regional pattern (for example, suggesting inferior or inferolateral STEMI). Reciprocal lead ST-segment depressions may also be present, further suggesting an acute STEMI. In these patients, the echocardiogram may show regional, rather than diffuse, hypokinesis (Sarda et al., 2001; Chan et al., 2005). When an acute STEMI cannot be ruled out, catheterization is usually indicated.

Acute myocarditis is a "don't-miss" diagnosis. Patients with myocarditis are at risk of developing fulminant heart failure and malignant ventricular arrhythmias leading to sudden cardiac death. The final chapter of this atlas (Critical Cases at 3 A.M.) includes a case where vital clues to acute myocarditis were missed, resulting in sudden cardiac death after discharge from the emergency department.

## Pericardial Effusion and Tamponade

Pericardial effusion should always be considered in patients who present with unexplained dyspnea (Blaivas, 2001). Shortness of breath is the most common presenting symptom in patients with pericardial tamponade, but it is often missed, as the diagnostic workup is directed at ruling out pulmonary embolism, heart failure, pneumonia and other causes. While bedside echocardiography is the definitive test for pericardial effusion and pericardial tamponade, the ECG often provides the first clues to the diagnosis.

The characteristic ECG findings in patients with pericardial tamponade include sinus tachycardia, low-voltage QRS complexes and, frequently, electrical alternans (Surawicz and Knilans, 2008; Spodick, 2003; Madias, 2008; Chan et al., 2005; Wagner and Strauss, 2014; Demangone, 2006).

Classically, the low voltage spares the P-wave (Chan et al., 2005; Surawicz and Knilans, 2008). There is, reportedly, a poor correlation between the ECG QRS voltage and the size of the pericardial effusion (Chan et al., 2005; Surawicz and Knilans, 2008).

**Box 5.2** ECG Signs of Pericardial Effusion

- Sinus tachycardia
- Low voltage QRS complexes
  - < 5 mm in all limb leads (refers to total R- and S-wave voltage) OR
  - < 10 mm in all precordial leads
- Electrical alternans
  - Cyclic (beat-to-beat) variation in the QRS amplitude or direction
  - Total electrical alternans (involving the P-wave as well as the QRS complex and T-wave), while rare, may be diagnostic of tamponade and has been associated with malignant effusions

**Box 5.3** Causes of Low Voltage

Cardiac causes
- Pericardial tamponade
- Myocarditis
- Infiltrative myocardial diseases or cardiomyopathy (e.g., amyloid)
- Congestive heart failure
- Chronic ischemic heart disease (s/p multiple myocardial infarctions leading to myocardial fibrosis)
- Myxedema

Extra-cardiac causes
- Emphysema
- Pneumothorax
- Obesity
- Pleural effusion
- Other fluid retention states (nephrotic syndrome, myxedema, anasarca)
- Normal variants

Electrical alternans, a cyclic variation in the amplitude or direction of the QRS complexes, has been attributed to a "swinging" or rotation of the heart in the fluid-filled pericardium. Fifty years ago, Littman called it "cardiac nystagmus" (Surawicz and Knilans, 2008). When there is electrical alternans that involves the P-wave, QRS complex and T-wave ("total electrical alternans"), it is said to be highly specific for pericardial tamponade.

Electrical alternans has also been associated with some supraventricular tachycardias, severe left ventricular failure and even extreme respiratory effort.

Low-voltage QRS complexes are not specific for pericardial tamponade (or for acute myocarditis). Other common causes of low-voltage QRS complexes are listed in the table (Chan et al., 2005; Surawicz and Knilans, 2008).

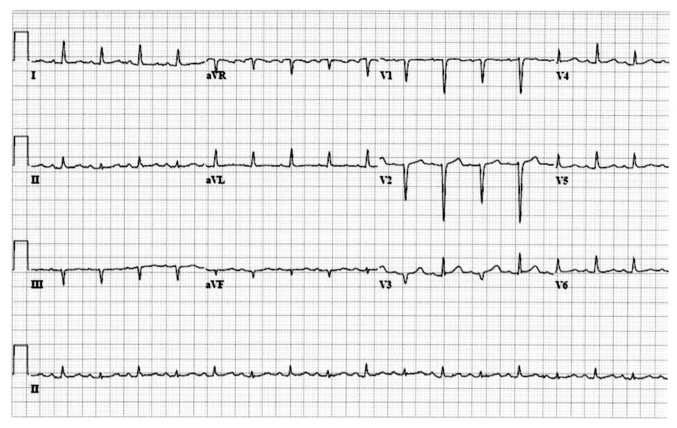

**ECG 5.2** A 73-year-old female with recurrent breast cancer presented with sudden shortness of breath.

## The Electrocardiogram

Not all patients with cancer and shortness of breath have a pulmonary embolism. This ECG has features that are practically pathognomonic for pericardial tamponade – specifically, sinus tachycardia, low-voltage QRS complexes in the limb leads and electrical alternans. Electrical alternans is most obvious in lead II and in precordial leads V1, V2 and V3. Lead V3 shows actual reversal of the polarity of the QRS complexes.

Technically, "low voltage" is present in the limb leads when the QRS complexes (including the R-wave and the S-wave) are less than 5 mm. In the precordial leads, the QRS complexes are said to have "low voltage" if the combined R-wave and S-wave voltage is less than 10 mm.

## Clinical Course

The echocardiogram showed a large pericardial effusion without clear tamponade physiology. A pericardial window was placed, and an 800 cc pericardial effusion was drained.

# The ECG in Chronic Obstructive Pulmonary Disease and Emphysema

While chronic obstructive pulmonary disease (COPD) and emphysema are not acute conditions, many of these patients present with acute dyspnea and chest pain; therefore, it is important to recognize the characteristic ECG features of these common, chronic conditions.

The most common ECG findings in emphysema are abnormal right axis deviation and other features of right ventricular enlargement, right atrial enlargement (P-pulmonale), low QRS voltage in the limb or precordial leads, the "Lead I sign" and poor R-wave progression (Wagner and Strauss, 2014; Surawicz and Knilans, 2008; Rodman et al., 1990; Goudis et al., 2015).

Here are some of the explanations for these ECG abnormalities in patients with emphysema:

## Low QRS Voltage (and the "Lead I Sign")

Low voltage is usually attributed to hyperinflation of the lungs, which impedes the surface electrodes' ability to record the depolarization currents. The "Lead I sign" includes such low voltage in lead I that the P-wave, QRS complex and T-wave are barely discernible (Surawicz and Knilans, 2008; Goudis et al., 2015).

## Right Ventricular Enlargement

The ECG signs of right ventricular enlargement are familiar and include right axis deviation and prominent R-waves in V1 (tall R, rSR' or qR). These abnormalities are the result of chronic hypoxia-induced pulmonary hypertension, which has led to right ventricular enlargement (cor pulmonale).

## Right Atrial Enlargement

Right atrial enlargement is common in patients with emphysema, the result of right ventricular failure and sometimes tricuspid valve insufficiency. Classically, the P-waves in the inferior leads are tall (> 2.5 small boxes), and as described in Chapter 1, they are peaked, "steepled" or "gothic" in appearance. The pattern is called "P-pulmonale." Not surprisingly, the P-wave in lead aVL is often inverted because this lead is electrically opposite to lead III (Goudis et al., 2015).

## Tachyardias

Tachycardias, including atrial fibrillation and multifocal atrial tachycardia, also occur commonly in patients with severe emphysema (Chan et al., 2005; Goudis et al., 2015). MAT is characterized by a rapid heart rate (> 100 beats per minute) and distinct but varying P-waves (at least three different non-sinus P-wave shapes and P-R intervals). MAT is a tachycardia attributed to enhanced automaticity (specifically, due to abnormal "triggered activity"). MAT usually occurs in older patients during acute respiratory failure due to COPD or congestive heart failure, especially in the presence of severe hypoxemia or acidemia. Electrolyte abnormalities (hypokalemia and hypomagnesemia), beta-adrenergic drugs, autonomic imbalances, coronary artery disease or other comorbidities may also contribute to these tachycardias (Goudis et al., 2015). In the past, MAT was frequently associated with theophylline toxicity.

## Poor R-Wave Progression

Poor R-wave progression is common in patients with COPD for at least three reasons (Goldberger et al., 2013; Goudis et al., 2015):

- *Clockwise rotation of the heart*: The enlarged right ventricle rotates in a "clockwise" direction along its longitudinal axis, as imagined by looking up at the heart from the patient's feet. As the enlarged right ventricle and right atrium rotate anteriorly in the chest,

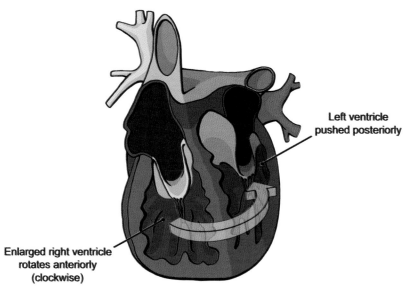

Left ventricle pushed posteriorly

Enlarged right ventricle rotates anteriorly (clockwise)

**Figure 5.1** Clockwise rotation of the heart in chronic emphysema. In emphysema, the right ventricle is enlarged, causing it to rotate anteriorly. This is called "clockwise" rotation, referring to the direction the heart rotates if viewed from the patient's feet. Clockwise rotation of the heart brings the right ventricle more anterior, while the left ventricle rotates in a posterior direction, away from the recording chest electrodes. Thus, in emphysema, the electrical activation of the left ventricle proceeds in a more posterior direction than is normal. This is one of the explanations for poor R-wave progression in emphysema.

they displace the larger left ventricle posteriorly, away from the recording chest electrodes.[1] See Figure 5.1.

- *Hyperinflation of the lungs*: Hyperinflation reduces the amplitude of the R-waves and contributes to poor R-wave progression simply because the emphysematous lung is a poor transmitter of electrical impulses.

- *Downward displacement of the heart in the thorax*: In patients with emphysema and hyperinflated lungs, the heart becomes "vertical." That is, the heart descends toward the epigastrium. The low-lying position of the heart means that the recording precordial electrodes are relatively superior to the main mass of the left ventricle. In effect, these precordial electrodes "miss" the electrical depolarization waves of the heart, leading to poor R-wave progression.

A clinical note: the low, vertical displacement of the heart also results in the epigastric location of the "point-of-maximal impulse" (PMI); commonly, the heart sounds are heard best with the stethoscope placed in the patient's epigastrium.

Figure 5.2 is a chest x-ray from a patient with emphysema. The precordial leads are placed in the proper position, but the normal position of the chest leads is relatively superior to the electrical center of the left ventricle. Thus, the exploring precordial leads may "miss" recording the main R-wave deflections of the left ventricle. Rerecording the ECG after moving the precordial leads one to two interspaces lower may yield a more normal-looking tracing.

As reviewed in other chapters, none of these ECG findings is specific for chronic emphysema. Poor R-wave progression is also common in patients with prior anterior wall myocardial infarction, dextrocardia and other

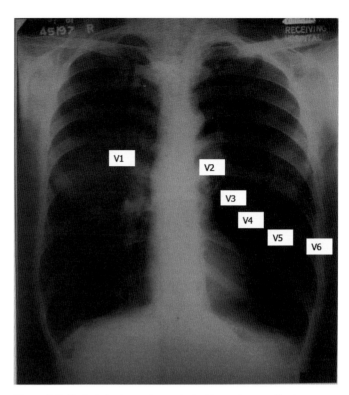

**Figure 5.2** Typical chest x-ray in a patient with emphysema. The lungs are hyperinflated, and the diaphragm and the heart are displaced inferiorly. The recording chest electrodes remain in their normal positions, but now they are too high to record the main electrical currents of the left ventricle. The result is low-voltage QRS complexes and poor R-wave progression.

conditions (or as an artifact if the precordial leads are placed too high on the chest). Low-voltage ECGs are common in myocarditis, pericardial tamponade and other conditions.

---

[1] Sometimes, in patients with severe emphysema, the QRS axis cannot be determined; the most common pattern is an S1-S2-S3 configuration, with prominent S-waves in leads I, II and III (Wagner, 2014; Surawicz, 2008; Goudis, 2015). This "indeterminate" axis is caused by the same anatomical and electrical changes outlined in Figure 5.1. Because the LV has rotated posteriorly, the overall electrical depolarization vector is now directed posteriorly. The axis is now "posterior" and cannot be determined based on the standard, frontal plane limb leads.

ECG 5.3 demonstrates several common findings of chronic obstructive pulmonary disease.

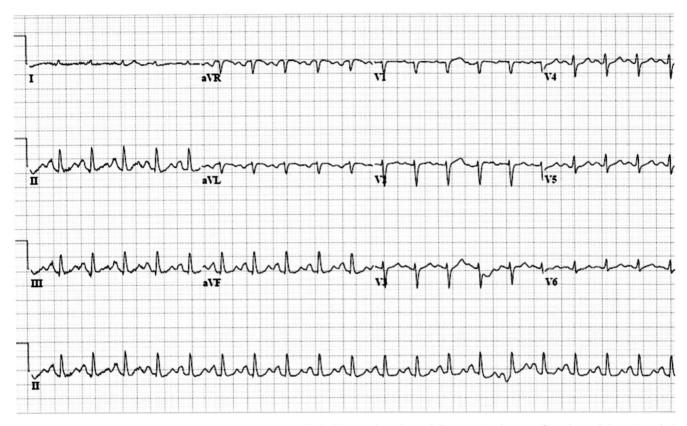

**ECG 5.3** A 64-year-old woman was found in cardiopulmonary arrest. She had been evaluated recently for worsening shortness of breath, cough, laryngitis and other upper respiratory tract infection (URI) symptoms. After resuscitation and endotracheal intubation, the following ECG was obtained.

## The Electrocardiogram

There are no acute findings on the ECG, apart from sinus tachycardia. However, the tracing is filled with features of chronic lung disease. These include right atrial enlargement (note the tall P-waves in leads II, III and aVF accompanied by "reciprocal" P-wave inversion in lead aVL); low precordial lead voltage; poor R-wave progression; and the "Lead I sign" (very low voltage in lead I with indistinct, barely discernible P-wave, QRS and T-wave in this lead).

This patient had chronic obstructive pulmonary disease, and her arrest was due to an acute, hypoxic "COPD exacerbation."

# Self-Study Electrocardiograms

**Case 5.1** A 52-year-old man with a recent diagnosis of small cell lung carcinoma developed severe shortness of breath while in the intensive care unit. He was markedly tachypneic, and his blood pressure was 110/90. His heart sounds were "distant."

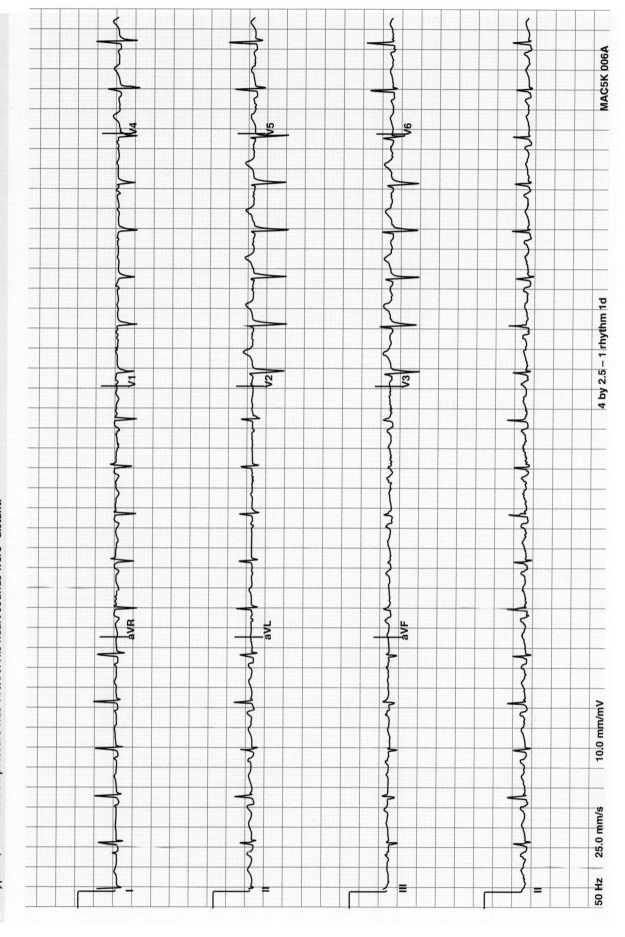

50 Hz | 25.0 mm/s | 10.0 mm/mV | 4 by 2.5 – 1 rhythm 1d | MAC5K 006A

**Case 5.2** A 70-year-old female presented to the emergency department with dizziness and shortness of breath. Her systolic blood pressure was 60.

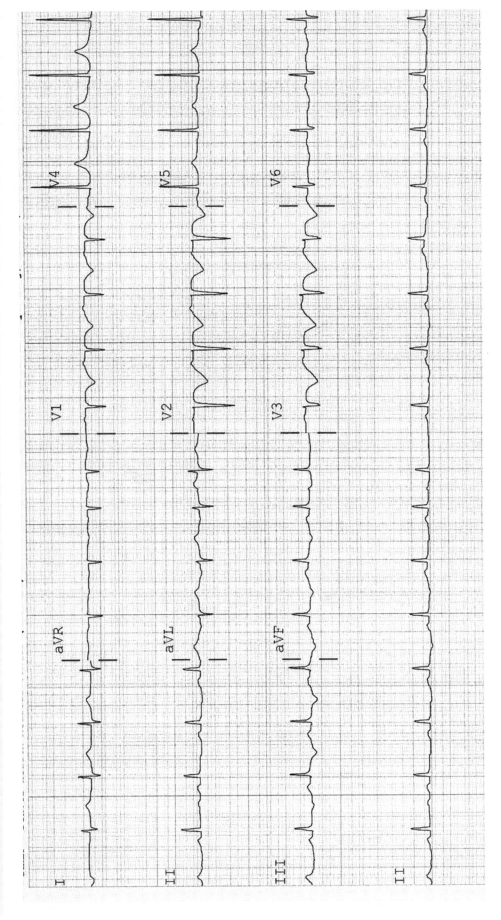

**Case 5.3** A 28-year-old female presented with severe chest pain, shortness of breath and abdominal pain, steady for an entire day. Her blood pressure was 117/55, her heart rate was 128, and an S3 gallop was heard on cardiac examination. She had been seen 5 days earlier for headache, fevers and myalgias after administration of the meningococcal vaccine. In the ED, her initial troponin was 32.

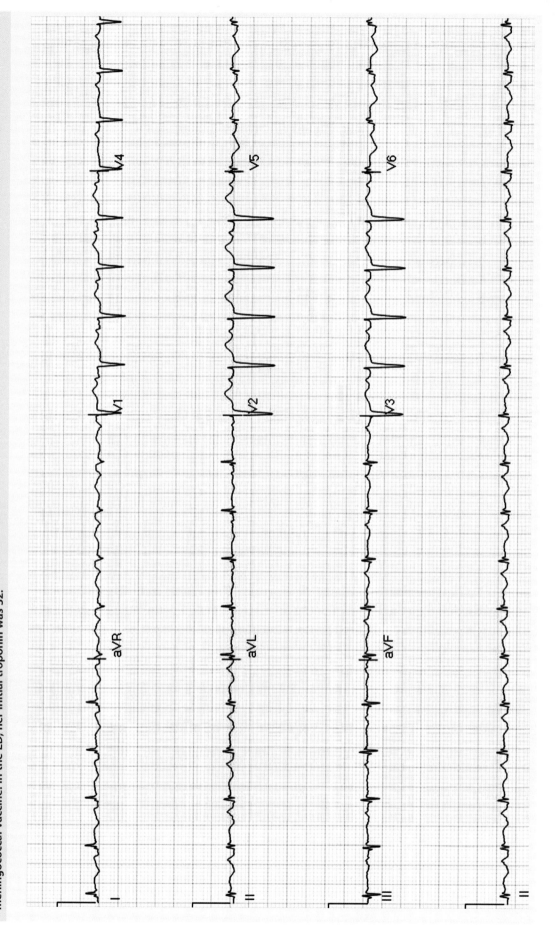

**Case 5.4** A 64-year-old woman presented with mild cough and shortness of breath.

**Case 5.5** A 31-year-old man presented with cough and shortness of breath. He has long-standing cystic fibrosis.

**Case 5.6** A 67-year-old man was walking at the airport when he suddenly "slumped over." He recovered before arrival of the paramedics. He also reported several episodes of exertion-related chest tightness several days earlier while traveling in Mexico. Prior to the syncopal episode, he experienced mild dizziness and shortness of breath. In the emergency department, he was stable, alert and joking with staff.

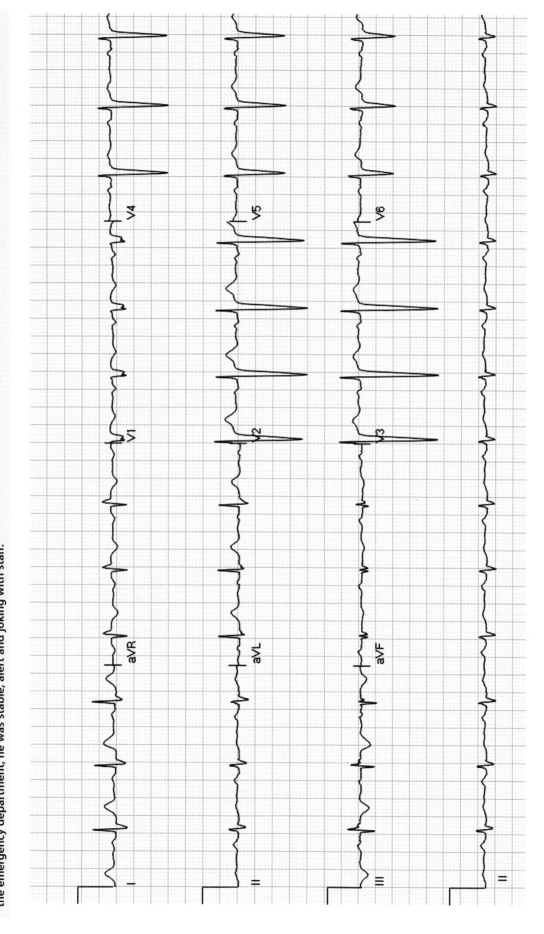

**Case 5.7** A 67-year-old retired musician with a history of diabetes endorsed shortness of breath for several weeks. His shortness of breath worsened the morning of his emergency department visit, and he had a near-syncopal episode. He reported he had undergone "an extensive workup for his shortness of breath" 1 week before.

**Case 5.8** Same patient – 3 days later, after treatment with anticoagulants, just prior to discharge from the hospital.

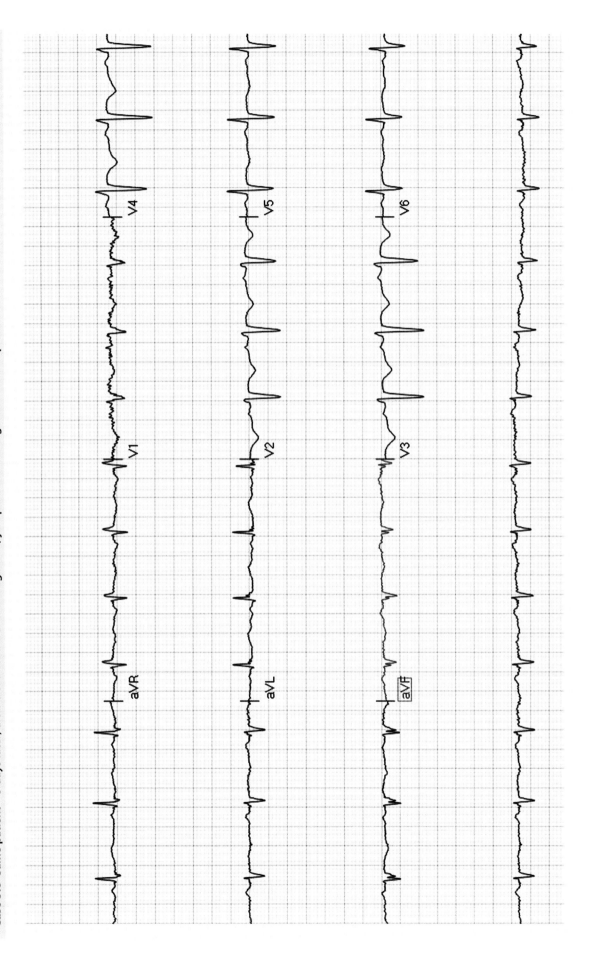

**Case 5.9** A 56-year-old female came to the hospital for routine blood tests. She was noted to be tachypneic (RR = 24). She had mild chest wall tenderness on physical examination.

ucasian

tion: 1

| | |
|---|---|
| Vent. rate | 108 BPM |
| PR interval | 132 ms |
| QRS duration | 76 ms |
| QT/QTc | 304/407 ms |
| P-R-T axes | 45  49  25 |

Sinus tachycardia
Otherwise normal ECG
No previous ECGs available

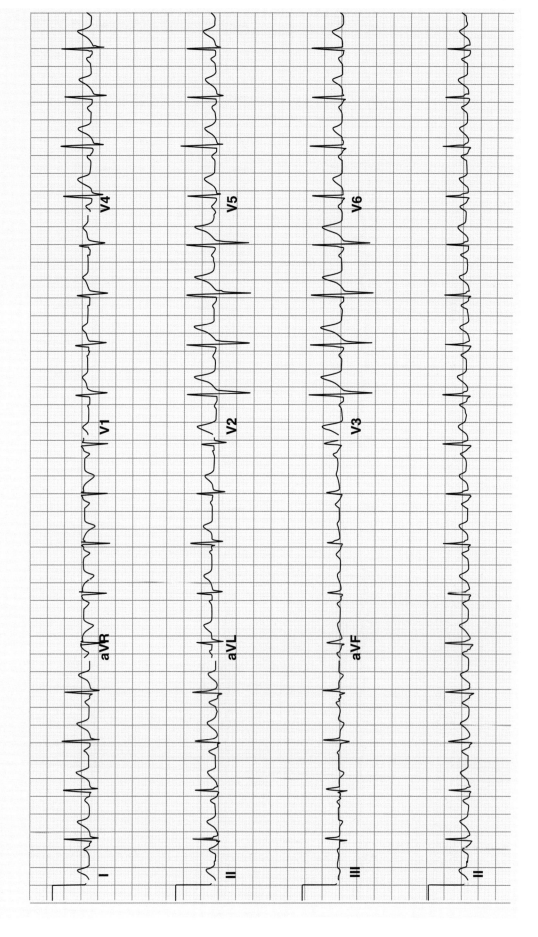

**Case 5.10** A 74-year-old female presented with shortness of breath and left lower extremity pain and swelling since a flight from South America 4 days earlier. On presentation, she was cyanotic. A bedside echocardiogram showed right ventricular dilatation with septal bowing but no pericardial effusion. She was intubated in the emergency department and sent for an emergent CT-PE study.

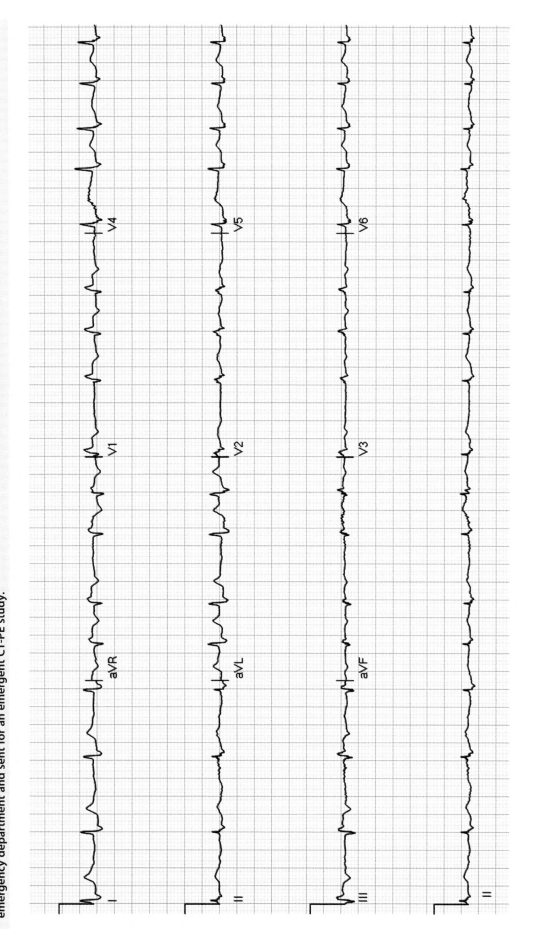

**Case 5.11** A 67-year-old female with a 1-year history of invasive primary lung carcinoma presented with 7–10 days of increasing shortness of breath and fatigue. In the emergency department, she was very slightly tachypneic.

**Case 5.12** A 42-year-old man presented with shortness of breath and left-sided chest pain of sudden onset. He also reported a recent sore throat. In the emergency department, he was relatively comfortable, with stable vital signs except for a tachycardia.

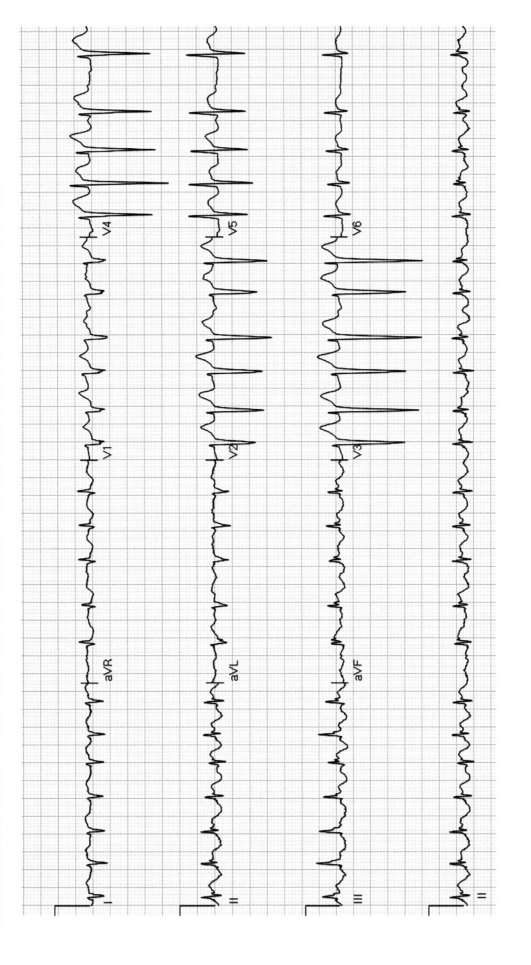

**Case 5.13** A 70-year-old man presented to the emergency department with shortness of breath.

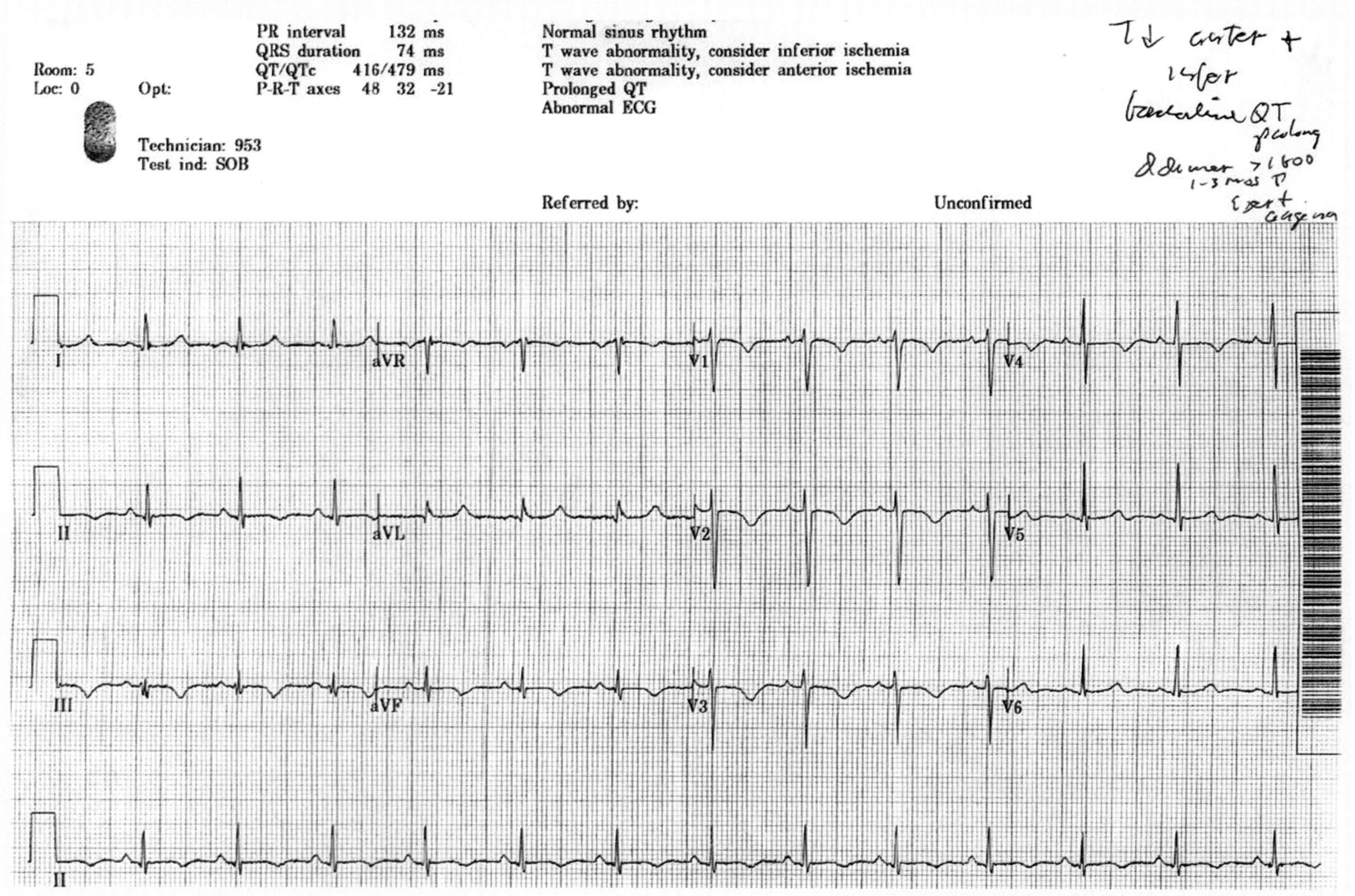

Room: 5
Loc: 0
Opt:
PR interval 132 ms
QRS duration 74 ms
QT/QTc 416/479 ms
P-R-T axes 48 32 -21
Normal sinus rhythm
T wave abnormality, consider inferior ischemia
T wave abnormality, consider anterior ischemia
Prolonged QT
Abnormal ECG
Technician: 953
Test ind: SOB
Referred by:
Unconfirmed
I
aVR
V1
V4
II
aVL
V2
V5
III
aVF
V3
V6
II

**Case 5.14** A 44-year-old man with a dilated cardiomyopathy and chronic congestive heart failure presented with gradually worsening shortness of breath.

**Case 5.15** A 22-year-old female presented with 2–3 days of cough and shortness of breath. She was treated 2 days earlier for acute bronchitis at an outside clinic, where she received nebulized albuterol.

oom:0902
oc:1002

| | | |
|---|---|---|
| Vent. rate | 135 | BPM |
| PR interval | 130 | ms |
| QRS duration | 96 | ms |
| QT/QTc | 298/447 | ms |
| P-R-T axes | 61  67 | -67 |

Sinus tachycardia
T wave abnormality, consider inferior ischemia
T wave abnormality, consider anterolateral ischemia
Abnormal ECG
When compared with ECG of 24-MAR-2015 09:48,
Vent. rate has increased BY 71 BPM
Non-specific change in ST segment in in anterior leads
T wave inversion now evident in in inferior leads
T wave inversion now evident in Anterolateral leads

## Self-Study Electrocardiograms

### Case 5.1 A 52-year-old man with a recent diagnosis of small cell lung carcinoma developed severe shortness of breath while in the intensive care unit. He was markedly tachypneic, and his blood pressure was 110/90. His heart sounds were "distant."

### The Electrocardiogram

The ECG is remarkable for low QRS voltage in the limb leads and the precordial leads. There is also subtle electrical alternans, best seen in the lead II rhythm strip in the lead VI. Pericardial tamponade is a relatively common diagnosis in patients with unexplained dyspnea. This patient also presented with a narrow pulse pressure, and he had distant heart sounds and jugular venous pressure elevation. That is, clinical findings of Beck's triad were present (hypotension, distant heart sounds and elevated jugular venous pressure). Jugular venous pressure elevation may be absent in tamponade, especially in patients with volume contraction.

### Case 5.2 A 70-year-old female presented to the emergency department with dizziness and shortness of breath. Her systolic blood pressure was 60.

### The Electrocardiogram

The ECG has at least three major features that are suggestive of an acute pulmonary embolism (PE) in addition to the mild sinus tachycardia. First, there is an abnormal right axis deviation. (The S-wave in lead I is distinctly abnormal for her age.) Second, there are marked T-wave inversions in the right precordial leads (after sinus tachycardia, right precordial T-wave inversions are the most common ECG abnormality in patients with acute PE). Third, there are T-wave inversions in the inferior leads. Concurrent T-wave inversions in the anterior and inferior leads are highly suggestive of acute PE.

### Clinical Course

Her final diagnosis was "large saddle pulmonary emboli."

### Case 5.3 A 28-year-old female presented with severe chest pain, shortness of breath and abdominal pain, steady for an entire day. Her blood pressure was 117/55, her heart rate was 128, and an S3 gallop was heard on cardiac examination. She had been seen 5 days earlier for headache, fevers and myalgias after administration of the meningococcal vaccine. In the ED, her initial troponin was 32.

### The Electrocardiogram

Understandably, the emergency medicine physician felt that she was suffering from an acute lateral wall STEMI (based on the ST-segment elevations in leads I and V5–V6). T-wave inversions are also present in these leads. However, the other abnormalities – sinus tachycardia and marked, diffuse low-voltage QRS complexes – should also have prompted consideration of another explanation for her dyspnea and chest pain (and S3 gallop).

### Clinical Course

This young woman had acute viral myocarditis. The patient's pain did not subside in the emergency department. She underwent an echocardiogram, which showed posterior, inferior and lateral hypokinesis. Because of the regional pattern of the wall motion abnormalities, she also underwent a coronary angiogram, which showed normal coronary arteries. However, she had severely elevated resting left-sided pressures requiring diuresis in the angiography suite.

Her troponin remained elevated for several days, always in the range of 35–65.

Acute myocarditis should always be suspected when a patient (especially a young patient with a viral prodrome) has sinus tachycardia and a low-voltage ECG.

Diffuse ST-T-wave changes, including ST-segment elevations, are common in myocarditis. Premature atrial or ventricular beats and conduction disturbances (even bundle branch block) are also common. The critical test is the echocardiogram. However, sometimes the ECG and the echocardiogram suggest that there is a regional at-risk territory, as in this case, and catheterization is necessary.

Acute myocarditis is a "don't-miss" diagnosis because even young patients may develop malignant arrhythmias or fulminant congestive heart failure.

## Case 5.4   A 64-year-old woman presented with mild cough and shortness of breath.

### The Electrocardiogram

This tracing illustrates several abnormalities that are common in emphysema. First, there is striking p-pulmonale (right atrial enlargement), manifested by tall, "gothic" P-waves (> 2.5 small boxes) in leads II, III and aVF (and accompanied by reciprocal P-wave inversion in lead aVL). Second, the ECG demonstrates the "Lead I sign" (low voltage and a nearly isoelectric P-wave, QRS complex and T-wave in lead I). Third, there is poor (nearly absent) R-wave progression. Poor R-wave progression is a common finding in patients with emphysema. As discussed earlier, the principal causes of poor R-wave progression in emphysema are hyperinflation of the lungs, clockwise rotation of the heart due to right ventricular enlargement and descent of the heart in the thorax.

## Case 5.5   A 31-year-old man presented with cough and shortness of breath. He has long-standing cystic fibrosis.

### The Electrocardiogram

The ECG was unchanged from numerous prior tracings. Sinus tachycardia is present. The other abnormalities are all consistent with chronic hypoxic lung disease. There is a right axis deviation and right atrial enlargement (RAE). RAE is recognized by the classic pattern of P-pulmonale: there are tall P-waves in the inferior leads (they are > 2.5 small boxes high, with a peaked, gothic or steepled appearance), and the P-wave in lead aVL is inverted (a reciprocal change). The "Lead I sign" is present (the voltage in lead I is markedly reduced, making the P-wave, T-wave and QRS complex hard to discern). There is also poor R-wave progression, deep S-waves in leads V5 and V6 and an rSR' pattern in lead V1, all consistent with right ventricular enlargement.

## Case 5.6   A 77-year-old man was walking at the airport when he suddenly "slumped over." He recovered before arrival of the paramedics. He also reported several episodes of exertion-related chest tightness several days earlier while traveling in Mexico. Prior to the syncopal episode, he experienced mild dizziness and shortness of breath. In the emergency department, he was stable, alert and joking with staff.

### The Electrocardiogram

No old comparison ECGs were available, and the official ECG reading was limited to "Inferior MI, age undetermined." But there are other, critical abnormalities. First, the QRS axis is abnormally rightward for his age. The S-wave in lead I is not very deep, but it should not be there in a 67-year-old patient. Second, lead III features a Q-wave and an inverted T-wave. Thus, there is a classic S1-Q3-T3. While "indeterminate age inferior MI" is also a likely diagnosis, with absent voltage in lead aVF, the tracing also suggests the possibility of acute pulmonary embolism. Poor R-wave progression is also present.

### Clinical Course

His CT-PE showed "extensive, bilateral pulmonary emboli with right heart strain."

## Case 5.7   A 67-year-old retired musician with a history of diabetes endorsed shortness of breath for several weeks. His shortness of breath worsened the morning of his emergency department visit, and he had a near-syncopal episode. He reported he had undergone "an extensive workup for his shortness of breath" 1 week before.

### The Electrocardiogram

In addition to sinus tachycardia, there is a small rSR' in lead V1, and there is an abnormal S-wave in lead I. As we have emphasized throughout this chapter, the axis is not technically rightward at all, but this S-wave is unquestionably abnormal for his age. And lead V1 (which monitors the right side of the heart) shows an abnormal rSR' pattern. He may also have an S1-Q3-T3, although this is harder to interpret in light of the evidence of a prior inferior wall infarction. Nonetheless, the constellation of findings is highly suggestive of acute PE.

## Clinical Course

This patient's d-dimer was 3,430, and a CT-PE study was positive for "extensive bilateral acute and chronic pulmonary emboli, with elevated pulmonary artery pressures and right heart strain." A left femoral vein DVT was also diagnosed. He was treated with anticoagulants (but not thrombolytics). His follow-up ECG (see next figure) showed resolution of these ECG abnormalities, likely reflecting improvement in the right heart strain and pulmonary hypertension.

## Case 5.8   Same patient – 3 days later, after treatment with anticoagulants, just prior to discharge from the hospital.

The ECG is consistent with an inferior myocardial infarction of indeterminate age and a left anterior fascicular block. However, the sinus tachycardia, abnormal RAD and rSR' in V1 are gone. He has developed T-wave inversions in the anterior precordial leads; these returned to normal after 1 week.

## Case 5.9   A 56-year-old female came to the hospital for routine blood tests. She was noted to be tachypneic (RR = 24). She had mild chest wall tenderness on physical examination.

### The Electrocardiogram

The ECG computer algorithm is not quite up to the task. There is a mild sinus tachycardia along with a small (but probably abnormal-for-age) S-wave in lead I and a Q-wave and inverted T-wave in lead III. Thus, the familiar S1-Q3-T3 pattern is present.

### Clinical Course

In the ED, she was mildly hypoxemic (pulse oximetry reading 89 percent). As it turns out, her "routine blood tests" included a follow-up INR, as she had recently started warfarin treatment for a lower extremity thrombophlebitis. Her chest x-ray demonstrated an area of decreased vascularity in the right middle lung field. She had a lung ventilation-perfusion study that was positive for an acute PE.

## Case 5.10   A 74-year-old female presented with shortness of breath and left lower extremity pain and swelling since a flight from South America 4 days earlier. On presentation, she was cyanotic. A bedside echocardiogram showed right ventricular dilatation with septal bowing but no pericardial effusion. She was intubated in the emergency department and sent for an emergent CT-PE study.

### The Electrocardiogram

The ECG is consistent with several life-threatening diagnoses. First, there is atrial fibrillation with a controlled ventricular response, a right bundle branch block and an S1-Q3-T3 pattern. Obviously, this suggests an acute pulmonary embolism with extensive clot and right heart strain and is consistent with her history.

At the same time, she has ST-segment elevations in lead III, with ST-segment depressions in the high lateral leads; it would be reasonable to diagnose an acute inferior wall STEMI. There are ST-segment elevations in V1, consistent with RV infarction.

Additionally, there is marked ST-segment elevation in lead aVR; this finding can be seen in acute pulmonary embolism. But the ECG demonstrates ST-segment elevations in aVR, which are at least as high as the ST-segment elevation in lead V1, plus ST-segment depressions in the left facing leads (I, II, aVL and V5–V6); all of this is also consistent with an acute left main coronary artery (LMCA) occlusion.

Finally, there is diffuse low voltage of the QRS complexes, even raising the possibility of pericardial effusion and tamponade or myocarditis.

### Clinical Course

This is a very challenging ECG, and it shows the value of point-of-care ultrasonography. In fact, she had a massive PE, first confirmed by a bedside echocardiogram. Her CT report was alarming: "There is a large burden of pulmonary embolism involving bilateral main pulmonary arteries (with occlusion of pulmonary arterial supply to right middle and lower lobes) and essentially all visualized segmental and subsegmental branches. There is evidence of significant right heart strain including enlarged right heart chambers, bowing of the interventricular septum into the left ventricle, and reflux of contrast into the inferior vena cava and hepatic veins."

This patient sustained a cardiac arrest in the emergency department, and despite aggressive resuscitation efforts, cooling and multiple pressors, she expired.

## Case 5.11 A 67-year-old female with a 1-year history of invasive primary lung carcinoma presented with 7–10 days of increasing shortness of breath and fatigue. In the emergency department, she was very slightly tachypneic.

### The Electrocardiogram

The most striking abnormality is the low voltage, present in the limb and precordial leads. This is enough to raise the suspicion of pericardial effusion. On this tracing, there is no electrical alternans. There is a right axis deviation, which was present on old ECG tracings.

### Clinical Course

Her echocardiogram confirmed the presence of a large pericardial effusion with moderate right-sided collapse. She underwent a pericardiocentesis with placement of a pericardial drain. Overall, 400 cc of serosanguinous fluid was drained, which was negative for malignant cells.

The most common presenting symptom in pericardial effusion is shortness of breath. Other causes of low-voltage QRS complexes include emphysema, myocarditis, infiltrative cardiomyopathy and, sometimes, obesity.

## Case 5.12 A 42-year-old man presented with shortness of breath and left-sided chest pain of sudden onset. He also reported a recent sore throat. In the emergency department, he was relatively comfortable, with stable vital signs except for a tachycardia.

### The Electrocardiogram

The ECG is abnormal. Atrial fibrillation is present, with a rapid ventricular response. There is a marked right axis deviation. And there are ST-segment elevations in leads II, III and aVF; while the ST-segments in the reciprocal leads are normal, the regional pattern is still suggestive of an inferior wall STEMI. The marked right axis deviation could also suggest an acute PE.

The other striking abnormality is the low voltage in the limb leads. The combination of low-voltage QRS complexes and tachycardia should always raise the possibility of acute myocarditis or pericardial effusion. One lead (V3) suggests electrical alternans.

### Clinical Course

The decision was made to obtain an echocardiogram, which showed global, diffuse hypokinesis plus an akinetic inferior wall. There was no pericardial effusion. Serial troponin levels were between 1 and 5.5. He was taken to the catheterization laboratory, where the coronary arteries were completely normal, and the only finding was an elevated left ventricular end diastolic pressure of 25 mm Hg.

The echocardiogram and electrocardiographic findings are both consistent with a diagnosis of diffuse as well as focal myocarditis. One month later, his echocardiogram was normal.

The combination of low-voltage QRS complexes, ST- and T-wave changes and tachycardia must always raise the suspicion of acute myocarditis. Classically, there are ST-segment elevations in multiple leads; however, in some cases, the ST-segment elevations may be regional and indistinguishable from an acute STEMI. The troponin levels are usually elevated in acute myocarditis, but unlike in the case of a STEMI, they are often high on presentation, and they may remain high throughout the illness.

Emergent echocardiography is often helpful in distinguishing myocarditis from an acute STEMI, although "focal" (that is, regional) myocarditis may make it hard to tell one from the other.

## Case 5.13  A 70-year-old man presented to the emergency department with shortness of breath.

### The Electrocardiogram

The computer reports *"T-wave abnormality, consider inferior ischemia; T-wave abnormality, consider anterior ischemia."*

The computer algorithms are not adept at pattern recognition. T-wave inversions do not always signal ischemia. In a patient with chest pain or dyspnea, concurrent T-wave inversions in the anterior and inferior regions of the heart are highly suggestive of acute PE (and they are quite unlikely to represent ischemia in two disparate vascular regions of the heart). On this tracing, QT prolongation is present, but it was also present on prior ECGs. Despite the absence of tachycardia or an abnormal right axis deviation, this ECG should prompt an evaluation for acute PE.

### Clinical Course

His d-dimer was more than 1,600 (as the emergency department physician noted on the original tracing). A V/Q lung perfusion scan demonstrated large bilateral pulmonary emboli.

## Case 5.14  A 44-year-old man with a dilated cardiomyopathy and chronic congestive heart failure presented with gradually worsening shortness of breath.

### The Electrocardiogram

Sinus tachycardia, T-wave inversions and probable left atrial enlargement are present. However, the most striking abnormality is the electrical alternans.

In this case, the QRS voltage is not low, and the diagnosis is not pericardial tamponade. Electrical alternans may be seen in patients with severe left ventricular failure. This patient had a well-established dilated cardiomyopathy; at the time of this ECG, his estimated ejection fraction was 10–20 percent.

## Case 5.15  A 22-year-old female presented with 2–3 days of cough and shortness of breath. She was treated 2 days earlier for acute bronchitis at an outside clinic, where she received nebulized albuterol.

### The Electrocardiogram

Once again, the computer algorithm is incorrect and cannot be trusted. The ECG should immediately suggest pulmonary embolism. She has a sinus tachycardia. There are inferior and anterior T-wave inversions (suggestive of acute PE with significant right heart strain rather than simultaneous inferior and anterior ischemia). An rSR' ("incomplete RBBB") is evident in V1. The ST-segment is also mildly elevated in aVR.

### Clinical Course

The CTPE findings were not surprising: "Moderate to large volume predominantly central bilateral pulmonary embolism involving both upper lobes, both lower lobes and the right middle lobe. Evidence for associated right heart strain with dilated right heart chambers, flattening of the septum and reflux of contrast into the IVC and hepatic veins."

She remained hemodynamically stable. Her BNP was mildly elevated, but her troponin was normal. She was admitted to the hospital. She was treated initially with heparin and then transitioned to a low molecular weight heparin. She recovered uneventfully.

## References

Blaivas M. Incidence of pericardial effusion in patients presenting to the emergency department with unexplained dyspnea. *Acad Emerg Med.* 2001; **8**:1143–1146.

Chan T. C., Brady W. J., Harrigan R. A. et al. *ECG in emergency medicine and acute care*. Philadelphia, PA: Elsevier Mosby, 2005.

Chan T. C., Vilke G. M., Pollack M., Brady W. J. Electrocardiographic manifestations: Pulmonary embolism. *J Emerg Med.* 2001; **21**:163–270.

Demangone D. ECG manifestations: Noncoronary heart disease. *Emerg Med Clin N Am.* 2006; **24**:113–131.

Digby, G. C., Kukla, P., Zhan, Z. Q. et al. The value of electrocardiographic abnormalities

in the prognosis of pulmonary embolism: A consensus paper. *Ann Noninvasive Electrocardiol.* 2015; **20**:207–223.

Ferrari E., Imbert A., Chevalier T. et al. The ECG in pulmonary embolism. Predictive value of negative T-waves in precordial leads – 80 case reports. *Chest.* 1997; **111**:537–543.

Geibel A., Zehender M., Kasper W. et al. Prognostic value of the ECG on admission in patients with acute major pulmonary embolism. *Eur Respir J.* 2005; **25**:843–848.

Goldberger A. L., Goldberger Z. D., Shvilkin A. *Goldberger's clinical electrocardiography.* Eighth edition. Philadelphia, PA: Elsevier Saunders, 2013.

Goudis C. A., Konstantinidis A. K., Ntalas I. V., Korantzopoulos P. Electrocardiographic abnormalities and cardiac arrhythmias in chronic obstructive pulmonary disease. *International J Cardiol.* 2015; **199**:264–273.

Madias J. E. Low QRS voltage and its causes. *J Electrocardiol.* 2008; **41**:498–500.

Marriott H. J. L. *Emergency electrocardiography.* Naples, FL: Trinity Press, 1997.

Petrov D. B. Appearance of right bundle branch block in electrocardiograms of patients with pulmonary embolism as a marker for obstruction of the main pulmonary trunk. *J Electrocardiography.* 2001; **34**:185–188.

Pollack M. L. ECG manifestations of selected extracardiac diseases. *Emerg Med Clin N Am.* 2006; **24**:133–143.

Rijnbeek P. R., Van Herpen G., Bots M. L et al. Normal values of the electrocardiogram for ages 16–19 years. *J Electrocardiol.* 2014; **47**:914–921.

Rodman D., Lowenstein S. R., Rodman T. The electrocardiogram in chronic obstructive lung disease. *J Emerg Med.* 1990; **8**:607–615.

Sarda L., Colin P., Boccara F. et al. Myocarditis in patients with clinical

presentation of myocardial infarction and normal coronary angiograms. *J Am Coll Cardiol.* 2001; **37**:786–792.

Spodick D. H. Acute cardiac tamponade. *N Engl J Med.* 2003; **349**:684–690.

Stephen J. M. Interpretation and clinical significance of the QRS axis of the electrocardiogram. *J Emerg Med.* 1990; **8**:757–763.

Surawicz B., Knilans T. K. *Chou's electrocardiography in clinical practice.* Sixth edition. Philadelphia, PA: Elsevier Saunders, 2008.

Wagner G. S., Strauss D. G. *Marriott's practical electrocardiography.* Twelfth edition. Philadelphia, PA: Lippincott, Williams & Wilkins, 2014.

# Confusing Conditions: ST-Segment Depressions and T-Wave Inversions

## Key Points

- Patients with chest pain, dyspnea or other symptoms consistent with an acute coronary syndrome (ACS) often do not have an obvious STEMI on their presenting ECG. Sometimes, the initial ECG only shows "nonspecific ST-depressions" or "T-wave abnormalities."

- The differential diagnosis of ST-segment depressions includes acute coronary syndrome (non-STEMI or unstable angina), ST-segment depressions that are reciprocal to a less-obvious STEMI, pulmonary embolism, left ventricular hypertrophy with repolarization abnormalities (strain pattern), digitalis effect, various cardiomyopathies, electrolyte disturbances and other miscellaneous conditions.

- ST-segment depressions that are horizontal or downsloping and ST-depressions that are ≥ 0.5 mm in V2–V3 or ≥ 1.0 mm in other leads are most likely due to ischemia. ST-depressions are especially diagnostic of acute ischemia (or non-STEMI) if they are present in two or more contiguous leads or are found in multiple ECG leads or if they are dynamic (appearing or increasing during episodes of chest pain and disappearing during asymptomatic periods). In ischemia, the T-waves may or may not be inverted.

- The "digitalis effect" includes a sagging ST-segment depression, said to resemble "Salvador Dalí's mustache" or the cables of a suspension bridge. Other ECG manifestations of digitalis effect include bradycardia or PR-segment lengthening, reduced-amplitude or even inverted T-waves, QT-interval shortening and the appearance of U-waves.

- ST-segment depressions and T-wave inversions are also common in patients with left ventricular hypertrophy (LVH). LVH is recognized by a combination of criteria, including increased QRS amplitude in left-facing limb and precordial leads, left axis deviation, poor R-wave progression, left atrial enlargement and widening of the QRS complex. The "strain pattern" is characterized by ST-segment depressions and T-wave inversions in these high-voltage, left-facing leads. Characteristically in patients with LVH, the ST-segments descend gradually into an inverted T-wave. The inverted T-wave usually has *asymmetric limbs* with a much sharper terminal

upstroke. The ST-segments are frequently elevated in the right precordial leads (V1–V3), leading to overdiagnosis of acute anterior wall STEMI.

- The differential diagnosis of T-wave inversions includes: pulmonary embolism; intracranial hemorrhage; myocardial ischemia (coronary T-waves, or Wellens' syndrome); cardiomyopathies or myocarditis; electrolyte abnormalities, especially hypokalemia; and normal variants.

- Ischemic T-wave inversions are classically symmetric. Often, they appear in an anatomic (regional) pattern. Even minor T-wave inversions may be significant if they are disproportionate to the voltage of the QRS complex.

- T-wave inversions may signify acute intra-cerebral hemorrhage. Often, the inverted T-waves are wide and bizarre with asymmetric and widely splayed limbs ("grotesque T-wave inversions"). QT prolongation, U-waves and bradycardia are often present.

- After sinus tachycardia, T-wave inversions in the right precordial leads (V1, V2 and V3) are the most common ECG abnormality in patients with pulmonary embolism. They correlate with more extensive pulmonary vascular clot burden and acute right ventricular dysfunction. T-wave inversions that appear simultaneously in the anterior and inferior leads are a strong clue to acute pulmonary embolism.

In earlier chapters of this atlas, we covered several important electrocardiographic emergencies, including inferior, anterior and posterior wall ST-elevation myocardial infarctions (STEMIs) and various causes of shortness of breath – in particular, pulmonary embolism, myocarditis and pericardial effusion. In most cases of STEMI, the diagnosis comes quickly: ST-segment elevations are present on the initial ECG; there is a regional (that is, anatomic or coronary vascular) distribution; and usually, the ST-elevations are accompanied by reciprocal ST-segment depressions in the opposite-facing leads.

But these are the easy cases. Frequently, our patients present with chest pain or dyspnea, and the ECG demonstrates only ST-segment depressions or T-wave inversions. How should we respond? Are these ST-segment depressions important? Or are they simply "nonspecific ST-T-wave changes," signifying nothing? How do we know if there is acute disease?

Emergency and critical care clinicians must have an organized approach to patients who have chest pain, dyspnea or similar symptoms, where the electrocardiogram demonstrates ST-segment depressions or T-wave inversions *without clear evidence of a STEMI.*

In this chapter, we consider the following causes of ST-T changes: acute coronary syndrome (non-STEMI or unstable angina), ST-segment depressions that are reciprocal to a nonobvious STEMI, pulmonary embolism, left ventricular hypertrophy with repolarization abnormalities ("strain pattern"), digitalis effect, intracranial hemorrhage and electrolyte disturbances (Chan et al., 2005; Pollehn et al., 2001).

We do not consider the myriad case reports of ST-segment deviations and T-wave inversions purportedly caused by cholecystitis, food impaction, pancreatitis, pneumothorax and other miscellaneous conditions.

The various nonischemic causes of ST-segment elevations and prominent (upright) T-waves that masquerade as STEMIs ("coronary mimics") are considered in Chapter 7.

## ST-Segment Depressions

ST-segment depressions may represent subendocardial ischemia in the region of the myocardium directly beneath the exploring leads. In patients with chest pain, dyspnea or similar symptoms, this is a primary consideration. At the same time, as emphasized throughout this atlas, ST-segment depressions may be reciprocal to a STEMI taking place in a myocardial zone that is anatomically and electrically opposite to the leads with the ST-depressions (Birnbaum, Wilson et al., 2014). Frequently, these ST-segment depressions are the only clue to a STEMI that is otherwise not obvious.

Apart from acute coronary syndromes (unstable angina, non-STEMI and STEMI), the differential diagnosis of ST-segment depressions also includes digitalis effect, left ventricular hypertrophy (with repolarization abnormalities, or "strain"), electrolyte abnormalities and, frequently, "nonspecific ST-segment changes."

## ST-Segment Depressions Reciprocal to an Acute ST-Elevation Myocardial Infarction

Whenever ST-segment depressions are present on the ECG, the most important first step is to verify that these ST-segment depressions are not reciprocal to an acute STEMI, even one that was not at first obvious. Don't be fooled. As illustrated in Chapters 2, 3 and 4 and throughout this atlas:

- ST-segment depressions in leads I and aVL may be early warnings of an inferior wall STEMI;
- ST-segment depressions in the inferior leads may signal an early high lateral STEMI; and
- ST-segment depressions in precordial leads V1–V4 (maximal in V2–V3) means that an acute posterior wall STEMI, often due to left circumflex artery occlusion, may be present, especially if the T-waves in these leads are "bolt" upright. As highlighted in Chapter 4, Posterior Wall Myocardial Infarction, this is a "STEMI equivalent" and

a clear indication for "cath lab activation" (Smith et al., 2002; Pride et al., 2010; Birnbaum, 2014; Nikus et al., 2014; Ayer and Terkelsen, 2014). See Chapter 4 for clues that can help differentiate anterior wall subendocardial ischemia (unstable angina or non-STEMI) from a true posterior wall STEMI.

- ST-segment depression in multiple inferior and lateral leads, when accompanied by ST-segment elevations in lead aVR, is also a "STEMI equivalent," indicating a high likelihood of left main coronary artery obstruction, or its equivalent (Birnbaum, Nikus et al., 2014; Nikus et al., 2014; Nikus et al., 2010).

## ST-Segment and T-Wave Changes Due to Ischemia or Non-STEMI

ST-segment depressions and T-wave inversions may be caused by coronary insufficiency in the absence of ST-elevation myocardial infarction. These patients are most likely to have either unstable angina or, if cardiac biomarkers are positive, a non-ST elevation MI (non-STEMI) (Amsterdam et al., 2014). In patients with acute coronary syndromes, ST-segment depressions usually represent *subendocardial ischemia*; as explained by Nikus, "when ischemia is confined primarily to the subendocardium, the overall ST vector typically faces the inner ventricular layer and the ventricular cavity, such that the surface ECG leads show ST-segment depressions" (Nikus et al., 2010).

Following is a brief summary of the ECG features that are most suggestive of subendocardial ischemia or a non-STEMI (Wagner and Strauss, 2014; Chan et al., 2005; Pollehn et al., 2001; Amsterdam et al., 2014; Smith et al., 2002).

### ST-Segment Depressions Indicating Subendocardial Ischemia or Non-STEMI

- The ST-segments are horizontal or downsloping;
- The ST-segment depressions are present in two or more contiguous leads;
- The ST-segment depressions are ≥ 0.5 mm in V2–V3 or ≥ 1 mm in other leads;
  - But lesser degrees of ST-segment depression or T-wave inversion may have diagnostic importance if they are large relative to a small-amplitude R-wave;
- The T-waves may or may not be inverted.

As emphasized repeatedly, before diagnosing ischemia or non-STEMI, it is critical to verify that the ST-segment depressions are not reciprocal to a subtle posterior, inferior, lateral or other STEMI.

### T-Wave Inversions Indicating Subendocardial Ischemia or Non-STEMI

- When present, the T-wave inversions are symmetric;
- The T-wave inversions, even if minor-appearing, are disproportionate to the low amplitude of the QRS complex; and
- The T-wave inversions are especially diagnostic if LVH is not present.

T-wave inversions may also occur during the evolutionary phase of acute STEMI. As described in Chapter 3, the T-waves are often tall and upright (hyperacute) in the first minutes of a STEMI, but they typically become inverted later, frequently while the ST-segments are still elevated[1] (Goldberger, 2006; Hayden et al., 2002; Goldberger, 1980).

As noted earlier, the ST-segment depressions and T-wave inversions summarized previously are especially diagnostic of an acute coronary syndrome if they are present in two or more contiguous leads. At the same time, ischemia-induced ST-segment depressions and T-wave inversion may be diffuse and not limited to a single anatomic region (Chan et al., 2005; Pollehn et al., 2001). Studies have shown that the sum of all the ST-segment depressions, across the entire ECG, is linearly related to the odds of early mortality in patients with an acute coronary syndrome (Smith et al., 2002).

These ST-T-wave changes are more likely to represent an acute coronary syndrome when they are dynamic, appearing or increasing during episodes of chest pain and abating during asymptomatic periods.

In general, acute coronary syndromes manifested only by ST-segment depressions or T-wave inversions are not an indication for routine, emergent thrombolysis. That is, unless the ST-segment depressions represent posterior wall STEMI or another "STEMI equivalent," as summarized in Chapter 3 and later in this chapter.

## Risk Stratification

Risk stratification of patients with possible acute coronary syndromes begins on presentation to the emergency department (or even in the prehospital setting) (Amsterdam et al., 2014). The following clinical and electrocardiographic findings are indicative of a patient at higher risk of early complications such as continuing angina, infarction, arrhythmias or death: an "unstable" or "up-tempo" pattern of chest pain (pain that is frequent, prolonged or occurring at resting or with minimal exertion); dynamic ST-T-wave changes (occurring or more pronounced with pain); ST-depressions in ≥ 3 leads; transient hypotension, ventricular ectopy, mitral insufficiency or signs of congestive heart failure; and an elevated troponin level. These unstable angina/NSTEMI patients are typically good candidates for aggressive medical therapy and, if indicated, early angiography.

## ST-Segment Depressions Due to Digitalis Effect

Digitalis, at therapeutic levels, causes a unique pattern of ST-segment depression known as the "digitalis effect." The depressed ST-segment has a sagging, upwardly concave, or scooped out, appearance that is said to resemble the cables of a suspension bridge or "Salvador Dalí's mustache" (see Figure 6.1). The T-wave may be upright, biphasic or inverted. Even at therapeutic doses, digitalis decreases sinus node automaticity and AV nodal

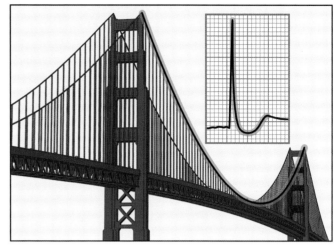

**Figure 6.1** Digitalis effect on the ECG.
The depressed ST-segment has a sagging, upwardly concave, or scooped out, appearance that is said to resemble the cables of a suspension bridge (or "Salvador Dalí's mustache"). The T-wave may be upright, biphasic or inverted.

conduction, and it may enhance AV junctional automaticity. Prominent U-waves and prolongation of the PR-segment may appear in patients with therapeutic levels of digitalis. Shortening of the QT interval and reduction in the T-wave amplitude are also common in the presence of therapeutic digoxin levels (Chan et al., 2005; Surawicz and Knilans, 2008; Delk et al., 2007; Ma et al., 2001; Hayden et al., 2002; Pollehn et al., 2001).

Digitalis effect may be differentiated from ischemia-induced ST-segment depressions in the following manner:

- In the setting of digitalis, the ST-segments are scooped or sagging ("Salvador Dalí's mustache" or the suspension bridge cables) with an upward concavity; the ST-depressions are most apparent in left-side leads with tall R-wave amplitude; and the QT-interval is often shortened.

- The ST-segment depressions caused by ischemia are likely to be flat or downsloping, often (but not always) with symmetric T-wave inversions. Ischemic T-wave inversions are usually found in a regional (anatomic) pattern; often, in ischemia, there is QT-segment prolongation (Pollehn et al., 2001).

The ECG manifestations of digitalis toxicity are quite different and may include both excitatory as well as inhibitory findings. The excitatory effects include accelerated junctional rhythms, atrial tachycardia with block, ventricular ectopy, ventricular tachycardia and bidirectional ventricular tachycardia (Yang et al., 2012; Surawicz and Knilans, 2008; Chan et al., 2005; Delk et al., 2007; Ma et al., 2001). Inhibitory effects include sinus bradycardia, AV nodal block and slowing and regularization of the ventricular response in atrial fibrillation.

---

[1] In the resolving phase of pericarditis, the T-waves also become inverted, but typically only after the elevated ST-segments have returned to baseline.

Examine ECG 6.1 for an example of the "digitalis effect."

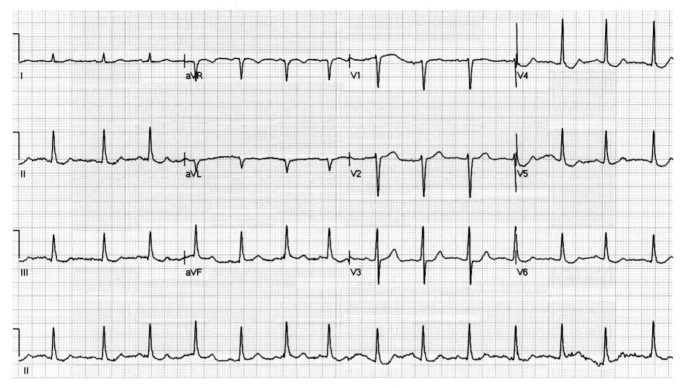

**ECG 6.1**   A 65-year-old female presented to the emergency department after a mechanical fall.

## The Electrocardiogram

The sagging, scooped and upwardly concave ST-segments (best seen in lead II and precordial leads V4–V6) are classic findings of digitalis effect. They resemble "Salvador Dalí's mustache."

There is no AV nodal block, ventricular ectopy, bradycardia, junctional rhythms or other ECG indication of a supra-therapeutic level of digitalis.

## Clinical Course

Her serum digoxin level was 1.3. There was no evidence of an acute coronary syndrome or other acute medical emergency.

## ST-Segment Depressions Accompanying Left Ventricular Hypertrophy

Left ventricular hypertrophy (LVH) appears commonly on routine electrocardiograms and in patients presenting with chest pain, dyspnea and other cardiovascular complaints. LVH usually represents chronic volume or pressure overload, caused by systemic hypertension, heart failure or valvular heart disease. Frequently, left ventricular hypertrophy is accompanied by ST-segment depressions and T-wave inversions. The combination is referred to as "LVH with repolarization abnormalities" or, formerly, "LVH with strain."

The "LVH with strain" pattern is a major reason for confusion and misdiagnosis. LVH is a common cause of overdiagnosis of STEMI and false-positive "cath lab activation" in patients with chest pain (Chan et al., 2005; Ayer and Terkelsen, 2014). In some studies, 30 percent of patients presenting to emergency departments with chest pain have LVH on their presenting ECGs (Chan et al., 2005). And, of course, electrocardiographic evidence of LVH is a risk factor for symptomatic coronary artery disease, development of congestive heart failure and premature death.

The problem for emergency and critical care clinicians is that the ECG pattern of "LVH with repolarization abnormalities" can masquerade as acute ischemia, anteroseptal STEMI, Wellens' warning and other acute coronary syndromes. And ECGs that demonstrate LVH, if not interpreted carefully, can just as easily hide an acute STEMI.

There are numerous published criteria and scoring systems for making the electrocardiographic diagnosis of left ventricular hypertrophy (Hancock et al., 2009; Surawicz and Knilans, 2008; Goldberger, 2006; Wagner and Strauss, 2014). Table 6.1

lists some of the commonly accepted QRS voltage criteria for LVH in the left column and other signs (repolarization abnormalities, left axis deviation, left atrial enlargement and others) in the right column.

The published diagnostic criteria for LVH have variable sensitivity and specificity for detecting LVH (compared with the gold standard of echocardiography or magnetic resonance imaging), and they also have varying ability to predict later cardiovascular complications (Hancock et al., 2009). For example, the precordial lead voltage criteria are much less specific for LVH in patients less than 35 years of age. Gender, race, body habitus, and, of course, lead placement also affect QRS amplitudes measured on the routine ECG (Wagner and Strauss, 2014; Goldberger, 2006).

However, the accuracy of the LVH scoring criteria is not our concern in emergency and critical care settings. Detecting LVH with optimal sensitivity and specificity is not the critical issue. Rather, what is important is that the ECG findings of "LVH with repolarization abnormalities" have to be differentiated from acute coronary syndromes and other cardiorespiratory emergencies. In addition, LVH and the "strain pattern" can hide acute STEMIs and other emergencies. For these reasons, treating physicians must be adept at determining whether "LVH with repolarization abnormalities" is the only abnormality – no matter what the ECG computer algorithm says.

For the most part, these ECG manifestations of LVH are easily explained. When left ventricular hypertrophy develops, the increased mass of the left ventricle rotates in a more leftward and posterior direction. Thus, (a) the QRS voltage is increased in the leftward-facing leads (I, aVL and V5–V6); (b) there is often poor R-wave progression; (c) the QRS voltage in lead V6 may be taller than the voltage in V5 (This abnormal finding is similar to the bedside observation that the point of maximal impulse [PMI] is shifted leftward and posteriorly); (d) the QRS duration is slightly widened, reflecting slower conduction through the thicker left ventricle; and (e) left atrial enlargement and left axis deviation are often present.

The ST-T-wave abnormalities ("strain pattern") represent repolarization changes brought on by left ventricular pressure overload (Wagner and Strauss, 2014; Surawicz and Knilans, 2008; Hayden et al., 2002; Pollehn et al., 2001; Demangone, 2006).

## A Closer Look at the "Strain Pattern"

When a patient's ECG demonstrates voltage criteria for LVH plus ST-segment depressions and T-wave inversions, the explanation might be "LVH with repolarization abnormalities" (the "strain pattern"). Or the patient might have LVH plus an acute coronary syndrome. How do we differentiate one from the other?

To get to the right diagnosis, we first need to appreciate the classic pattern of the repolarization abnormalities associated with LVH. Examine Figure 6.2.

In Figure 6.2, the first complex (A) demonstrates changes that are typical of myocardial ischemia (unstable angina or a non-STEMI). The ST-segment is normal in this example.

**Table 6.1**

| ECG Signs of Left Ventricular Hypertrophy | |
|---|---|
| **Voltage Signs** | **Other Signs** |
| Increased voltage over left-facing chest or limb leads<br>• Deepest S in V1 or V2 + tallest R in V5 or V6 is ≥ 35 mm<br>• S wave in V1 + R wave in V5 or V6 is ≥ 35 mm | Repolarization abnormalities<br>• Downsloping ST-segment depressions in the left-sided leads (leads I, aVL and V5–V6)<br>• T-waves are inverted and have asymmetric limbs (a gradual descent of the ST-segment into the inverted T-wave, followed by a rapid upstroke)<br>• ST-segment *elevation* in V2, V3, V4 |
| • R-wave ≥ 12 mm in limb leads I or aVL<br>• R-wave in V6 > 28 mm (or R-wave in V6 > V5) | • Left atrial enlargement<br><br>• Left axis deviation<br>• Poor R-wave progression<br>• QRS widening (usually slight but may even exceed 11 sec and resemble a LBBB) |

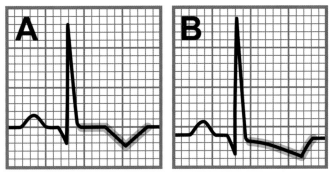

**Figure 6.2** Differentiating LVH with repolarization abnormalities from ischemia.

Complex B depicts the strain pattern (repolarization abnormalities) due to LVH. The hallmark is the presence of inverted T-waves *with asymmetric limbs* (Nable and Lawner, 2015). As described by Grauer and Curry, "The typical repolarization abnormalities of strain consist of ST-segment depression with asymmetric T-wave inversions, in which the gradual descent of the sagging ST segment blends imperceptibly with the first portion of the T-wave. The final ascending portion of the T wave has a much more rapid upslope as it returns to the baseline" (Grauer and Curry, 1987). The ascent of the T-wave may even "overshoot" the baseline of the ST-segment (Chan et al., 2005).

In LVH with strain, the T-wave is always inverted in association with the descending ST-segments. The ST-segment depressions should only be seen in the same left-facing leads (I, aVL, V5 and V6) where the QRS amplitude is abnormally large (Chan et al., 2005; Demangone, 2006).

The diagnosis of "LVH with strain" is more likely if left atrial enlargement, left axis deviation, poor R-wave progression and QRS widening are present. It goes without saying that ST-segment depressions and T-wave inversions should not automatically be attributed to "LVH and repolarization abnormalities" unless the left-sided leads show increased QRS voltage consistent with LVH. Furthermore, every effort should be made to compare the presenting ECG with prior tracings; "LVH with repolarization abnormalities" is stable over time.

However, flat or downsloping ST-segments are also commonly seen. The T-wave is symmetrically inverted. In patients with acute coronary syndromes, the ST-segment abnormalities and symmetric T-wave inversions are usually seen in a regional distribution (for example, in the anterior or inferior leads), although they may be "global," present in multiple leads. The ST-T-wave changes are often dynamic, coming and going with changes in the patient's chest pain or other symptoms. Patients with acute coronary syndromes may also have ST-segment depressions with upright (normal) T-waves.

ECG 6.2 illustrates classic findings of "LVH with repolarization abnormalities."

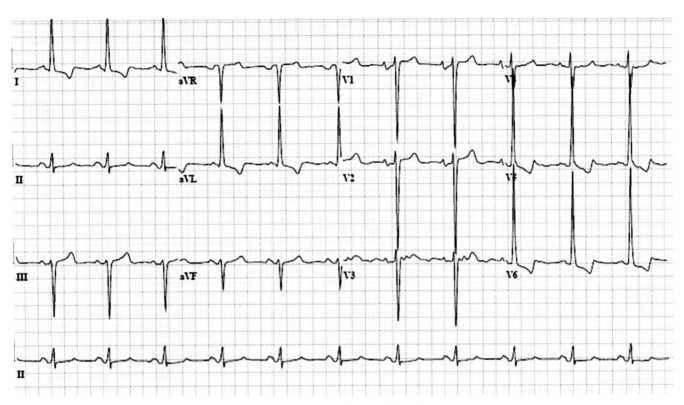

**ECG 6.2** A 57-year-old female presented to the emergency department with shortness of breath.

## The Electrocardiogram

The electrocardiogram does not explain the patient's presenting complaint of shortness of breath. All of the changes in this ECG are consistent with "left ventricular hypertrophy with repolarization abnormalities." For example, the left-facing limb lead voltage (leads I and aVL) is abnormally high (> 11 mm); the precordial lead voltage is also increased (for example, the sum of the S-wave voltage in lead V1 or V2 + the R-wave voltage in V5 or V6 is more than 35 mm); there is poor R-wave progression; left axis deviation is present; there is left atrial enlargement; and there is a classic strain pattern in leads I, aVL, V5 and V6 manifested by a downsloping ST-segment that blends into the inverted T-wave. As expected, the T-wave is inverted in an asymmetric fashion: the descending limb is gradual, the ascending limb is sharp, and the ascending limb even overshoots the baseline before it finally becomes electrically neutral.

Also, notice that the ST-segments are elevated in leads V2 and V3; these right precordial ST-segment elevations are probably reciprocal to the ST-segment depressions in leads V5 and V6, which, in the letting of LVH, are actually posterior, as well as lateral, leads. Not uncommonly, the ST-segments are elevated enough in leads V2 and V3 that they may suggest an acute anterior wall ST-elevation myocardial infarction.

## LVH Can Resemble Anteroseptal Infarctions (and Wellens' Syndrome)

When LVH and repolarization abnormalities are present on the ECG, it makes everything more difficult. The ST-segment depressions and T-wave inversions in the lateral precordial leads (V5 and V6) are often matched by ST-segment elevations in the right-sided precordial leads (especially V2 and V3).

Often, there is poor R-wave progression or frank loss of the initial R-waves in the anteroseptal leads. The ECG may suggest acute anteroseptal STEMI, old anteroseptal infarction, Wellens' warning or a variety of other abnormalities (Chan et al., 2005). The bottom line is that, in the presence of LVH with repolarization abnormalities, the ECG becomes much less specific. Consider the following case (ECG 6.3).

| | | | |
|---|---|---|---|
| Vent. rate | 62 | pbm | Normal sinus rhythm |
| PR interval | 148 | ms | Left ventricular anlargement with repolarization abnormality |
| QRS duration | 108 | ms | Nonspecific intraventricular block |
| QT/QTc | 434/440 | ms | Persistent Anterior T wave changes |
| P-R-T axes | 57 5 137 | | Abnormal ECG |

Techmician: 858

When compared with ECG of,
No significant change was found

Referred by:

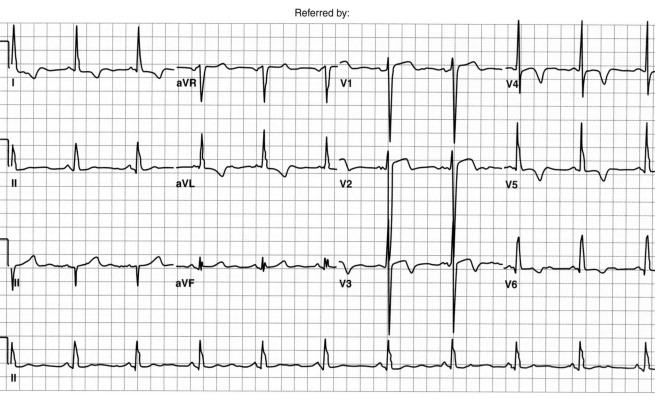

**ECG 6.3** A 56-year-old female with diabetes and chronic hypertension presented with atypical chest pain.

## The Electrocardiogram

The ECG demonstrates voltage criteria for LVH in the limb leads. (The R-wave voltage is > 11 mm in leads I and aVL.) The increased voltage in the precordial leads (the S-wave in V2 and R-wave in V5) also meets criteria for LVH. ST-segment depressions and T-wave inversions are present in the left-facing leads.

In leads I and aVL, the ST-segment depressions and T-wave inversions have the classic appearance of the strain pattern. However, the T-wave inversions in leads V5 and V6 are more symmetric, suggesting the possibility of cardiac ischemia. This is especially significant since the T-wave inversions in V4–V6 are not accompanied by any downsloping ST-segment depressions. An acute coronary syndrome is suggested.

Perhaps the most striking ECG abnormality is the presence of ST-segment elevations in leads V2 and V3, with terminal T-wave inversions, a pattern that is indistinguishable from Wellens' warning of impending (or recently reperfused) LAD occlusion.

The entire ECG is concerning for Wellens' warning and an early or impending STEMI, but it is also consistent with chronic, stable LVH and strain. In this case, all of the limb and precordial lead ST-T abnormalities were unchanged from prior tracings. Thus, the ECG represents a "false positive."

How might one approach a patient with chest pain and a similar ECG? If the history is especially concerning for an acute STEMI, then consideration of emergent reperfusion therapy is appropriate. In many other cases, it may be helpful to use other diagnostic tools, including: comparison with old ECG tracings; frequent, serial ECGs and troponin levels; and an emergent echocardiogram, to rule in, or rule out, regional wall motion abnormalities (Amsterdam et al., 2014).

These are challenging cases, especially when the presenting symptoms are vague or have resolved. The best strategy may be to analyze the ECG carefully, recognize that many of the changes that normally point to a STEMI are not specific in the presence of LVH and strain, admit we don't know for sure and consult with the interventional cardiology team.

## Clinical Course

The patient was admitted for observation. Old, baseline ECGs were obtained, which showed identical ST- and T-wave changes. There were no serum troponin elevations.

It is easy to see why "LVH with repolarization abnormalities" is such a common cause of false positive "cath lab" activations.

## T-Wave Inversions

The T-wave is a reflection of ventricular repolarization. The differential diagnosis of T-wave inversions is broad and includes an array of cardiac and noncardiac conditions (Hayden et al., 2002; Smith et al., 2002; Goldberger, 1980).

## Normal T-Wave Inversions

T-wave inversions may be normal in leads with negative QRS complexes (aVR, III, V1 and sometimes aVL) (Goldberger,

2006). Some young patients have large T-wave inversions in the right precordial leads (V1, V2 and V3). In some individuals the T-wave inversions persist into adulthood (the "persistent juvenile T-wave pattern") (Hayden et al., 2002; Goldberger, 2006; Goldberger, 1980). In some patients, inverted or biphasic T-waves may appear in the right precordial leads, along with ST-segment elevations in a pattern that resembles Wellens' syndrome or an acute anterior wall STEMI; this pattern is more common in athletes and young African American men, and it often disappears with exercise or other sympathetic stimulation (Hayden et al., 2002; Smith et al., 2002). T-wave inversions are also expected in patients with a right or left bundle branch block (secondary T-wave inversions), following premature ventricular contractions, in ventricular-paced rhythms, during or following tachycardias, in patients with the Wolff-Parkinson-White syndrome and in other cardiac and noncardiac conditions.

In emergency and critical care practice, it is important to consider the following conditions that may present with abnormal T-wave inversions.

## Acute Coronary Syndromes

T-wave inversions are routinely observed during the evolution of acute STEMIs, in the leads that show ST-segment elevations. The T-waves may become inverted at any time during the STEMI, but they typically invert while the ST-segments remain elevated (Smith et al., 2002). T-wave inversions may persist months or longer, and when accompanied by pathologic Q-waves, they may be indicative of a subacute or remote myocardial infarction.

T-wave inversions are also very common in acute ischemia in the absence of a STEMI (unstable angina or non-ST-elevation myocardial infarction). As highlighted earlier, narrow and symmetric T-wave inversions, sometimes in a regional (or anatomic) distribution but at other times global, are the hallmark of acute cardiac ischemia (Hayden et al., 2002; Amsterdam et al., 2014; Ayer and Terkelsen, 2014). The ST-segment may or may not be depressed.

Two specific syndromes are noteworthy.

- *Biphasic T-waves in the right or mid-precordial leads (typically V2–V4)*, where the terminal portion of the T-wave is inverted, may represent a critical LAD occlusion (Wellens' syndrome, Type A).
- *Acute, narrow, symmetric T-wave inversions in the precordial leads* may also presage an anterior wall STEMI, due to acute, total LAD occlusion (Wellens' syndrome, Type B).

As summarized in Chapter 3, both Wellens' patterns frequently represent an evolutionary phase of acute myocardial infarction, typically after some reperfusion of the occluded infarct-related artery has taken place. The infarct-related arteries remain at high risk for sudden reocclusion.

## Pulmonary Embolism

After sinus tachycardia, T-wave inversions in the right precordial leads (V1, V2 and V3) are the most common ECG abnormality in patients with pulmonary embolism. Right precordial T-wave inversions are associated with a larger clot burden, higher pulmonary artery pressures, and a higher short-term risk of hemodynamic instability. As discussed in Chapter 5, The Electrocardiography of Shortness of Breath, T-wave inversions that appear simultaneously in the anterior and inferior leads are a strong clue to acute pulmonary embolism. Acute right axis deviation, S1-Q3-T3 pattern or rSR' pattern in precordial lead V1 may also be present in patients with acute pulmonary embolism.

## Intracerebral Hemorrhage

T-wave inversions are commonly reported in patients with acute intracerebral hemorrhage. Sometimes, the T-waves are wide and bizarre, with asymmetric and widely splayed limbs ("grotesque T-wave inversions"). QT prolongation, U-waves and bradycardia are often present (Goldberger, 2006; Hayden et al., 2002; Catanzaro et al., 2008). The T-wave inversions, U-waves and QT interval prolongation probably represent altered ventricular repolarization due to an imbalance in autonomic nervous input to the heart.

After a brief history and physical examination, it is usually not difficult to determine if anterior T-wave inversions represent an acute coronary syndrome or a subarachnoid hemorrhage. However, as discussed in Chapters 3 and 7, it may be challenging to differentiate between these two etiologies in comatose survivors of out-of-hospital cardiac arrest (Yamashina et al., 2015; Lewandowski, 2014; Arnaout et al., 2015; Mitsuma et al., 2011).

## Stress Cardiomyopathy (Takotsubo Syndrome), Cardiomyopathy and Myocarditis

The takotsubo syndrome (stress cardiomyopathy or apical myocardial ballooning syndrome) and many other cardiomyopathies are associated with T-wave inversions. T-wave inversion is also common during the evolutionary phase of acute myocarditis (Hayden et al., 2002; Goldberger, 2006). Myocarditis is considered in detail in Chapter 5, The Electrocardiography of Shortness of Breath. The takotsubo syndrome, which often presents with ST-segment elevations, is considered in Chapter 7, Confusing Conditions: ST-Segment Elevations and Tall T-Waves (Coronary Mimics).

Review the clinical presentation and ECG for the following case (ECG 6.4): What is the appropriate differential diagnosis? Which etiologies are most likely?

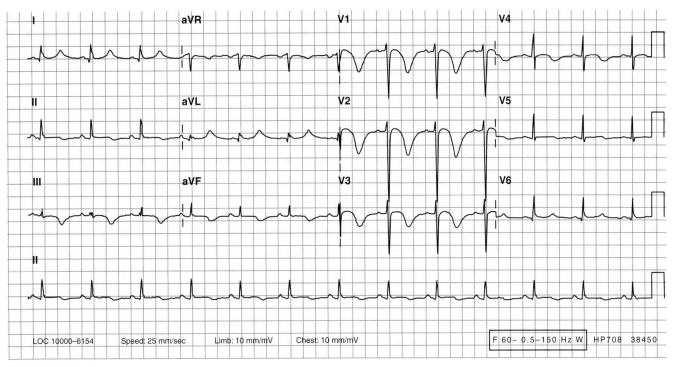

**ECG 6.4** A 47-year-old man presented to the emergency department with 4–5 days of stuttering, substernal, squeezing chest pain. His pain was associated with shortness of breath, nausea, diaphoresis, a nonproductive cough and mild dizziness. His triage vital signs were normal except for an initial heart rate of 112. His pulse oximetry reading was 86 percent on room air.

## The Electrocardiogram

The computer reading was straightforward: "Sinus tachycardia; QT interval long for rate; Anterior T-wave abnormality, possible ischemia; Inferior T-wave abnormality, possible ischemia; Artifact in lead(s) II, III, aVF."

Given his history and this ECG, anterior wall ischemia was judged most likely, and he was transferred to a regional medical center for emergent coronary angiography. The angiogram report read, "normal, nonocclusive coronary study." It was not unreasonable to consider that these symmetric T-wave inversions might represent an acute coronary syndrome, possibly a critical LAD occlusion ("coronary T-waves" or Wellens' syndrome, pattern B). Ischemia is made more likely by the finding of a prolonged QT-interval.

At the same time, the T-waves are inverted simultaneously in the anterior and inferior leads, making an acute pulmonary embolism with right heart strain just as likely.

## Clinical Course

In this patient, other causes of deep T-wave inversions (electrolyte abnormalities such as hypokalemia, subarachnoid hemorrhage, takotsubo cardiomyopathy and other causes) did not seem likely. This patient's troponin was 0.05 and did not rise.

A CTPE study revealed large, bilateral pulmonary emboli with "a large clot burden and evidence of right heart strain." A transthoracic echocardiogram demonstrated "a flattened septum that bowed into the left ventricle, compatible with right ventricular pressure and volume overload, and moderate right ventricular dilatation."

As highlighted in Chapter 5, The Electrocardiography of Shortness of Breath, inverted T-waves in the right precordial leads (V1–V4) are probably the most common ECG finding in acute, severe PE, and they are predictive of a larger clot and hemodynamic burden and a higher risk of in-hospital complications (hypotension requiring pressor support, cardiac arrest and mortality). New T-wave inversions that appear simultaneously in the anterior and inferior leads are hallmarks of acute PE.

# Self-Study Electrocardiograms

**Case 6.1** A 64-year-old man presented with chest pain.

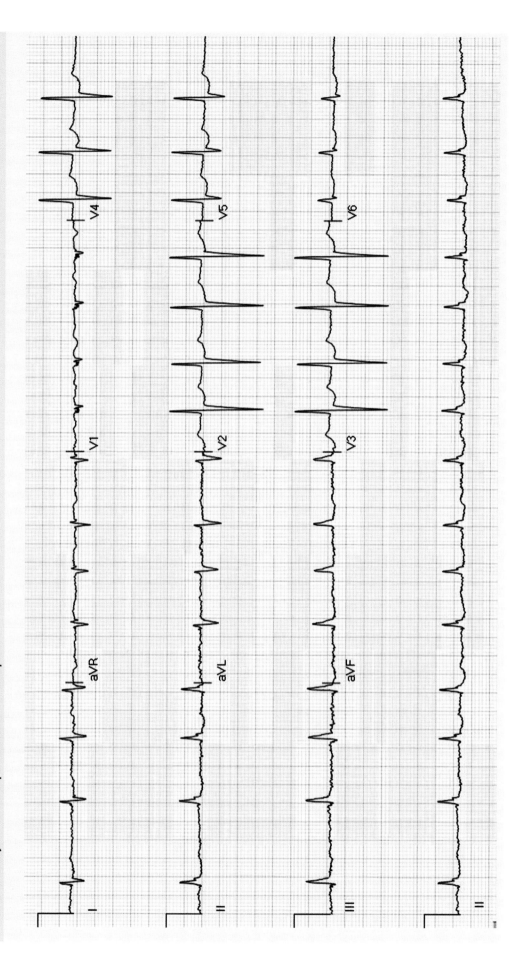

**Case 6.2** A 71-year-old man presented to the emergency department after a near-syncopal episode.

**Case 6.3** A 35-year-old man presented with 1 week of increasing effort-related chest pain, with radiation to his neck and throat. In the ED, his pain kept recurring at rest despite administration of intravenous nitroglycerin. His initial troponin was 0.22.

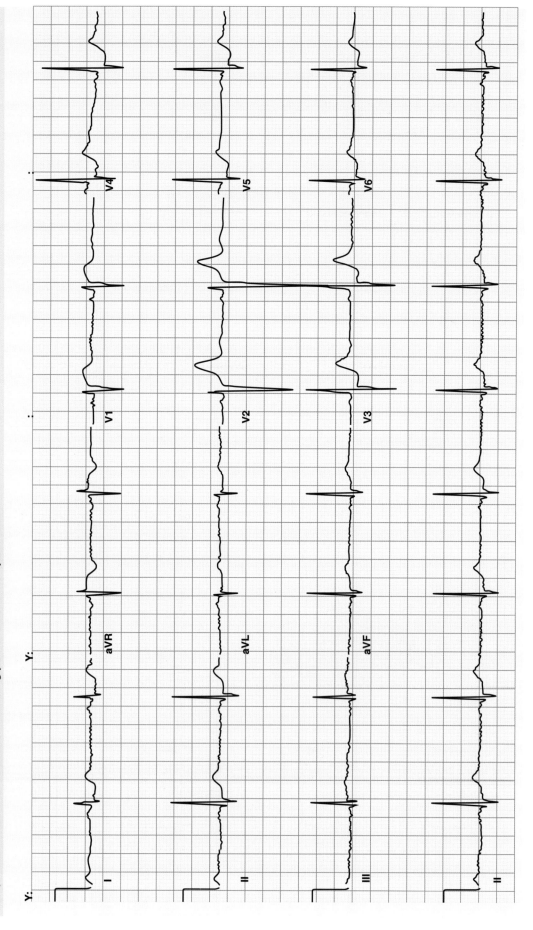

**Case 6.4** A 54-year-old female was visiting the zoo when she had the sudden onset of chest pain, shortness of breath and near-syncope.

Technician: 380

Confirmed By

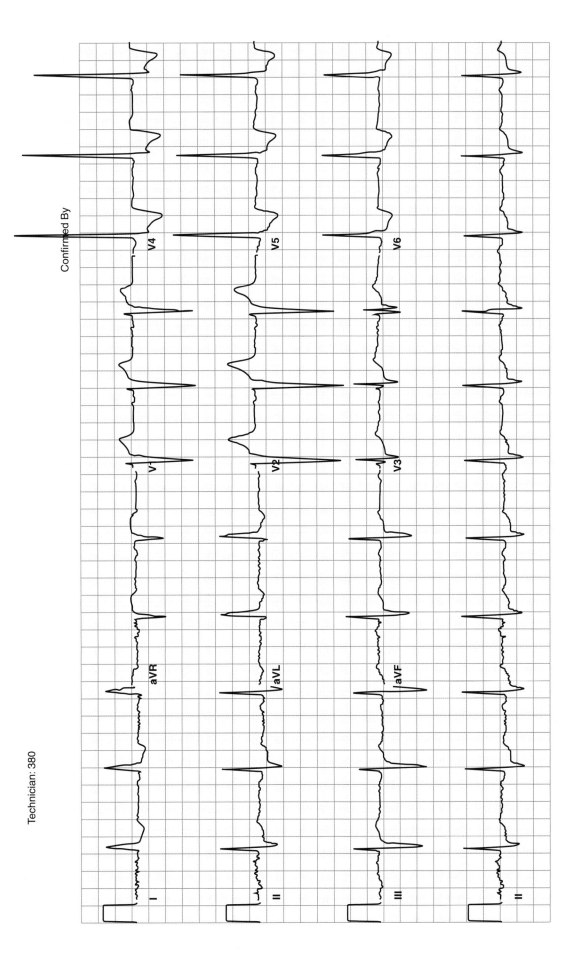

**Case 6.5** A 57-year-old man presented with 3 hours of substernal chest pain that radiated to his jaw. His initial troponin was mildly elevated at 0.44.

Male          Unknown

Room:S42
Loc:1002

| | | BPM |
|---|---|---|
| Vent. rate | 58 | |
| PR interval | 128 | ms |
| QRS duration | 96 | ms |
| QT/QTc | 418/410 | |
| P-R-T axes | 36  -29 | -12 |

Sinus bradycardia
Nonspecific ST abnormality
Abnormal ECG
When compared with ECG of
No significant change was found

14:23,

Referred by:   SELF              Reviewe

Y:                    Y:

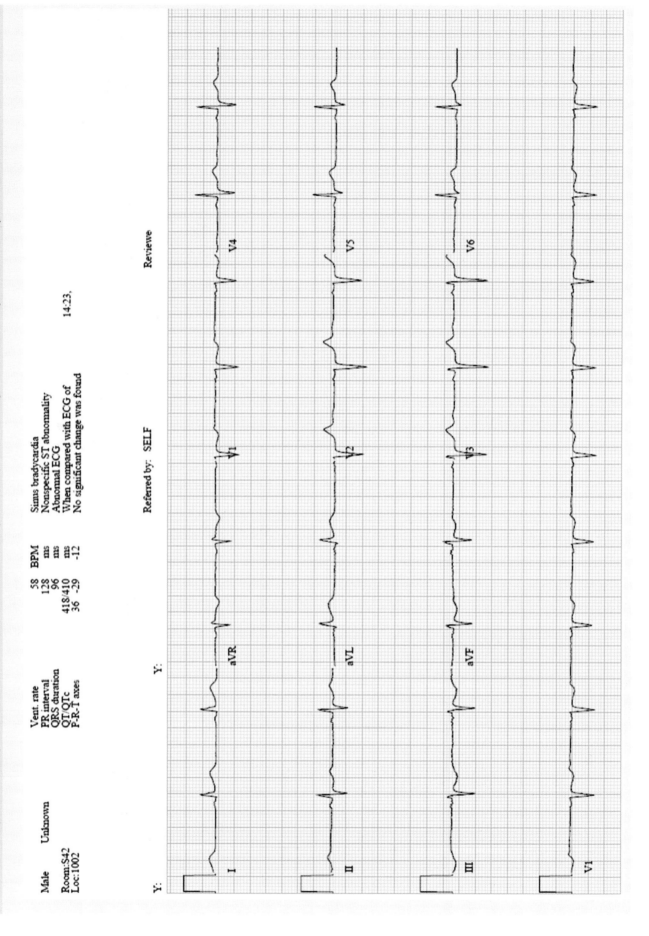

**Case 6.6** A 42-year-old female presented because of recurrent episodes of chest pain. She had a history of alcohol dependence and a long history of severe, erosive esophagitis and gastritis. Three years earlier, she had a normal coronary angiogram. She presented to the ED with "atypical chest pain and epigastric pain." Her pain resolved in the ED after receiving nitroglycerin, morphine and beta blockers.

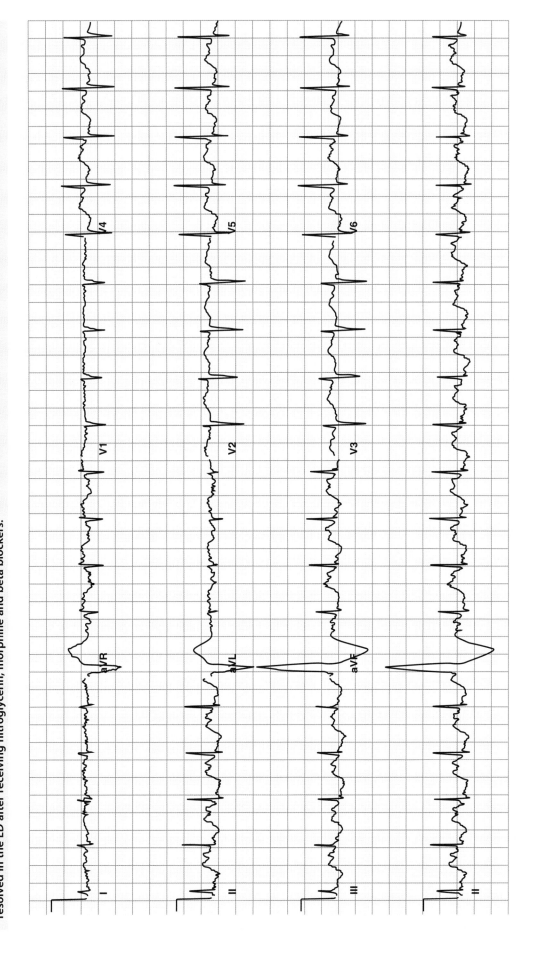

**Case 6.7** A 51-year-old man with a history of chronic hypertension presented with a diffuse occipital headache. He denied chest pain or shortness of breath. He had not been taking his antihypertensive medications for the past month.

**Case 6.8** A 23-year-old female with hemoglobin SS sickle cell disease presented with a painful crisis. On the second hospital day, she developed chest pain and shortness of breath. Her hemoglobin was 6.2. Her troponin level was 0.43.

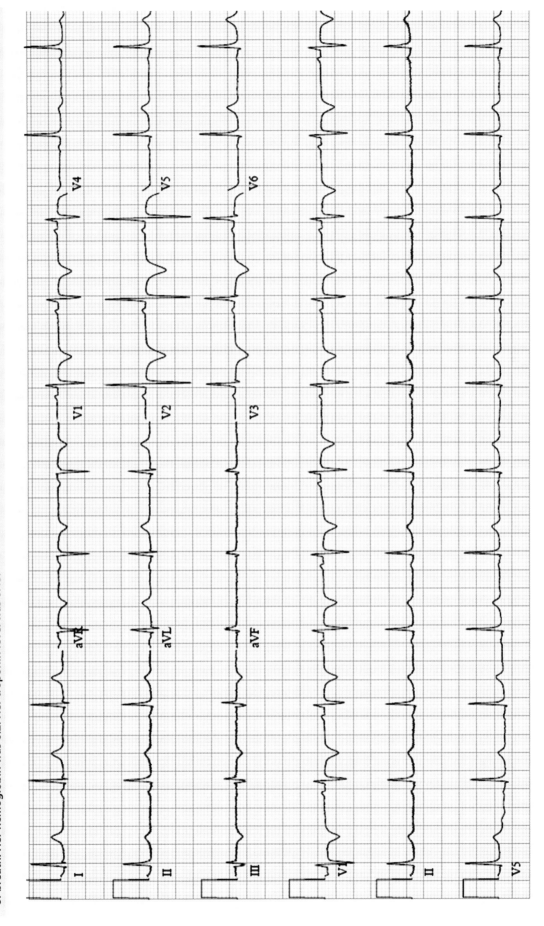

**Case 6.9** A 73-year-old female presented with weakness and altered mental status.

**Case 6.10** A 48-year-old female presented with squeezing chest pain while at rest. Her blood pressure was 198/105. This ECG was taking during an episode of chest pain.

Case 6.10 (Continued) Same patient: Baseline ECG obtained 3 months earlier.

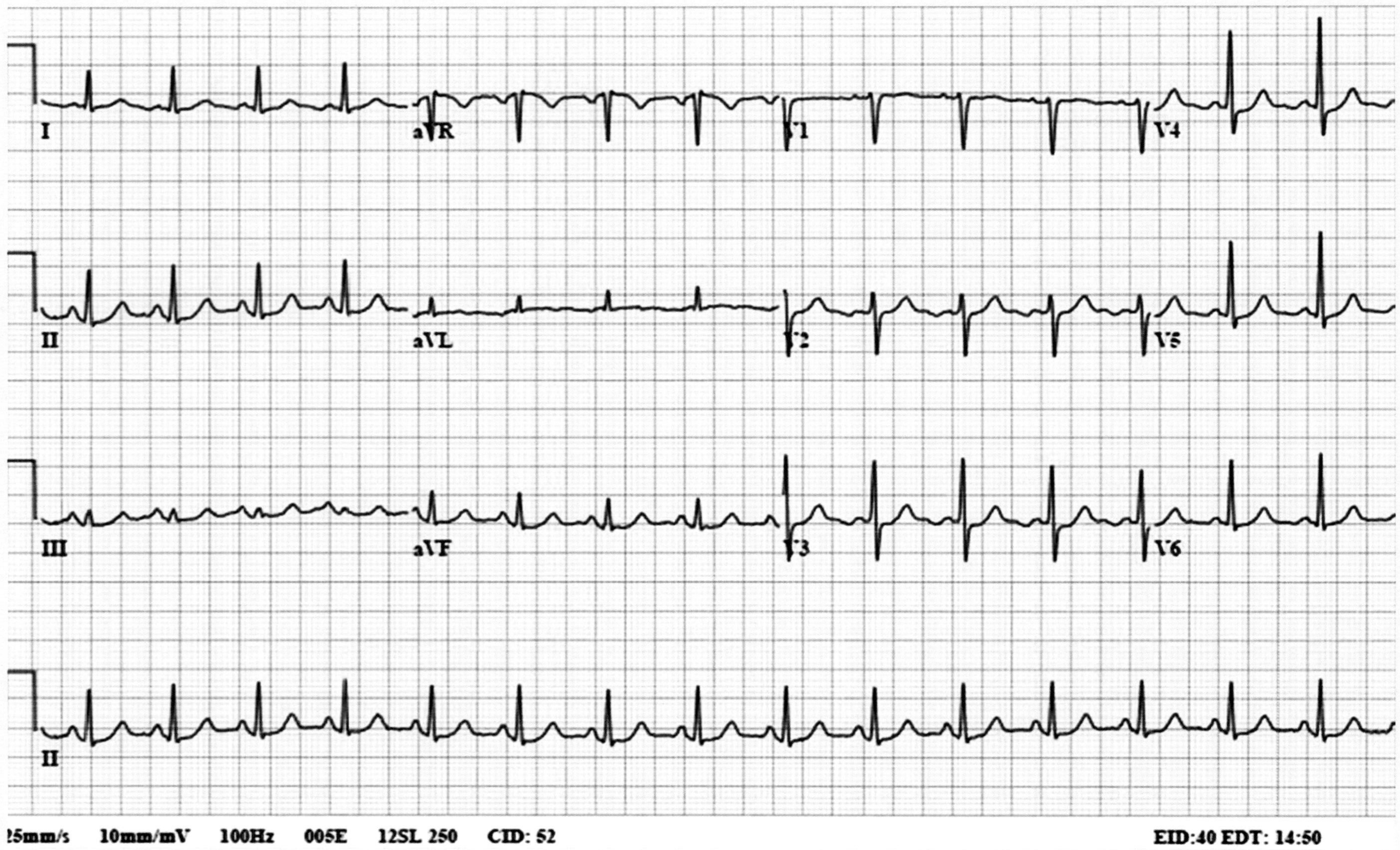

I  aVR  V1  V4

II  aVL  V2  V5

III  aVF  V3  V6

II

25mm/s   10mm/mV   100Hz   005E   12SL 250   CID: 52          EID:40 EDT: 14:50

**Case 6.10 (Continued)** Same patient on the second day after her visit for chest pain. Taken during an episode of squeezing chest pain.

**Case 6.11** A 66-year-old female with a history of hypertension presented with blurry vision and a brief syncopal episode.

**Case 6.12** A 69-year-old man was skiing when he experienced sudden upper back pain followed by a syncopal episode and then a cardiopulmonary arrest.

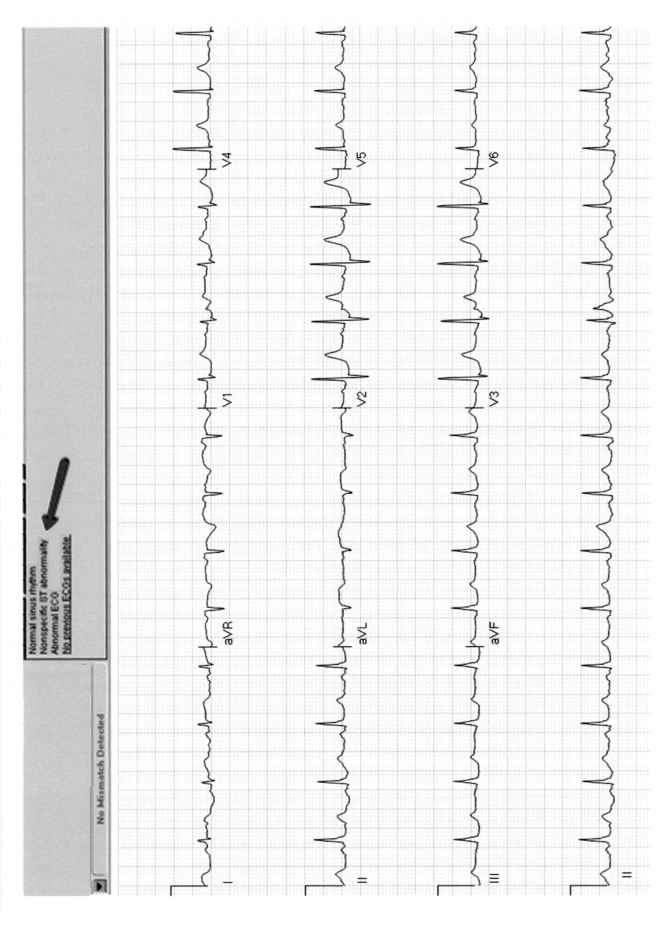

No Mismatch Detected

Normal sinus rhythm
Nonspecific ST abnormality
Abnormal ECG
No previous ECGs available

**Case 6.13** A 61-year-old man presented with chest pressure, shortness of breath and increasing cough and sputum production. He reported dyspnea walking just 30–40 feet. On examination, he had a mild tachycardia. He was also tachypneic and had diminished breath sounds and soft expiratory wheezes in all lung fields.

Male        Unknown

Room:S65
Loc:1002

| PR interval | 124 | ms |
| QRS duration | 94 | ms |
| QT/QTc | 398/528 | ms |
| P-R-T axes | 61   63 | -76 |

Technician:
Test ind:

OTHER:

Sinus tachycardia
Possible Left atrial enlargement
ST & T wave abnormality, consider inferior ischemia
ST & T wave abnormality, consider anterior ischemia
Prolonged QT
Abnormal ECG
No previous ECGs available

Referred by:

OTHER:

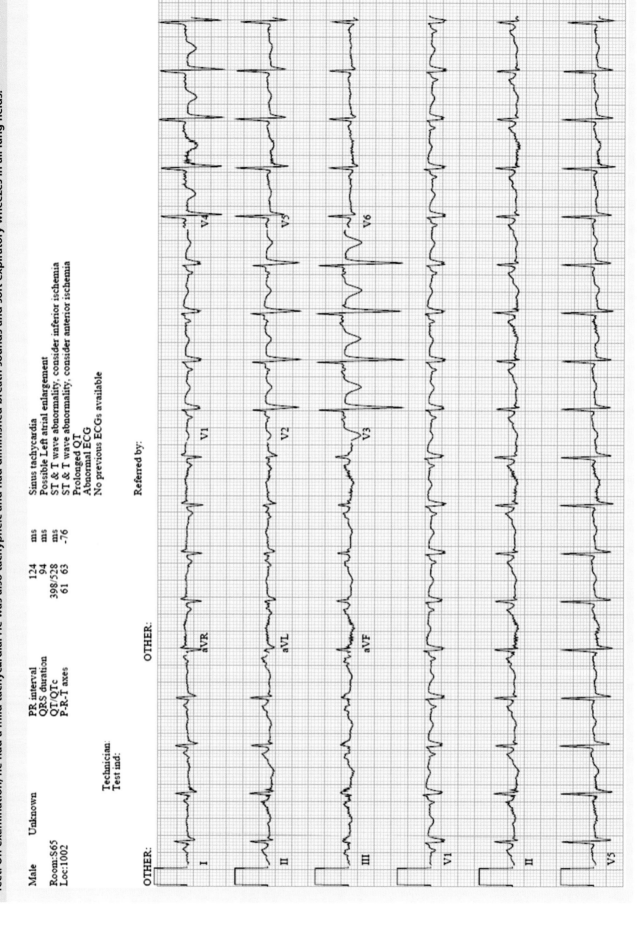

**Case 6.14** A 62-year-old female reported a history of lower extremity deep venous thrombosis and pulmonary emboli, hyperlipidemia, hypertension and mild renal insufficiency. She presented with 1 week of worsening chest pain, occurring at rest, with radiation to her neck and both arms. Her initial troponin was mildly elevated at 0.23, and her chest x-ray was normal. Her INR was supra-therapeutic. Her triage blood pressure was 185/81. Otherwise, her vital signs and physical examination were normal.

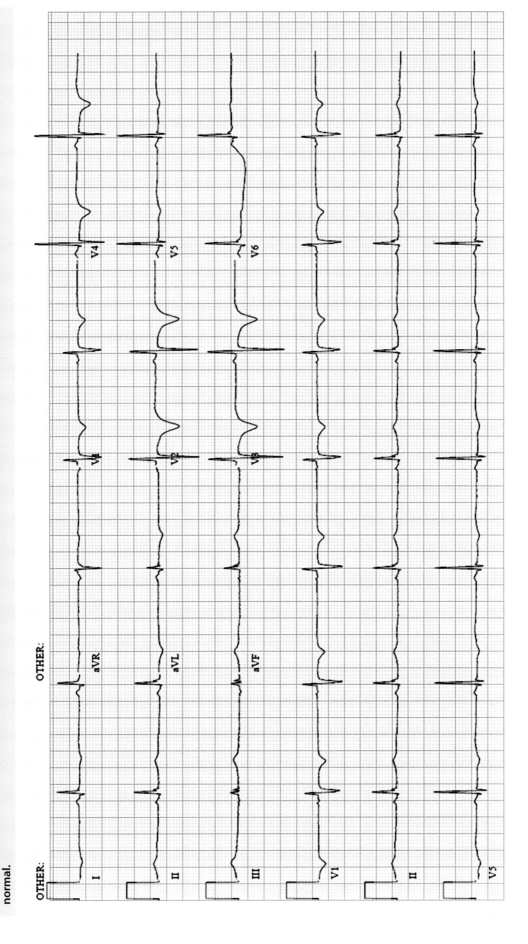

**Case 6.15** A 78-year-old man 20 years status-post coronary artery bypass surgery, presented with 1 day of exertional chest pain after stopping his clopidogrel bisulfate 5 days earlier for a screening colonoscopy. His chest pain then occurred at rest, and there was radiation to both shoulders. His troponin in the emergency department was 0.00.

**Case 6.16** A 68-year-old female endorsed blurry vision and generalized weakness, worsening over the past 6 months. She reported a history of cataracts, chronic congestive heart failure and hyperlipidemia. The computer reading said, "Sinus bradycardia, minimal voltage criteria for LVH, and nonspecific ST and T-wave abnormality."

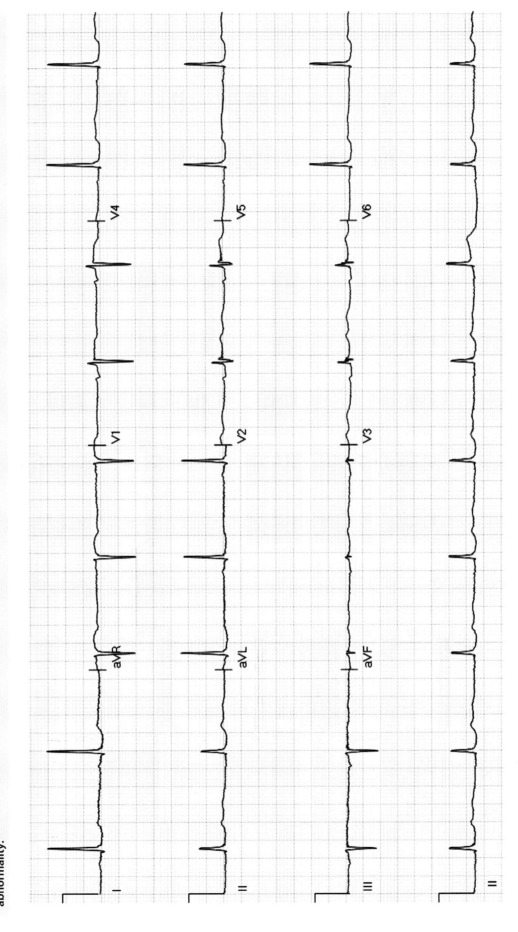

**Case 6.17** A 52-year-old man with known lung cancer and coronary artery disease presented with chest pain and shortness of breath.

OTHER:

OTHER:

**Case 6.18** A 56-year-old man with a history of smoking and a family history of coronary artery disease presented to the ED with chest pain, tightness around his sternum and anxiety; the chest discomfort awoke him from sleep at 1 A.M. He had normal vital signs and a normal physical examination. His initial troponin was 2.15. His pain resolved with NTG but then quickly returned. The repeat troponin was 4.59.

Room:367
Loc:1002

01b

| Vent. rate | 103 | BPM |
| PR interval | 130 | ms |
| QRS duration | 98 | ms |
| QT/QTc | 372/487 | ms |
| P-R-T axes | 58 -50 | 234 |

Sinus tachycardia
Left anterior fascicular block
Left ventricular hypertrophy with repolarization abnormality
Inferior infarct , age undetermined
Anterolateral infarct , age undetermined
Marked ST abnormality, possible anterior subendocardial injury
Abnormal ECG
No previous ECGs available

Referred by:  SELF

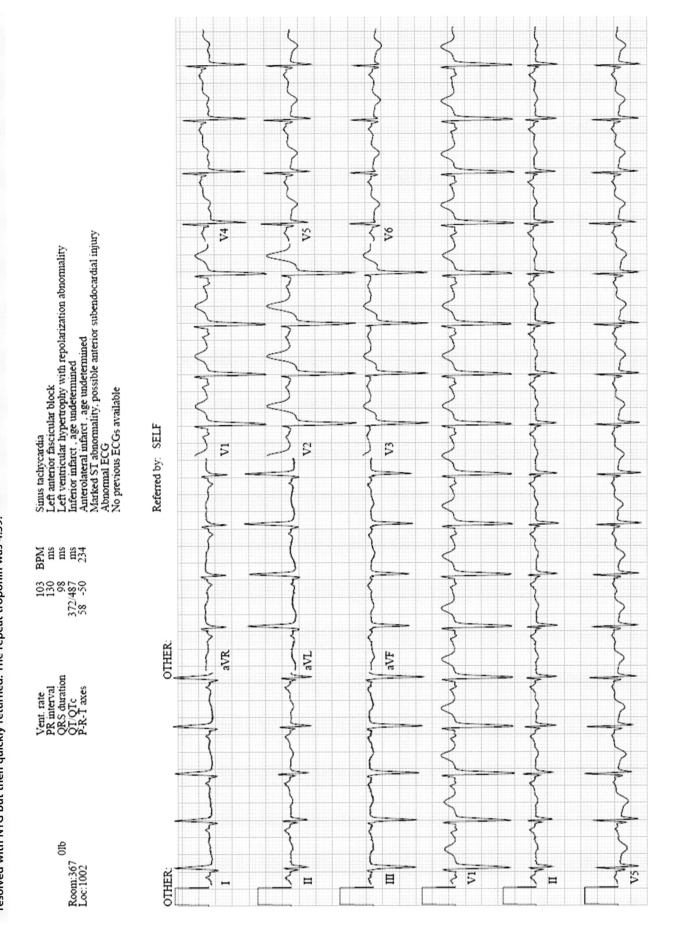

**Case 6.18 (Continued)** Same patient – repeat ECG taken 3 hours later.

## Self-Study Electrocardiograms

### Case 6.1   A 64-year-old man presented with chest pain.

#### The Electrocardiogram
The electrocardiogram shows atrial fibrillation with a controlled ventricular response (HR = 95) along with rounded, sagging ST-segment depressions in lead II and in the precordial leads that are most consistent with digitalis effect. There is also an abnormal right axis deviation that was unchanged from earlier tracings.

#### Clinical Course
This patient's serum digoxin level was 1.26, slightly above the laboratory's therapeutic range. His history included COPD, atrial fibrillation, congestive heart failure and anemia.

### Case 6.2   A 71-year-old man presented to the emergency department after a near-syncopal episode.

#### The Electrocardiogram
The ECG demonstrates classic findings of left ventricular hypertrophy with repolarization abnormalities ("strain"). The QRS voltage is increased in the left-facing precordial leads and in lead I (refer to the criteria listed earlier in this chapter). Deep S-waves are present in the right precordial leads (V1–V3). The QRS complex is slightly widened (to 0.114 seconds). The ST-segment and T-wave changes in the lateral precordial leads are classic for "LVH with strain": the ST-segment descends gradually and merges "imperceptibly" into the inverted T-wave. The inverted T-wave is asymmetric with a gradual descending limb and a sharp ascending limb.

The ST-segments are elevated in the right precordial leads. But in the setting of LVH, this finding is not specific for anterior wall STEMI. As highlighted in this chapter (and again in Chapter 7, **Confusing Conditions: ST-Segment Elevations and Tall T-Waves (Coronary Mimics)**), LVH is the most common reason for false-positive "cath lab" activations.

The reason for this patient's syncopal episode is not readily apparent on this tracing. However, the ECG was also consistent with a possible old inferior myocardial infarction (abnormally deep Q-wave in III, diminished R-wave amplitude in II and aVF and T-wave inversions in III and aVF), raising the possibility of ventricular tachycardia as the cause of his syncope. Therefore, he was admitted for cardiac monitoring and further care.

### Case 6.3   A 35-year-old man presented with 1 week of increasing effort-related chest pain, with radiation to his neck and throat. In the ED, his pain kept recurring at rest despite administration of intravenous nitroglycerin. His initial troponin was 0.22.

#### The Electrocardiogram
Despite the patient's young age, this is clearly a very high-risk presentation. The first concern is the tempo of his pain, which is increasing in frequency and duration and is now occurring while at rest despite nitroglycerin. Second, his troponin is already elevated. And perhaps most important, his ECG shows horizontal or downsloping ST-segment depressions in six different leads (I, aVL and V3, V4, V5 and V6). Thus, there is evidence of anterior, lateral and high lateral ischemia. In this case, the T-waves remain upright (making LVH with "strain" a very unlikely explanation for the ST-segment depressions). As noted earlier, in patients with unstable angina or a non-STEMI, the acute prognosis worsens linearly with the number of leads that demonstrate ST-segment depressions.

In addition, the astute electrocardiographer will note that there are prominent ST-segment elevations in lead aVR, suggesting acute left main coronary artery obstruction (or a significant "equivalent," such as thrombotic obstruction involving two or three major coronary arteries).

#### Clinical Course
Emergent angiography was warranted in this patient, given the severity of his pain, the extent of his ST-segment depressions and the worrisome ST-segment elevation in lead aVR.

The patient was taken to the catheterization suite, where he had a 100 percent proximal LAD occlusion and a 100 percent proximal obtuse marginal artery occlusion. He developed hypotension and required an intra-aortic balloon pump.

## Case 6.4 A 54-year-old female was visiting the zoo when she had the sudden onset of chest pain, shortness of breath and near-syncope.

### The Electrocardiogram

The tracing shows voltage criteria for LVH with classic repolarization abnormalities. The precordial lead voltage meets criteria for LVH, the QRS complex is moderately widened, and the ST-segment and T-wave pattern in leads V5 and V6 are typical of the "strain" pattern. (There is downsloping ST-segment depression and an asymmetric T-wave inversion.)

This patient's symptoms are certainly concerning for a cardiorespiratory catastrophe. The ECG is important, but not because it is diagnostic. Rather, it is important because *it does not explain her symptoms.*

### Clinical Course

The clinicians confidently read this ECG as showing LVH with repolarization abnormalities, which did not explain her severe chest pain, dyspnea and near-syncope.

When patients present with chest pain or dyspnea and have a normal or nondiagnostic ECG – as in this case – it is critical to consider posterior wall STEMI (because the 12-lead ECG is often silent), pulmonary thromboembolism, thoracic aortic dissection and other cardiorespiratory or even gastrointestinal emergencies. It is not enough to state, "ST-T-wave changes, possible acute coronary syndrome, admit for medical management, heparin, nitrates and serial ECGs and troponin levels."

The finding of LVH on the ECG is commonly caused by chronic hypertension, making thoracic aortic dissection more likely. This patient developed progressive dyspnea and hypoxemia in the emergency department. She was intubated and transferred to the catheterization laboratory, where a pacemaker and intra-aortic balloon pump were inserted. She had a cardiac arrest and could not be resuscitated. The catheterization revealed an acute aortic dissection.

## Case 6.5 A 57-year-old man presented with 3 hours of substernal chest pain that radiated to his jaw. His initial troponin was mildly elevated at 0.44.

### The Electrocardiogram

This case was also presented in Chapter 3. Despite the reassuring interpretation by the computer algorithm, this ECG does not show a "nonspecific ST abnormality." The "nonspecific ST abnormalities" are actually mild ST-segment depressions that are confined to leads II, III and aVF. Therefore, they are regional. These inferior ST-segment depressions are accompanied by ST-elevations in the high lateral leads, especially lead aVL.

The emergency medicine team was not fooled and made the correct diagnosis. The ED note said, "ECGs reviewed. Concern is for high lateral infarct with reciprocal inferior changes ... although patient does not meet [conventional cath lab] activation criteria, we think this is an acute STEMI, and activation is indicated, especially with his ongoing pain."

### Clinical Course

His troponin level peaked at 87. He was taken immediately for coronary angiography, which revealed a 100 percent occluded left circumflex artery. He became pain-free after placement of a stent. As highlighted in this chapter and throughout this atlas, in approaching the patient whose ECG demonstrates "ST-segment depressions," it is critical to consider first whether these ST-segment depressions are reciprocal to a true STEMI, even a STEMI that was not at first obvious.

## Case 6.6 A 42-year-old female presented because of recurrent episodes of chest pain. She had a history of alcohol dependence and a long history of severe, erosive esophagitis and gastritis. Three years earlier, she had a normal coronary angiogram. She presented to the ED with "atypical chest pain and epigastric pain." Her pain resolved in the ED after receiving nitroglycerin, morphine and beta blockers.

### The Electrocardiogram

This patient's history is not uncommon in emergency medicine practice – a patient with chest pain, gastrointestinal disease, alcohol dependence and an electrocardiogram with diffuse ST-segment and T-wave abnormalities. Sinus tachycardia is present along with a short PR interval and a premature ectopic complex. There are diffuse ST-segment depressions involving the inferior, anterior and lateral leads. One additional abnormality is the markedly prolonged QT interval (the QTc = 552 msec).

Diffuse anterior, inferior and lateral ("concentric") myocardial ischemia is possible (and she also has ST-segment elevation in lead aVR).

### Clinical Course

The treating physicians did not feel that her symptoms were suggestive of an acute coronary syndrome. Given the diffuse ST-T-wave changes, QT-interval prolongation and ectopy, they felt that a metabolic disturbance should also be considered. In fact, her serum potassium and magnesium levels were both low (2.0 and 1.0, respectively). After intravenous fluids and electrolyte replacement, her ST-segment depressions, ventricular ectopy and QT prolongation resolved.

## Case 6.7 A 51-year-old man with a history of chronic hypertension presented with a diffuse occipital headache. He denied chest pain or shortness of breath. He had not been taking his antihypertensive medications for the past month.

### The Electrocardiogram

The ECG demonstrates T-wave inversions in the anterior and lateral precordial leads and in the inferior limb leads. The QT interval is markedly prolonged, and U-waves are present in some leads. In another clinical setting, concurrent T-wave inversions in the anterior and inferior leads should suggest acute pulmonary embolism. However, this patient presented with an acute headache.

### Clinical Course

The CT scan confirmed the diagnosis of an acute subarachnoid hemorrhage.

## Case 6.8 A 23-year-old female with hemoglobin SS sickle cell disease presented with a painful crisis. On the second hospital day, she developed chest pain and shortness of breath. Her hemoglobin was 6.2. Her troponin level was 0.43.

### The Electrocardiogram

Symmetric T-wave inversions are present in leads V1–V3, suggesting anterior wall ischemia. The ST-segments are not depressed. There are no voltage or other criteria to suggest LVH. The T-wave inversion in lead III may be normal.

The symmetric T-wave inversions, with normal, isoelectric ST-segments, are most suggestive of ischemia, although pulmonary thromboembolism has to be considered. Her history did not suggest acute intracerebral hemorrhage.

### Clinical Course

Her chest pain and ECG abnormalities were felt to be most consistent with demand ischemia in the setting of her profound anemia. After transfusion and further treatment for her sickle cell anemia, her ECG returned to normal. Her troponin levels also trended downward to normal.

## Case 6.9 A 73-year-old female presented with weakness and altered mental status.

### The Electrocardiogram

The ECG demonstrates atrial fibrillation and ST-segment depressions in the lateral leads. The ST-segments are scooped, rounded and upwardly concave, and they have the contour of "Salvador Dalí's mustache" (and are most consistent with "digitalis effect"). She also has LVH.

### Clinical Course

This patient was taking digoxin to help manage her chronic atrial fibrillation. Her mental status change was evaluated with CT scan and MRI, which revealed a subacute cerebellar infarction. Her serum digoxin level was in the therapeutic range.

## Case 6.10    A 48-year-old female presented with squeezing chest pain while at rest. Her blood pressure was 198/105. This ECG was taken during an episode of chest pain.

### The Electrocardiogram

The ECG demonstrates a normal sinus rhythm with a mild sinus arrhythmia. There are diffuse ST-segment depressions in leads II aVF and, especially, in leads V2–V6. The ST-segment depressions are horizontal and are deeper than 2 mm in precordial leads V3–V6. This is not a "strain pattern," since there are no voltage-related or other features of left ventricular hypertrophy. In addition, the T-waves remain upright; in LVH the downsloping ST-segments almost always end in an inverted T-wave. The ST-segments are horizontal with a sharp junction before the take-off the T-wave; the pattern does not suggest digitalis effect. These are also not simply "nonspecific ST-T-wave changes." Note that the ST-segment depressions are actually very marked when you consider the small amplitude of the R-waves in the affected leads.

This ECG is consistent with subendocardial ischemia, indicating unstable angina or non-STEMI (UA/NSTEMI) and typically signifying acute atherosclerotic plaque rupture. When the ST-segment depressions exceed 2 mm and when three or more leads are involved, the changes are even more specific for UA/NSTEMI.

For comparison, her baseline ECG (taken 3 months earlier, while she was asymptomatic) is shown.

## Case 6.10    Same patient: Baseline ECG obtained 3 months earlier.

The baseline ECG was normal, except for a sinus tachycardia. An additional ECG was taken during the current visit while she was having chest pain (next tracing).

## Case 6.10    Same patient on the second day after her visit for chest pain. Taken during an episode of squeezing chest pain.

This second ECG, also obtained while she was experiencing chest pain, shows deep, symmetric T-wave inversions across the precordium. Note how deep the T-wave inversions are when compared with the very modest height of the R-waves. These are suggestive of an acute coronary syndrome (ACS), either unstable angina or a non-STEMI. These are "coronary T-waves" (Wellens' syndrome, Type B), and they are suggestive of critical LAD disease. While these changes often appear during pain-free intervals and may represent reperfusion of an occluded epicardial coronary artery, the culprit artery (the LAD) remains at risk for additional plaque rupture and reocclusion. In this case, the occurrence and recurrence of ST-segment depressions and T-wave inversions during episodes of pain clearly represent "dynamic ST-T-wave changes," and these are characteristic of an acute coronary syndrome in a patient at high risk.

### Clinical Course

She underwent urgent (but not immediate) coronary angiography, which revealed three-vessel coronary artery disease. Stents were placed. Her final discharge diagnosis was non-STEMI.

## Case 6.11    A 66-year-old female with a history of hypertension presented with blurry vision and a brief syncopal episode.

### The Electrocardiogram

The initial ECG, showing deep T-wave inversions in precordial leads V1–V4, prompted concern for acute anterior wall ischemia, a pulmonary embolism or, possibly, an intracranial hemorrhage. The QT-interval is also prolonged (QTc = 520 msec). Her serum electrolytes were normal, except for a mildly depressed magnesium (1.2). Her troponin remained normal throughout her hospital course.

### Clinical Course

She had a catheterization on the day of admission, which demonstrated only mild, nonobstructing coronary atherosclerosis. An echocardiogram demonstrated apical ballooning, consistent with takotsubo cardiomyopathy. On further history, she denied any recent losses or social-situational stresses. Her ECG remained abnormal at the time of discharge. Takotsubo is not uncommon, and patients often present with chest pain, syncope or any other vague or nonspecific symptom. The ECG, which may demonstrate deep T-wave inversions or ST-segment elevations, often suggests an acute coronary syndrome. Although the echocardiogram often demonstrates the telltale apical hypokinesis and ballooning, serum troponin levels may be elevated; depending on the presenting symptoms, coronary angiography is often needed to rule out coronary obstruction. Takotsubo is often called a "stress-induced cardiomyopathy" or, sometimes, the "broken heart syndrome." Takotsubo cardiomyopathy is discussed further in Chapter 7.

## Case 6.12  A 69-year-old man was skiing when he experienced sudden upper back pain followed by a syncopal episode and then a cardiopulmonary arrest.

### The Electrocardiogram

The computer reading is falsely reassuring. This ECG demonstrates much more than simply "nonspecific ST abnormality." ST-segment depressions are present in III and aVF and in precordial leads V1–V3.

When interpreting an ECG with ST-segment depressions, remember the first rule: *First, consider whether the ST-segments are reciprocal to a STEMI.* In this case, the ST-segment depressions, primarily in leads V1–V3 and accompanied by sharply upright T-waves, are highly suggestive of a posterior wall STEMI. The R-wave in V2 is also abnormally tall. (The R:S ratio is > 1.0.)

And what should we make of the inferior wall ST-segment depressions, which are most marked in lead III? We start by examining the lead that is electrically opposite to lead III: there is unmistakable ST-segment straightening and elevation in aVL. Lead I shows a similar abnormality. This patient is in the throes of an acute STEMI of the high lateral and posterior wall.

### Clinical Course

His initial troponin level was 4.0. Because of his complaint of severe upper back pain, a CT-angiogram of the chest was obtained, and it was negative for an acute thoracic aortic dissection.

He had a subsequent cardiac arrest in the emergency department and underwent open chest cardiac massage and a pericardiocentesis. He survived. While angiography was not performed, a stress echocardiogram prior to discharge demonstrated (predictably) severe akinesis in the distribution of the left circumflex artery. The echocardiogram also demonstrated a pericardial effusion, felt to be due to prolonged CPR. This ECG shows classic changes of an acute posterior and high lateral wall STEMI, almost always representing an acute occlusion of the LCA or one of its branches.

## Case 6.13  A 61-year-old man presented with chest pressure, shortness of breath and increasing cough and sputum production. He reported dyspnea walking just 30–40 feet. On examination, he had a mild tachycardia. He was also tachypneic and had diminished breath sounds and soft expiratory wheezes in all lung fields.

### The Electrocardiogram

This emergency medicine team interpreted this ECG as showing "sinus tachycardia, possible right atrial enlargement, pulmonary disease pattern, also T-wave inversions inferiorly consistent with ischemia, anterior T-wave inversions consistent with ischemia." As you can see, the computer offered a similar (and erroneous) interpretation.

In this case, both the clinician and the computer failed at "pattern recognition." Sinus tachycardia is present, and the axis is abnormally rightward for this patient's age. (Notice the S-wave in lead I.) Neither of these findings is specific for pulmonary embolism, and the right axis deviation could be chronic in this patient with COPD. However, as highlighted in Chapter 5 and repeatedly in this chapter, T-wave inversions in the right precordial leads are a common sign of extensive PE. And the combination of T-wave inversions in the anterior and inferior leads is much more likely to be PE than ischemia of two walls. The ECG, in this patient with chest pain, dyspnea and tachycardia, is highly suggestive of PE with acute right heart strain and elevated pulmonary artery pressures.

### Clinical Course

A chest x-ray was ordered, and it demonstrated a right lower lobe consolidation and a pleural effusion, "concerning for pneumonia with parapneumonic effusion." The admitting diagnosis was pneumonia with a possible obstructing endobronchial mass. Therefore, a chest CT scan was obtained. Of note, the patient's chest x-ray findings (volume loss, lung consolidation and ipsilateral pleural effusion) are also highly suggestive of acute pulmonary embolism.

The CT demonstrated a "large burden of pulmonary embolism with right main and left lobar occlusive emboli, resulting in a right-sided pleural effusion and opacities suggestive of developing pulmonary infarctions of the right lower lobe, lingual and areas of the left lower lobe." His echocardiogram demonstrated a "flattened septum, consistent with right ventricular pressure overload, and moderate dilatation and hypokinesis of the right ventricle."

He was treated with intravenous heparin and improved rapidly, although his hospital course was complicated by bouts of atrial fibrillation. His ECG on the third hospital day showed a completely normal QRS axis (no S-wave in lead I) and resolution of the sinus tachycardia and T-wave inversions in the inferior leads. Minor anterior precordial T-wave inversions persisted.

## Case 6.14    A 62-year-old female reported a history of lower extremity deep venous thrombosis and pulmonary emboli, hyperlipidemia, hypertension and mild renal insufficiency. She presented with 1 week of worsening chest pain, occurring at rest, with radiation to her neck and both arms. Her initial troponin was mildly elevated at 0.23, and her chest x-ray was normal. Her INR was supra-therapeutic. Her triage blood pressure was 185/81. Otherwise, her vital signs and physical examination were normal.

### The Electrocardiogram

The ECG shows sinus bradycardia along with marked T-wave inversions in precordial leads V1–V4. These T-wave inversions are deep and symmetric, most consistent with anterior wall ischemia ("coronary T-waves" or Wellens' syndrome Type B). PE is always in the differential diagnosis when T-wave inversions are present in the right precordial leads.

### Clinical Course

Her troponin level trended upward slightly and peaked at 0.39. She was admitted with a diagnosis of acute non-STEMI; her catheterization (performed on the third hospital day) demonstrated a long 90 percent stenosis of the proximal left anterior descending artery, involving the first septal branch. A bare metal stent was placed.

The differential diagnosis of the T-wave inversions in the anterior precordium includes acute pulmonary thromboembolism, even in the absence of a sinus tachycardia or an abnormal right axis deviation. The other causes of T-wave inversions include subarachnoid hemorrhage, electrolyte abnormalities, normal variants and takotsubo or another cardiomyopathy.

## Case 6.15    A 78-year-old man 20 years status-post coronary artery bypass surgery, presented with 1 day of exertional chest pain after stopping his clopidogrel bisulfate 5 days earlier for a screening colonoscopy. His chest pain then occurred at rest, and there was radiation to both shoulders. His troponin in the emergency department was 0.00.

### The Electrocardiogram

The initial ECG shows only mild ST-segment depressions in leads V4–V6 and mild ST-segment depression in lead I. Digitalis effect, electrolyte abnormalities and myocardial ischemia might be considered in this case. Importantly, there is no ST-segment elevation in aVR and, after careful inspection, no evidence that the lateral wall ST-segment depressions are reciprocal to a subtle STEMI. The mostly horizontal ST-segment depressions, appearing in a regional distribution (V4–V6), are most suggestive of lateral wall subendocardial ischemia.

### Clinical Course

The repeat serum troponin level was 0.61, and the troponin peaked at 1.29. A repeat ECG, obtained 3 hours later, when the patient was free of pain, showed complete resolution of the lateral wall ST-segment depressions.

Coronary angiography showed diffuse three-vessel native coronary artery occlusions. There was a high-grade occlusion of a previously placed stent in a saphenous vein graft in the proximal obtuse marginal artery (OM), which was felt to be the culprit obstructing lesion (and the explanation for the lateral ST-segment depressions). A new drug-eluting stent was placed with good perfusion. The final diagnosis was non-STEMI due to diffuse coronary artery disease and graft occlusion.

## Case 6.16    A 68-year-old female endorsed blurry vision and generalized weakness, worsening over the past 6 months. She reported a history of cataracts, chronic congestive heart failure and hyperlipidemia. The computer reading said, "Sinus bradycardia, minimal voltage criteria for LVH, and nonspecific ST and T-wave abnormality."

### The Electrocardiogram

The computer reading was partially correct: However, the only suggestion of LVH is the abnormal voltage in limb leads I and aV (> 11 mm). The sagging, smooth, upwardly concave ST-segment depressions (resembling "Salvador Dalí's mustache") and

U-waves are highly suggestive of digitalis effect. Typically, the ST-depressions of digitalis effect are most pronounced in the left-sided leads, where there is high voltage. Sinus bradycardia is also present, consistent with digitalis effect (or even toxicity).

### Clinical Course

Her digoxin level was in the low therapeutic range (0.9). Her potassium was low at 2.9. Her vision problems were attributed to cataracts, rather than digitalis poisoning, and she was referred for evaluation by an ophthalmologist.

## Case 6.17 A 52-year-old man with known lung cancer and coronary artery disease presented with chest pain and shortness of breath.

### The Electrocardiogram

The ECG has numerous abnormalities. Most obvious are the tall, peaked T-waves in the anterior precordial leads, compatible with either acute, early anterior wall STEMI (hyperacute T-waves) or hyperkalemia.

In the lateral precordial leads (V5 and V6), the ST-segments are depressed, and the T-waves are inverted; in combination with the large voltage in the precordial leads, the pattern is consistent with LVH and repolarization abnormalities. The QRS is widened, and left atrial enlargement is present, also consistent with LVH.

There is also ST-segment depression in the inferior leads (especially II and aVF).

What do we make of these diffuse abnormalities? Perhaps the most critical question is what is the significance of ST-segment depressions in the lateral precordium combined with the hyperacute right precordial T-waves? Does all of this represent only LVH with strain or acute ischemia or even a STEMI equivalent? Operationally, should we refer this patient emergently for coronary angiography?

As highlighted in Chapter 3, it is usually a good idea to examine lead aVR (the once "forgotten lead") where there is prominent ST-segment elevation. In combination with the inferior (lead II) and lateral ST-segment depressions, this can indicate a severe obstruction of the left main coronary artery or its "equivalent" (severe LAD or three-vessel disease).

### Clinical Course

The emergency department clinicians wondered if the prominent T-waves in the right precordial leads and the ST-segment depressions in the lateral leads were new. They retrieved an ECG taken 11 days earlier, which showed LVH with only minor repolarization abnormalities, but the T-waves were not peaked. Furthermore, the ST-segments were only mildly depressed, and the T-waves were upright. Lead aVR was essentially normal.

The team recognized these findings as indicating a high possibility of LMCA or LAD obstruction or obstruction of multiple coronary arteries (left main equivalent). The patient's serum troponin level did not rise above 2.18. Clinically, he remained stable. Coronary angiography was performed emergently. Not surprisingly, there was severe coronary artery disease, including a severe, 90 percent stenosis of the proximal LAD, chronic total occlusion of the right coronary artery, a 95 percent stenosis of the left circumflex artery and a 99 percent stenosis of a large obtuse marginal. He underwent coronary artery bypass grafting. He did well and was discharged after a 1-week hospital stay.

## Case 6.18 A 56-year-old man with a history of smoking and a family history of coronary artery disease presented to the ED with chest pain, tightness around his sternum and anxiety; the chest discomfort awoke him from sleep at 1 A.M. He had normal vital signs and a normal physical examination. His initial troponin was 2.15. His pain resolved with NTG but then quickly returned. The repeat troponin was 4.59.

### The Electrocardiogram

There are significant ST-segment depressions in the anterior precordial leads (V2–V4), which the computer interprets as "possible anterior subendocardial injury." There is also a mild sinus tachycardia, a left anterior fascicular block, an inferior wall infarction of indeterminate age and, possibly, an anterior wall infarction of indeterminate age.

The emergency medicine team and the cardiology consultants focused, properly, on the ST-segment depressions in precordial leads V2–V4 and the T-wave inversions in V5 and V6. The emergency medicine and cardiology notes in the electronic record were almost identical: "Patient does not have ST-elevation MI. There are ST-depressions in the V2 and V3 leads. Therefore, this is not STEMI, but given elevated troponin, he has NSTEMI."

This interpretation is too simplistic. In fact, it is incorrect. There is not a STEMI as classically defined, but the presence of regional ST-segment depressions must always prompt a careful search for evidence of a reciprocal STEMI. In this case, the ECG

227

suggests a "STEMI equivalent"– that is, an acute posterior wall STEMI. As we highlighted in Chapter 4, Posterior Wall Myocardial Infarction, the hallmark of acute posterior STEMI is the "reciprocal sign" on the 12-lead ECG. The classic features are found in the right precordial leads (V1–V3): ST-segment depressions are present, accompanied by tall, upright T-waves.

### Clinical Course

The ED clinicians ordered posterior leads, but they were negative in this case. (No repeat posterior lead ECGs were obtained.) However, the echocardiogram demonstrated extensive lateral and posterior wall hypokinesis. Most posterior STEMIs actually involve a substantial amount of the lateral wall of the left ventricle. A repeat ECG was obtained 3 hours later, demonstrating more marked right precordial ST-segment depressions.

## Case 6.18 Same patient – repeat ECG taken 3 hours later.

### The Electrocardiogram

The repeat ECG demonstrates more pronounced ST-segment depressions and very tall T-waves along with a suggestion of an evolving lateral wall STEMI. (V5 and V6 show mild ST-segment elevation and abnormal straightening along with more pronounced T-wave inversions.)

### Clinical Course (Continued)

This patient's troponin peaked at 73 on the second hospital day. His catheterization was not performed until the third hospital day, probably because the treating team felt his diagnosis was a non-STEMI. There was diffuse three-vessel disease, with the most severe obstruction (80 percent stenosis) in the left circumflex artery. According to the catheterization report, this was felt to be the infarct-related artery. He underwent a successful three-vessel coronary artery bypass graft.

The combination of ST-segment depressions and upright T-waves in the right precordial leads (V1–V3) must always suggest a true posterior wall STEMI. At the very least, posterior ECG leads, serial ECGs and a bedside echocardiogram should be obtained before this pattern is attributed to "non-STEMI."

Unfortunately, delayed recognition of true posterior STEMI and delay in reperfusion in these patients are quite common. As highlighted in Chapter 4, Posterior Wall Myocardial Infarction, in one large study of patients with posterior wall STEMIs, mostly due to left circumflex artery occlusion, the median "door-to-balloon time" was 29 hours. In three-fourths of patients, the anterior ST-depressions were misclassified as NSTEMI or unstable angina. Most importantly, delayed reperfusion was associated with worse clinical outcomes.

## References

Amsterdam E. A., Wenger N. K. et al. AHA/ACC Guideline for the management of patients with non-ST elevation acute coronary syndromes. *J Am Coll Cardiol.* 2014; **64**:e139–228.

Arnaout M., Mongardon N., Deye N. et al. Out-of-hospital cardiac arrest from brain cause: Epidemiology, clinical features and outcome in a multicenter cohort. *Crit Care Med.* 2015; **43**:453–460.

Ayer A., Terkelsen C. J. Difficult ECGs in STEMI: Lessons learned from serial sampling of pre- and in-hospital ECGs. *J Electrocardiol.* 2014; **47**:448–458.

Birnbaum Y., Nikus K., Kligfield P. et al. The role of the ECG in diagnosis, risk estimation and catheterization laboratory activation in patients with acute coronary syndromes: A consensus document. *Ann Noninvasive Electrocardiol.* 2014; **19**:412–425.

Birnbaum Y., Wilson J. M., Fiol M. et al. ECG diagnosis and classification of acute coronary syndromes. *Ann Noninvasive Electrocardiol.* 2014; **19**:4–14.

Cantanzaro J. N., Meraj P. M., Sheng S. et al. Electrocardiographic T-wave changes underlying acute cardiac and cerebral events. *Am J Emerg Med.* 2008; **26**:716–720.

Chan T. C., Brady W. J., Harrigan R. A. et al. *ECG in emergency medicine and acute care.* Philadelphia, PA: Elsevier Mosby, 2005.

Delk C., Holstege C. P., Brady W. J. Electrocardiographic abnormalities associated with poisoning. *Am J Emerg Med.* 2007; **25**:672–687.

Demangone D. ECG manifestations: Noncoronary heart disease. *Emerg Med Clin N Am.* 2006; **24**:113–131.

Goldberger A. L. *Clinical electrocardiography: A simplified approach.* Seventh edition. St. Louis, MO: Elsevier/ Mosby, 2006.

Goldberger A. L. Recognition of ECG pseudo-infarct patterns. *Mod Concepts Cardiovasc Dis.* 1980; **49**(3):13–18.

Grauer K., Curry R. W. ECG of the month: Left ventricular hypertrophy. *Cardiovasc Rev and Rep.* 1987; November:69–71.

Hancock E. W., Deal B. J., Mirvis D. M. et al. AHA/ACCF/HRS recommendations for the standardization and interpretation of the electrocardiogram. Part V: Electrocardiogram changes associated with cardiac chamber hypertrophy. A scientific statement from the American Heart Association, Electrocardiography and Arrhythmias Committee; Council on Clinical Cardiology; the American College of Cardiology Foundation; and the Heart Rhythm Society. *J Amer Col Cardiol.* 2009; **53**:992–1002.

Hayden G. E., Brady W. J., Perron A. D. et al. Electrocardiographic T-wave inversion: Differential diagnosis in the chest pain patient. *Am J Emerg Med.* 2002; **20**:252–262.

Lewandowski P. Subarachnoid hemorrhage imitating acute coronary syndrome as a cause of out-of-hospital cardiac arrest – case report. *Anesthesiology Intensive Therapy.* 2014; **46**:289–292.

Ma G., Brady W. J., Pollack M., Chan T. C. Electrocardiographic manifestations: Digitalis toxicity. *J Emerg Med.* 2001; **20**:145–152.

Mitsuma W., Ito M., Kodama M. Clinical and cardiac features of patients with subarachnoid hemorrhage presenting with out-of-hospital cardiac arrest. *Resuscitation.* 2011; **82**:1294–1297.

Nable J. V., Lawner B. J. Chameleons: Electrocardiogram imitators of ST-segment elevation myocardial infarction. *Emerg Med Clin N Am.* 2015; **33**:529–537.

Nikus K., Birnbaum Y., Eskola M. et al. Updated electrocardiographic classification of acute coronary syndromes. *Current Cardiol Rev.* 2014; **10**: 229–236.

Nikus K., Pahlm O., Wagner G. et al. Electrocardiographic classification of acute coronary syndromes: A review by a committee of the International Society for Holter and Non-invasive Cardiology. *J Electrocardio.* 2010; **43**:91–103.

Pollehn T., Brady W. J., Perron A. D. Electrocardiographic ST segment depression. *Am J Emerg Med.* 2001; **19**: 303–309.

Pride Y. B., Tung P., Mohanavelu S. et al. Angiogoraphic and clinical outcomes among patients with acute coronary syndromes presenting with isolated anterior ST-segment depression. *J Amer Coll Cardiol Intv.* 2010; **3**:806–811.

Smith S. W., Zvosec D. L., Sharkey S. W., Hentry T. D. *The ECG in acute MI. An evidence-based manual of reperfusion therapy.* Philadelphia, PA: Lippincott Williams & Wilkins, 2002.

Surawicz B., Knilans T. K. *Chou's electrocardiography in clinical practice.* Sixth edition. Philadelphia, PA: Elsevier Saunders, 2008.

Wagner G. S., Strauss D. G. *Marriott's practical electrocardiography.* Twelfth edition. Philadelphia, PA: Lippincott, Williams & Wilkins, 2014.

Yamashina Y., Yagi T., Isshida A. et al. Differentiating between comatose patients resuscitated from acute coronary syndrome-associated and subarachnoid hemorrhage-associated out-of-hospital cardiac arrest. *J Cardiol.* 2015; **65**:508–513.

Yang E. H., Shah S., Criley J. M. Digitalis toxicity: A fading but crucial complication to recognize. *Am J Med.* 2012; **125**:337–343.

# Confusing Conditions: ST-Segment Elevations and Tall T-Waves (Coronary Mimics)

## Key Points

- Not all ST-segment elevations signify an acute myocardial infarction. Indeed, noncoronary ST-segment elevations are common. Many such patients have diagnoses other than acute STEMI, most often left ventricular hypertrophy (LVH), left bundle branch block (LBBB), left ventricular aneurysm, pericarditis or the early repolarization pattern (ERP). These conditions often masquerade as ST-elevation myocardial infarction and are referred to as "pseudo-infarct patterns" or "coronary mimics." Misdiagnosis, which may lead to unnecessary reperfusion therapy, is common.

- In differentiating benign ST-segment elevation from STEMI, the contour of the ST-segment may be helpful. Or the shape of the ST-segment may be misleading. Benign-appearing (that is, smooth and upwardly concave) ST-segment elevations can still represent an acute STEMI.

- The early repolarization pattern (formerly called "benign early repolarization") is common in young, healthy patients. The hallmark of ERP is the presence of diffuse ST-segment elevation, most commonly in the precordial leads. Other features of ERP include preservation of the upward concavity of the elevated ST-segments; a smooth blending of the elevated ST-segment into the ascending limb of a tall, upright (sometimes "hyperacute-appearing") T-wave; and prominent J-point elevation with a notched, "fish-hook" appearance. ERP can usually be differentiated from acute STEMI because the ST-segment elevations in ERP are not limited to a regional (anatomic) distribution, and they are not accompanied by reciprocal ST-segment depressions. Still, when the ST-elevations are limited to the anterior precordial leads, it can be challenging to differentiate ERP from a subtle, anterior wall STEMI. A small subset of ERP patients may be at higher risk of developing polymorphic ventricular tachycardia and sudden cardiac death.

- Acute pericarditis is characterized by even more diffuse ST-segment elevations, almost always involving the precordial and limb leads. The ST-segments are usually smooth and concave upward and seldom exceed 5 mm in amplitude. The T-waves are less prominent (more "humble") than in ERP. PR-segment depression is common (except in leads aVR and V1, where PR-segment elevation is often seen).

- Patients with electrocardiographic signs of LVH often have ST-segment elevations in the right precordial leads; there should also be high-amplitude R-waves and ST-segment depressions accompanied by T-wave inversions in the left-facing leads. Other features of LVH include poor R-wave progression, left axis deviation, QRS widening and left atrial enlargement. The ST-segment elevations in leads V1–V3 must be differentiated from acute coronary syndromes. The elevated ST-segment can mimic ominous patterns of acute LAD occlusion, including Wellens' sign.

- ST-segment elevations in the right precordial leads are also routine in left bundle branch block (LBBB). In some cases, acute anterior wall STEMI may be differentiated from the secondary ST-segment elevations of the LBBB by applying the Sgarbossa criteria (or by obtaining serial ECGs, by performing bedside echocardiography or by comparing the presenting ECG to baseline tracings).

- Other causes of noncoronary ST-segment elevations include hypothermia, hyperkalemia, takotsubo cardiomyopathy and the Brugada syndrome. Examples are provided in this chapter.

- Prominent T-waves are also a common ECG finding, especially in the precordial leads. The differential diagnosis includes, in addition to the "hyperacute T-waves" of an acute coronary syndrome, ERP, hyperkalemia, LVH, bundle branch block, hypertrophic cardiomyopathy and other conditions.

## Pseudo-Infarct Patterns (Coronary Mimics)

In earlier chapters of this atlas, we have covered several important electrocardiographic emergencies, including inferior, anterior and posterior wall ST-elevation myocardial infarctions (STEMIs) and various causes of shortness of breath (pulmonary emboli, pericardial effusion, myocarditis and the classic, everyday electrocardiographic appearance of COPD). In Chapter 6, we described a group of "confounding and confusing conditions" – patients with chest pain, shortness of breath or other cardiovascular symptoms whose ECGs demonstrate only ST-segment depressions or T-wave inversions. Some of these patients have "nonspecific ST-T-wave changes" without any acute disease. In other cases, the ST- and T-wave changes represent an acute coronary syndrome (unstable angina or non-STEMI), pulmonary embolus, digitalis effect, an electrolyte disturbance or left ventricular hypertrophy with repolarization abnormalities (the "strain" pattern).

One topic is left: ST-segment elevations that do not represent myocardial infarctions. Some patients will have acute pericarditis. In other cases, the ST-segment elevations represent a stable pattern of early repolarization (early repolarization pattern, or ERP). Noncoronary ST-segment elevations may also be caused by hypothermia, myocarditis, left ventricular aneurysm, left ventricular hypertrophy, left bundle branch block, hyperkalemia, Brugada syndrome, myocarditis, takotsubo cardiomyopathy or other cardiomyopathies (Huang, and Birnbaum 2011; Goldberger, 1980; Birnbaum, Nikus et al., 2014; Birnbaum, Wilson et al., 2014; Nable and Lawner, 2015; Pollak and Brady, 2012). These conditions often masquerade as ST-elevation myocardial infarction and are referred to as "pseudo-infarct patterns" or "coronary mimics" (Pollak and Brady, 2012; Nable and Lawner, 2015; Wang et al., 2003). In one recent review, these STEMI imitators were called "chameleons" (Nable and Lawner, 2015).

We should emphasize that ST-segment elevations in the right precordial leads are extraordinarily common, even on routine ECGs, in patients without any symptoms or "syndrome" (Huang and Birnbaum, 2011; Tran et al., 2011). ST-segment elevations can be seen in leads V1, V2 and V3 in young and old patients and in health as well as in disease. In one study of 6,014 healthy men ages 16–58 years of age, 91 percent had ST-elevations of 1–3 mm in at least one precordial lead (most commonly in lead V2) (Wang et al., 2003; His et al., 1960; Huang and Birnbaum, 2011; Tran et al., 2011). For this reason (as emphasized in Chapter 6), even minor ST-segment depressions in precordial leads V1–V3 must be considered abnormal and taken seriously.

As noted in Chapter 6, the literature also includes large numbers of case reports where the ST-segment elevations are "caused" by a pneumothorax, cholecystitis, intestinal ischemia, food impaction or even drinking cold (or hot) water. For the most part, these are anecdotal case reports, and no serious attempt is made to demonstrate causality.

## Coronary Mimics: ST-Segment Elevations That Are *Not* Myocardial Infarction

In large series of patients presenting to emergency departments with chest pain, noncoronary ST-segment elevations (pseudo-infarct patterns) are common. Many such patients have diagnoses other than acute STEMI, most often left ventricular hypertrophy, left bundle branch block, left ventricular aneurysm, pericarditis or ERP (Wang et al., 2003; Brady et al., 2001; Nable and Lawner, 2015; Pollak and Brady, 2012).

Misdiagnosis is common, even among experienced electrocardiographers; unnecessary thrombolytic therapy or percutaneous angioplasty is often administered (Tran et al., 2011; Jayroe et al., 2009; Huang and Birnbaum, 2011).

The following table summarizes the most common noncoronary causes of ST-segment elevations.

**Pseudo-Infarct Patterns: Noncoronary Causes of ST-Segment Elevations**

- Early repolarization pattern
- Acute pericarditis
- Myocarditis
- Hypothermia (Osborn J-waves)
- Left ventricular hypertrophy (limited to V1–V3, reciprocal to the lateral wall ST-segment depressions)
- Left bundle branch block
- Left ventricular aneurysm
- Brugada syndrome
- Hyperkalemia ("dialyzable injury current;" typically V1–V3)
- Takotsubo cardiomyopathy

## The Shape of the ST-Segment: Concave Upward, "Smiley Faces" and J-Point Elevation

In differentiating benign ST-segment elevation from STEMI, the contour of the ST-segment may be helpful. For example, in many patients with ERP, acute pericarditis or left ventricular hypertrophy, the normal, concave-upward contour of the ST-segment is usually preserved. And in the majority of STEMIs, the ST-segment becomes abnormally straight or acquires a downwardly concave or dome-shaped pattern (Brady et al., 2001).

However, *upward concavity does not rule out a STEMI* (Brady et al., 2001; Smith, 2006; Birnbaum, Wilson et al., 2014; Huang and Birnbaum, 2011; Chung et al., 2013; Tran et al., 2011). ST-segments that are straight or dome-shaped (concave downward) may be very specific for STEMI, but this

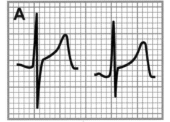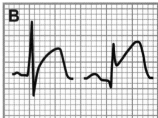

**Figure 7.1** The shape of the ST-segment elevation.
The ST-segment elevations in Panel A appear reassuring; indeed, this smooth, upwardly concave morphology is classically associated with more benign, non-acute coronary syndrome etiologies such as early repolarization pattern, left ventricular hypertrophy or pericarditis. The patterns in Panel B are usually more sinister, with ST-segments that are straighter, have lost their upward concavity or are concave downward. However, as highlighted in this section, a reassuring, concave-upward ST-segment *does not exclude acute STEMI*.

pattern is not at all sensitive, and its absence cannot be used to exclude the diagnosis of STEMI. Furthermore, saying that the ECG shows *only J-point elevation* (and is, therefore, benign) is a false argument. Most acute STEMIs also have J-point elevation, and sometimes, STEMIs have concave upward ("smiley face") ST-segments. These patterns are "overlapping, not distinct" (Brady et al., 2001; Birnbaum, Wilson et al., 2014; Chung et al., 2013).

As highlighted throughout this atlas, the key to recognizing an acute STEMI, even if the ST-segments have a benign shape, is the presence of a regional (anatomic) pattern to the ST-segment elevations and reciprocal ST-segment depressions. These two features make a STEMI much more likely (although focal myocarditis may also represent with regional ST-segment elevations).

So, does the shape of the ST-segment matter? Yes, sometimes – but not as much as previously thought. If there is a regional pattern to the ST-segment elevations, this matters more. Regional ST-segment elevations with reciprocal ST-segment depressions signify a STEMI and trump "shapeliness" every time.

## "Looking Backward": Reviewing the Patient's Old ECGs

When patients present with ST-segment elevations, the first step is always to rule out (or rule in) an acute STEMI. When the clinical or electrocardiographic diagnosis is less clear, we also know to search for old ECG tracings to ascertain whether the ST-segment elevations are new or are more pronounced.

However, while critical, this approach is not foolproof. Changes in lead placement can cause variability in the position of the ST-segments. And some nonischemic patterns of ST-segment elevations may also fluctuate over time, depending on the patient's heart rate, body position, autonomic tone or other factors. For example, the ST-segment elevations of ERP tend to be less dramatic at higher heart rates, and the features of ERP may even disappear over time (Adhikarla et al., 2011; Birnbaum, Wilson et al., 2014). The patterns of the Brugada syndrome have a tendency to show spontaneous variability in addition to fluctuations caused by multiple different medications and changes in sympathetic-parasympathetic balance (Huang and Birnbaum, 2011; Birnbaum, 2014; Pollak and Brady, 2012).

This is only a cautionary note; reviewing baseline ECGs remains a vital step in patients with chest pain, dyspnea, abdominal pain, dizziness or other suggestive symptoms, if the diagnosis of STEMI is not clear.

## Early Repolarization Pattern

The early repolarization pattern (ERP) has, for many decades, been referred to as "benign early repolarization." ERP is a common ECG pattern that can be recognized, in most cases, by a constellation of electrocardiographic findings (Huang and Birnbaum, 2011; Nable and Lawner, 2015; Pollak and Brady, 2012):

### Early Repolarization Pattern: The ECG

- Diffuse precordial ST-elevations with preservation of the normal upward concavity.
- ST-segment elevations that are more common and more dominant in the anterior or lateral precordial leads (especially V4); often (30–50 percent of cases) there are concurrent ST-segment elevations in the inferior leads.
- An upwardly concave, rising ST-segment that blends into the ascending limb of a tall, upright (and sometimes peaked) T-wave.
- Prominent J-point elevation with a notched, "fish-hook" pattern – especially in leads V3 and V4.
- ST-elevations that typically do not exceed 3 mm in the precordial leads or 0.5–1 mm in the limb leads.
- Absence of a regional (anatomic) pattern to the ST-elevations – and absence of reciprocal ST-segment depressions.
- PR-segment depression may occur, although less frequently than in pericarditis.
- Some ECG features of ERP may overlap with the "athletic heart syndrome," including sinus bradycardia, heart block (first or second degree), junctional rhythms and pronounced sinus arrhythmia.

ERP may be present in more than 10 percent of the population. ERP is much more common in young individuals, and it is more common in males (Huang and Birnbaum, 2011; Pollak and Brady, 2012; Klatsky et al., 2003). We should be cautious in suggesting the diagnosis of ERP in patients older than age 50.

The mechanism of ERP is, surprisingly, unclear. The ST-segment elevations may represent "nonhomogeneous repolarization of the ventricles," with an imbalance in repolarization between the epicardium and endocardium or among different anatomic regions of the heart (Huston et al., 1985; Eastaugh, 1985). Increased parasympathetic tone probably plays a causative role. "Early repolarization" has never been proven, but the name persists (Huang and Birnbaum, 2011).

The ST-segment elevations of ERP most commonly appear in the anterior precordial leads, especially leads V3 and V4. In 30–50 percent of cases, similar ST-segment elevations may be present in the inferior limb leads. However, ST-segment elevations restricted to the inferior leads alone is not common in ERP and must be considered suspicious of an acute coronary syndrome or another etiology. Most importantly, ERP causes prominent ST-elevations but does not cause reciprocal ST-segment depressions.

## Is Early Repolarization Always "Benign"?

The traditional name "benign early repolarization" implied that the condition has no prognostic significance. Indeed, ERP is more common in young persons, overlaps with the "athletic heart syndrome" and has always been considered a sign of good health (Adler et al., 2013). ERP is more common in individuals younger than age 40 who are physically active (Klatsky et al., 2003).

In recent years, the view that "early repolarization" is always "benign" has changed (Patton et al., 2016; Antzelevitch et al., 2017). Large epidemiologic studies (as well as case reports) have suggested that some patients with this pattern – especially those with ST-segment elevations involving the inferior, as well as the anterior, leads – carry a higher risk of sudden cardiac death due to ventricular fibrillation (VF), even in the absence of other structural heart disease (Wu et al., 2013; Tikkanen, 2009; Adler et al., 2013). Patients with more "horizontal" or "descending" (as opposed to "ascending") ST-segment elevations and patients with greater J-point elevation (≥ 2 mm), especially in multiple leads, may also be at higher risk of sudden VF (Rosso et al., 2008; Wu et al., 2013; Huang and Birnbaum, 2011; Tikkanen et al., 2009; Antzelevitch et al., 2011; Antzelevitch et al., 2017; Patton et al., 2016; Benito et al., 2010).

Whether the association between the ERP pattern and malignant ventricular arrhythmias is causal, and whether this observation should affect clinical decision-making, is unclear (Adler et al., 2013). The overall risk of a malignant ventricular arrhythmia in asymptomatic, healthy patients with the incidental finding of ERP is low. Possibly, the finding of early repolarization changes involving both the anterior and inferior leads has greater significance in patients who present with syncope, those with a family history of sudden cardiac death, those with coronary or other structural heart disease, those with a prolonged QT interval, or those resuscitated from out-of-hospital cardiac arrest. Patients who present with syncope should always be asked whether there is a family history of SCD, and this certainly applies to patients whose ECG demonstrates early repolarization.

Some investigators have proposed the term "J-wave syndrome" in view of the higher risk associated when the early repolarization pattern is present in multiple leads. When the ECG demonstrates marked J-point elevation, and especially if the elevated ST-segments are horizontal or downsloping (rather than steeply upsloping), it may even represent a variation of the Brugada syndrome and carry similar arrhythmogenic risks (Benito et al., 2010; Antzelevitch et al., 2011; Antzelevitch et al., 2017; Patton et al., 2016). Indeed, there is a growing consensus that the J-wave syndromes (including Brugada as well as some high-risk early repolarization patterns) have similar ECG patterns, genetic substrates and arrhythmogenicity.

## Early Repolarization Pattern and Other Healthy Heart Patterns

The early repolarization pattern probably overlaps with other normal juvenile patterns (Huang and Birnbaum, 2011). In particular, young athletes often have anterior precordial ST-elevations that are indistinguishable from ERP. The ERP pattern in healthy athletes likely represents a state of increased parasympathetic tone. The common features of the athletic heart syndrome, including resting sinus bradycardia, sinus arrhythmia, first- or second-degree AV block and, of course, diffuse ST-segment elevations (with J-point elevations and tall T-waves), are also features of ERP. Classically in these patients, the J-point and ST-segment elevations, and the prolonged PR-segment, revert to normal during exercise (Somers et al., 2002; Goldberger, 1980).

Review ECG 7.1, which illustrates classic features of ERP.

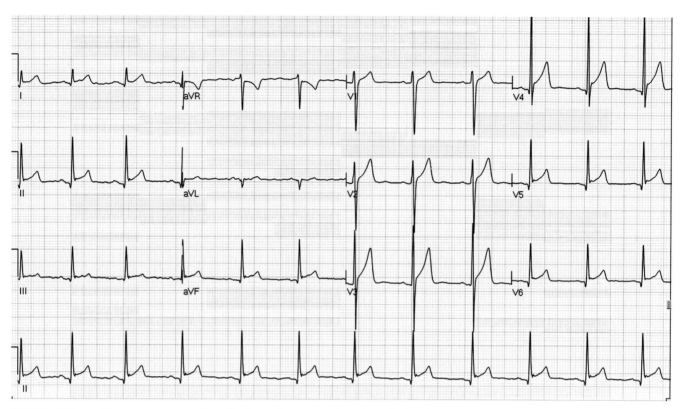

**ECG 7.1** A 25-year-old man was transported from the airport after a syncopal episode. He had no chest pain or dyspnea. A "cardiac alert" was called by the paramedics because of the ST-elevations on the prehospital ECG.

## The Electrocardiogram

The ECG is consistent with early repolarization. There are diffuse precordial and inferior wall ST-segment elevations with preservation of the normal upward concavity and prominent, upright T-waves. A prominent J-point notch (the "fish hook") is present in several leads, including lead V4. The ST-segment elevations are upsloping. There is no anatomic or regional pattern, and there are no worrisome reciprocal ST-segment depressions. There is slight PR-segment depression, which occurs in ERP, albeit less often than in acute pericarditis.

## Clinical Course

The patient underwent a thorough evaluation for dizziness and near-syncope and was discharged from the emergency department. What is unknown in a patient with a complaint of syncope and an ECG that demonstrates ERP involving the precordial and limb leads is whether additional evaluation is needed. At the very least, it is prudent to inquire about prior syncopal episodes or a family history of sudden death.

## Acute Pericarditis (Myopericarditis)

In textbooks, it is easy to recognize the patient with acute pericarditis: he or she is young and healthy and has chest pain that is sharp, pleuritic and positional (improved by sitting up and leaning forward). More often than not, there is a preceding cough or febrile illness. And careful auscultation reveals a one-, two- or three-component pericardial friction rub (LeWinter, 2014; Demangone, 2006).

But in actual clinical practice, acute pericarditis can resemble acute coronary syndromes. The patient may be young or old. Shortness of breath is common. Diaphoresis may be present. The pain of pericarditis may be heavy, pressure-like or squeezing, and occasionally, the pain may radiate to the arms (Spodick, 2003). And in both conditions, the troponin levels may be elevated on presentation. In pericarditis, troponin elevations reflect subepicardial myocarditis (myopericarditis) (Nable and Lawner, 2015; Pollak and Brady, 2012). For these reasons, the ECG plays a critical role in differentiating pericarditis from ACS or other significant cardiorespiratory emergencies.

Here are the most common ECG findings in patients with acute pericarditis (Huang and Birnbaum, 2011; Nable and Lawner, 2015; Demangone, 2006). Because the pericardium is electrically silent, these changes reflect inflammation of the subpericardial myocardium (Pollak and Brady, 2012). Sometimes, pericarditis occurs without significant inflammation of the epicardium; one example is uremic pericarditis. In these cases, there is little if any alteration of the ECG (Rutsky and Rostand, 1989; Huang and Birnbaum, 2011).

### ECG Findings of Acute Pericarditis

- Global ST-segment elevations

  - Without a regional (coronary anatomic) pattern or reciprocal ST-segment depressions (except in aVR and V1).

  - Typically seen in all leads except aVR and V1 (leads that do not directly face epicardial surfaces).

  - Often most prominent in leads V5–V6 and limb leads II, III and aVF.

  - The normal upward concavity of the ST-elevations is usually preserved.

  - The ST-segment elevations typically do not exceed 5 mm.

- PR-segment depressions

  - These reflect sub-epicardial atrial injury or atrial repolarization abnormalities and are most common in lead II (also common in III, aVF and V4–V6).

  - Usually, the PR-segment is elevated in aVR and V1.

- T-waves

  - The T-waves are often small or "humble," especially when compared to the height of the elevated ST-segments.

  - In lead V6, an ST-segment amplitude: T-wave amplitude ratio ≥ 0.25 usually indicates pericarditis, not ERP.

  - The T-waves remain upright while the ST-segments are elevated, helping to distinguish acute pericarditis from a STEMI.

  - The T-waves often become inverted later, sometimes over hours or days but usually after normalization of the ST-segments.

As many as two-thirds of patients presenting with uncomplicated pericarditis have a small *pericardial effusion*. Larger effusions are less common (LeWinter, 2014). If there is a large pericardial effusion, other distinctive ECG changes may appear, including low-amplitude QRS complexes and electrical alternans. See Chapter 5 for additional discussion.

Severe *myocarditis* is often heralded by low-amplitude QRS complexes, sinus tachycardia, conduction system delays and ST-T-wave changes, including regional ST-segment elevations that may mimic an acute STEMI (Pollak and Brady, 2012). These were reviewed in Chapter 5, The Electrocardiography of Shortness of Breath.

## PR-Segment Depression

PR-segment depression in all leads except aVR and V1 is a common finding in acute pericarditis. The PR-segment is usually elevated in lead aVR. In contrast, PR-segment depression is uncommon in acute STEMI, although it can occur as a reflection of atrial infarction. PR-segment depression also occurs commonly in ERP, although it is usually less marked than in pericarditis. PR-segment depression may also be seen in various tachycardias (for example, sinus tachycardia and ectopic atrial tachycardias) and other high-catecholamine states.

This patient's chest pain was due to postoperative pericarditis. While the diagnosis cannot be confirmed solely from this lead II rhythm strip, he has striking PR-segment depression.

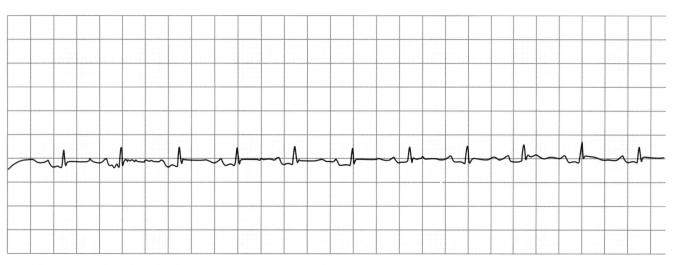

**ECG 7.2** A postoperative patient who developed chest pain and tachycardia.

235

## Complications of Acute Pericarditis and the Importance of Risk Stratification

Acute pericarditis may be complicated by atrial fibrillation or atrial tachycardias. However, acute pericarditis is seldom complicated by malignant ventricular tachycardias or conduction system delays unless there is underlying cardiac disease *or unless myocarditis is also present* (Spodick, 1976; Lange and Hillis, 2004).

Troponin elevations are common (occurring in at least 30 percent of cases of acute pericarditis) and usually represent myopericarditis. It is the accompanying myocarditis that presents a risk. Life-threatening arrhythmias and left ventricular dysfunction are the feared complications of myocarditis or myopericarditis, and these are most closely associated with wall motion abnormalities and cardiac enlargement on echocardiography.

High-risk pericarditis patients include those with fever, a subacute onset (over weeks), a large pericardial effusion or signs of pericardial tamponade, trauma, abnormal left ventricular wall motion, use of anticoagulants and those who are immunocompromised (Lange and Hillis, 2004; Imazio et al., 2007; Imazio et al., 2010). Elevated troponin levels and radiographic evidence of cardiac enlargement may also help select high-risk patients who require same-day echocardiography.

When faced with the patient, young or old, with clinical and electrocardiographic signs of pericarditis, the key questions are: Is the heart enlarged? Is left ventricular dysfunction (myocarditis) present? Is there evidence of a pericardial effusion or tamponade? For these reasons, emergent or urgent echocardiogram is recommended in all patients presenting with acute pericarditis (Spodick, 1976; LeWinter, 2014; Klein et al., 2013; Cheitlin et al., 2003). Acute myocarditis can have a fulminant course. (See Chapter 5, The Electrocardiography of Shortness of Breath.)

## Acute Pericarditis versus ST-Elevation Myocardial Infarction

The most important feature that differentiates acute STEMI versus acute pericarditis in a patient with chest pain and ST-segment elevations is the *regional (anatomic) pattern*. That is, in patients with STEMI, the ST-segment elevations usually correspond to a single coronary artery distribution, and there are ST-segment depressions in the opposite-facing leads.

In contrast, the ST-segment elevations in pericarditis are generalized and typically involve most of the precordial and limb leads. The only "reciprocal" ECG changes in pericarditis are in leads aVR and V1, where ST-segment depressions and PR-segment elevations are commonly seen. In addition, the ST-segment elevations in acute pericarditis usually do not exceed 5 mm, and they usually maintain their normal smooth, upward concavity.

Emergency clinicians should also examine the T-waves, PR-segments and QT interval:

- In patients with acute STEMI, it is common to see ST-segment elevations and T-wave inversions in the same leads on the same tracing. This rarely occurs in acute pericarditis, as the T-waves typically do not become inverted for one or more days. In acute pericarditis, the ST- and PR-segments usually normalize before T-wave inversion is seen.

- Tall, broad, bulky or "hyper-acute" T-waves should always raise concern for STEMI rather than acute pericarditis. In pericarditis, the T-waves are relatively "humble" relative to the ST-segment elevations. T-waves that "tower over" the R-waves in multiple precordial leads are likely to be "hyperacute," signaling an acute STEMI.

- PR-segment depressions are much more common in acute pericarditis, although they may occur in patients with acute myocardial infarction in the presence of atrial infarction.

- QT-prolongation also favors acute STEMI.

- The ST-T wave changes of acute STEMI evolve much more rapidly than the ST-T-wave changes of acute pericarditis.

A caveat: on rare occasions, an acute STEMI may involve the anterior and precordial leads. As discussed in Chapters 2 and 3, occlusion of a long "wraparound" LAD can result in a simultaneous ST-segment elevations in the anterior and inferior leads, which at times may resemble the global ST-segment elevations of pericarditis. As always, serial ECG tracings and echocardiography may be diagnostic.

## Early Repolarization versus Pericarditis

It is not always possible to differentiate ERP from pericarditis, absent a clear and compelling history or a pericardial friction rub. However, clues are often present:

- As noted earlier, PR-segment depression can occur in both conditions, although it is more marked and more frequent in acute pericarditis (Wang et al., 2003; Spodick, 1976 [NEJM]).

- The ECG pattern of ERP tends to remain stable over time (although, as noted earlier, the ST-elevations and J-point elevation may fluctuate with the patient's heart rate and autonomic nervous system balance, and the entire ERP pattern may disappear over a period of years).

- Acute pericarditis almost always causes "global" ST-segment elevations, involving the precordial and limb leads equally. As noted earlier, the ST-segment elevations of ERP are usually widespread in the precordial leads, while they spare the limb leads in more than half of all cases.

- The T-waves in ERP are unusually tall, and they may even appear peaked. In pericarditis, the T-waves are not so prominent; as noted earlier, they often appear "humble" relative to the elevated ST-segments. Later in the evolution of acute pericarditis (over a variable period of hours to days), the T-waves typically become inverted. In 1982, a paper was published in *Circulation* suggesting that the ratio of the ST-segment amplitude to the T-wave amplitude in lead V6 may help distinguish ERP from pericarditis. If the ST:T-wave ratio is $\geq 0.25$, the diagnosis of pericarditis is virtually certain (with a positive and negative predictive value both, reportedly, of 100 percent (Ginzton and Laks, 1982)).

- ERP is also more likely when there is sinus bradycardia or even AV block, reflecting heightened vagal tone (which may have a causal role).

The following ECG tracing has abnormal ST-segment elevations. Which is more likely – acute STEMI, pericarditis or ERP?

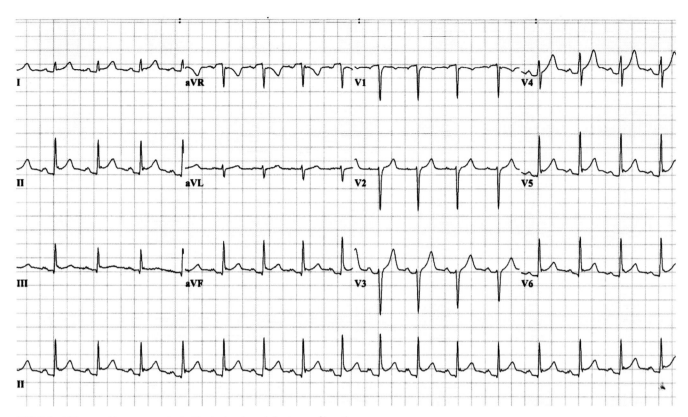

**ECG 7.3** A 33-year-old man presented with chest pain and shortness of breath.

## The Electrocardiogram

The ECG shows classic findings of acute pericarditis. There are global, concave-upward ST-segment elevations involving the precordial and limb leads. The T-wave is upright but is relatively small in lead V6 (the ratio of the ST-segment height: T-wave amplitude is greater than 0.25); this makes the diagnosis of pericarditis much more likely than ERP. And there is marked PR-segment depression in lead II and in other leads, accompanied by the expected PR-segment elevation in leads aVR and V1.

There is no localized, regional pattern to the ST-segment elevations, and there are no reciprocal ST-segment depressions (except for aVR and V1). Thus, acute STEMI is highly unlikely.

## Early Repolarization versus Subtle Anterior STEMI

ST-segment elevations in the anterior precordial leads are characteristic of BER. But they are also characteristic of acute anterior wall STEMI. How do we tell one from the other?

In a widely cited article, Smith et al. described 171 emergency department chest pain patients with ERP and 143 patients with subtle, nonobvious anterior wall STEMI (Smith et al., 2012). When the ECGs were compared, a single (albeit complex) equation was derived that accurately predicted an anterior wall STEMI: [1.196 × ST-segment elevation 60 msec after the J-point in lead V3 in mm] + [0.059 × QTc in msec] – [0.326 × R-wave amplitude in lead V4 in mm]. If the value of this equation was ≥ 23.4, it predicted anterior wall STEMI with strong test characteristics. Importantly, *J-point elevation, notching, T-wave amplitude and upward concavity of the ST-segments did not help in distinguishing ERP from STEMI.*

Online calculators are now available to help clinicians diagnose subtle anterior STEMI and differentiate STEMI from ERP. These electrocardiographic predictors could also be incorporated into the ECG computer algorithms. However, the bottom line is that, in patients with anterior wall ST-segment elevations, an acute STEMI is more likely if the R-wave amplitude is lower, the ST-segment elevation is higher, and the QTc is longer.

As always, diagnostic accuracy is aided by comparing the presenting to ECG to baseline tracings, obtaining serial ECGs and performing echocardiography.

Here is an example. Does this patient have ERP, acute pericarditis or an acute anterior STEMI?

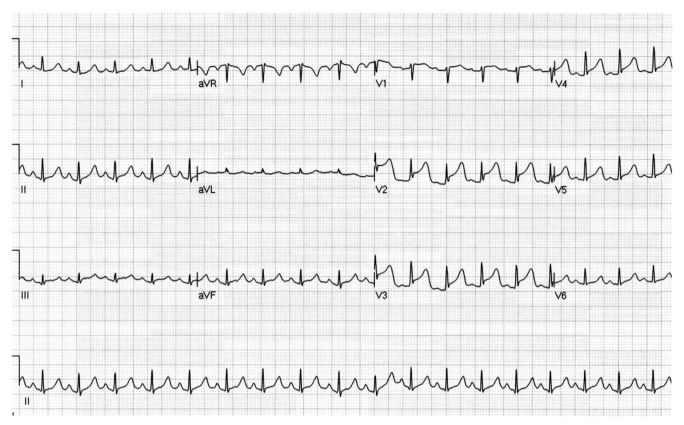

**ECG 7.4** A 43-year-old woman with a history of hypertension and hyperlipidemia presented with substernal chest pain, nausea and shortness of breath over the prior 2–3 days. Her blood pressure in the emergency department was 108/78.

## The Electrocardiogram

The patient presented with a compelling history, accompanied by hypotension. Her 12-lead ECG is compelling as well. There is sinus tachycardia. Also, the ECG demonstrates obvious ST-segment elevations in the anterior precordial leads (V2, V3 and V4), consistent with acute anteroseptal STEMI.

However, the QRS amplitude is low in the limb and precordial leads; combined with sinus tachycardia, this raises acute myocarditis as a possibility. To add to the confusion, there is PR-segment depression in numerous leads, which could indicate acute pericarditis (although PR-segment depression is also seen in the setting of a STEMI, attributed to atrial infarction).

Furthermore, can we exclude ERP, in light of the precordial lead ST-segment elevations? After all, the upward concavity of the ST-elevations is preserved, and there is marked J-point elevation with a "fish-hook" notch (for example, in V2, V3 and V4).

What is her diagnosis?

She has an acute anterior wall STEMI. The ST-segment elevations are regional, found almost exclusively in the territory of the LAD (precordial leads V2–V4). True, the ST-segment elevations in V2–V4 are concave upward, and there is even notching and J-point elevation; but as emphasized repeatedly, these features do not rule out acute STEMI. In addition, the ST-segment elevations are relatively dramatic

when compared with the modest amplitude of the precordial lead QRS complexes.

This particular STEMI is not so subtle, so we may not need to deploy the Smith equation. Nonetheless, if we measure the R-wave amplitude in V4, the QTc and the height of the ST-segment in V3 and deploy the Smith equation, the result is ≥ 29, indicative of a STEMI.

## Clinical Course

This patient was taken immediately to the catheterization laboratory, where (not surprisingly) the LAD was totally obstructed in the middle segment. Normal flow was restored by percutaneous coronary angioplasty.

## Left Ventricular Hypertrophy

The electrocardiographic features of left ventricular hypertrophy (LVH) were discussed extensively in Chapter 6. On the ECG, LVH is likely in the presence of high-amplitude R-waves in the left-facing leads (I, aVL, V5 and V6) and deep S-waves in the right-sided leads. LVH is usually accompanied by repolarization abnormalities (the "strain" pattern): gradually descending ST-segment depressions are present in the left-sided leads, accompanied by asymmetric T-wave inversions. There are several supporting ECG criteria for LVH: (a) poor R-wave progression, (b) QRS widening, (c) left axis deviation and (d) left atrial enlargement (Pollak and Brady, 2012).

Chapter 6 included a detailed discussion of "LVH with repolarization abnormalities" because the ST-T-wave changes in the left-facing leads must be differentiated from other causes of ST-segment depressions and T-wave inversions, especially an acute coronary syndrome. ST-segment depressions may be reciprocal to an acute STEMI, or they may represent subendocardial ischemia (unstable angina or a non-STEMI).

This chapter has focused on ST-segment elevations that are not caused by an acute STEMI. There is a good reason to include LVH. Many patients who have electrocardiographic signs of LVH *also have ST-segment elevations in the right precordial leads* that can be indistinguishable from the current of injury of an acute anterior wall STEMI (Armstrong et al., 2012). The ST-segment elevations in the right precordial leads are a normal and expected finding in LVH; they likely represent a reciprocal change to the ST-segment depressions in V5 and V6. When the hypertrophied LV rotates leftward and posteriorly, the anterior precordial leads V1–V3 actually become "reciprocal" to V5 and V6 (Huang and Birnbaum, 2011; Pollak and Brady, 2012).

Unlike the ST-elevations of an evolving acute STEMI, the ST-segment and T-wave changes of LVH remain relatively fixed over time (although changes in lead placement and other factors can lead to changes in the 12-lead ECG). Thus, serial ECGs may prove invaluable. Still, the right precordial ST-segment elevations of LVH are a common reason for false-positive STEMI diagnoses, often resulting in unnecessary reperfusion interventions (Nable and Lawner, 2015; McCabe et al., 2012; Armstrong et al., 2012).

In LVH, the elevated ST-segments often retain a smooth, upwardly concave and benign-looking contour. But not always. The ST-segment elevations in leads V2 and V3 can look ominous, exactly like Wellens' syndrome. Examples were provided in Chapter 6.

LVH with repolarization abnormalities is often so readily apparent on the 12-lead ECG that it prevents us from making other critical diagnoses. For example, Chapter 2, Inferior Wall Myocardial Infarction, included two examples of inferior wall STEMIs that were missed. Inferior wall STEMIs may be missed if the clinicians (and the computer) became so distracted by the diagnosis of LVH with strain that they never examine the rest of the ECG.

## Left Bundle Branch Block

ST-segment deviations (elevations and depressions) are routine in left bundle branch block (LBBB). Usually, in LBBB, the ST-segments and T-waves are displaced in a "discordant" direction; that is, they deviate in a direction that is opposite to the main deflection of the QRS complex (Rautaharju et al., 2009). In contrast, in acute ischemia or infarction, the ST-segments tend to deviate "concordantly" with the main direction of the QRS complex (Huang and Birnbaum, 2011).

When LBBB is present, the QRS complex in the right precordial leads is mostly directed in a negative direction. Therefore, the ST-segments are routinely elevated when LBBB is present; this is a normal, nonischemic "secondary" ST-segment deviation. Obviously, these ST-segment elevations,

which can be marked, can masquerade as, or can hide, an acute anterior wall STEMI.

National guidelines no longer recommend emergent reperfusion in every patient with a LBBB who presents with chest pain or similar symptoms. In fact, only a minority of such patients will have an acute STEMI (Nable and Lawner, 2015; O'Gara et al., 2013; Lawner and Nable, 2012). Serial ECG tracings, serial cardiac enzyme measurements and echocardiography may help in confirming or excluding the diagnosis of acute STEMI.

In addition, in many cases, acute anterior wall STEMI may be differentiated from the secondary ST-segment elevations of the LBBB by applying the Sgarbossa criteria. In patients with a LBBB (whether new, old or unknown) who present with chest pain or other symptoms suggesting an acute coronary syndrome, an evolving anterior wall STEMI is more likely if (a) there is ST-segment elevation ($\geq 1$ mm) in any lead in a direction *concordant* with the QRS complex (5 points); (b) there is ST-segment depression ($\geq 1$ mm) in precordial leads V1, V2 or V3 (3 points); or (c) there is extreme ST-segment elevation ($\geq 5$ mm) in any lead that is *discordant* to the QRS complex (2 points).

According to a 2008 meta-analysis by Tabas et al., a Sgarbossa score of 3 or more (indicating at least 1 mm of concordant ST-segment elevation or 1 mm of ST-segment depression in precordial leads V1–V3) is highly specific for STEMI. However, a Sgarbossa score of 2 ($\geq 5$ mm of discordant ST-segment elevation) is not specific (Tabas et al., 2008).

Importantly, the Sgarbossa algorithm is not sensitive enough to exclude the diagnosis of STEMI (Huang and Birnbaum, 2011; Sgarbossa, 1996; Nable and Lawner, 2015; Lawner and Nable, 2012; Pollak and Brady, 2012; Tabas et al., 2008). Even a Sgarbossa score of 0 has a low sensitivity and negative likelihood ratio and cannot be used to rule out myocardial infarction (Tabas et al., 2008).

Studies also suggest that the same Sgarbossa criteria (with similarly poor sensitivity but moderate specificity) may be applied to help in the diagnosis of acute STEMI where the ECG is confounded by the presence of a right ventricular pacemaker (Lawner and Nable, 2012; Pollak and Brady, 2012).

Right bundle branch block (RBBB) does not significantly distort the ST-segment; therefore, RBBB is less likely to obscure the diagnosis of a STEMI. Nonetheless, STEMIs may be missed in the presence of RBBB, as highlighted in Chapter 2, Inferior Wall Myocardial Infarction.

## Hypothermia

The ECG can provide valuable clues to hypothermia (Solomon et al., 1988; Salinsky and Worrilow, 2014; Vassallo et al., 1999; Mustafa et al., 2005). Depending on the patient's core temperature, the ECG may demonstrate muscle tremor or shivering artifacts. Dysrhythmias are common, especially slow atrial fibrillation, sinus bradycardia and ectopic atrial or junctional rhythms. QRS widening may occur, and often, the PR and QT intervals are also prolonged. Ventricular ectopy and ventricular fibrillation may occur.

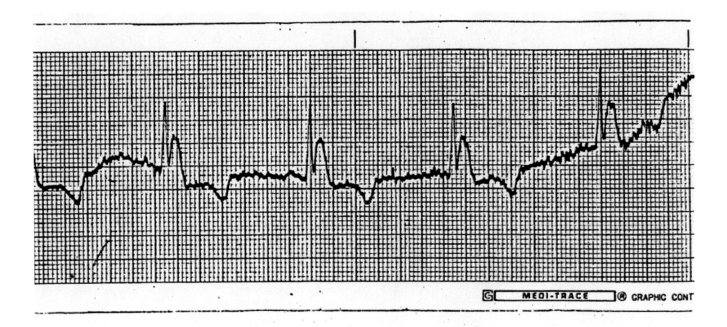

**ECG 7.5**  Rhythm strip from a patient with severe hypothermia

Most famously, a "J-wave of Osborn" may appear. The Osborn wave (or "camel hump") was originally described in 1953 as "a secondary wave following the S-wave so closely that it appears to be part of the QRS complex" (Osborn, 1953). Indeed, Osborn waves may be small, subtle upticks in the terminal portion of the S-wave, or they may be almost as tall as the R-wave, masquerading as bundle branch blocks, the Brugada pattern or even an acute STEMI (Salinsky and Worrilow, 2014).

Some (but not all) studies suggest that the height of the Osborn wave correlates with the degree of hypothermia; the Osborn wave does diminish with core rewarming. Physiologic studies suggest that the Osborn wave in hypothermia may result from an "increase in the epicardial potassium current, relative to the current in the endocardium during ventricular repolarization" (Krantz and Lowery, 2005).

An important point for the emergency or critical care electrocardiographer is that Osborn waves may resemble ST-segment elevations caused by an acute STEMI or other conditions. Early recognition of severe hypothermia will facilitate careful rewarming of the patient before the development of conduction system disturbances or ventricular fibrillation.

ECG 7.5 should immediately suggest hypothermia.

## The Electrocardiogram

Profound bradycardia is present, along with shivering (or electrical) artifact. The rhythm strip also has classic Osborn waves – "secondary waves following the S-wave so closely that [they] appear to be part of the QRS complex." It is easy to see how large Osborn waves may be mistaken for ischemic ST-segment elevations or even a wide complex rhythm.

The following 12-lead ECG was also recorded on a patient with severe hypothermia.

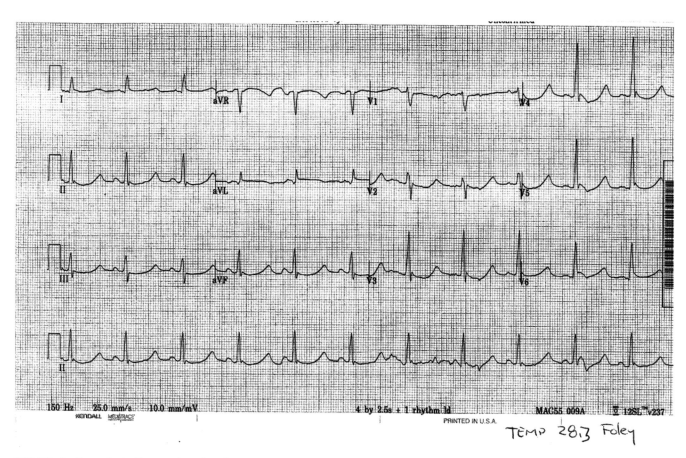

150 Hz    25.0 mm/s    10.0 mm/mV                                    4 by 2.5s + 1 rhythm ld                              MAC55 009A          12SL™ v237
KENDALL MEDITRACE                                                    PRINTED IN U.S.A.

TEMP 28.3 Foley

**ECG 7.6** Another patient with severe hypothermia

## The Electrocardiogram

In this tracing, there are only minor upticks at the end of the QRS complex; nonetheless, these are Osborn waves. There is also marked prolongation of the QTc internal. As noted on the bottom of the 12-lead ECG, this patient had severe hypothermia.

## Left Ventricular Aneurysm

Left ventricular aneurysms typically develop within 2 weeks after an anterior wall STEMI; they are less common after inferior wall STEMIs (Nable and Lawner, 2015). ST-segment elevations that persist more than 3 weeks following a STEMI suggest that ventricular dilatation and remodeling have occurred and that a left ventricular aneurysm is present (Pollak and Brady, 2012). The ST-elevations may mimic an acute STEMI (Meizlish et al., 1984; Huang and Birnbaum, 2011). Q-waves are also present in most cases.

## Takotsubo Cardiomyopathy (Apical Ballooning Syndrome)

Takotsubo cardiomyopathy is an interesting syndrome, characterized by a constellation of findings: chest pain as a presenting symptom, regional ST-segment elevations on the ECG and

troponin elevations. Frequently, T-wave inversions appear on the initial ECG or within hours of presentation (Kosuge and Kimura, 2014; Pelliccia et al., 2014; Nable and Lawner, 2015; Kurisu and Kihara, 2012; Sanchez-Jimenez, 2013).

Patients with takotsubo cardiomyopathy may present with chest pain that is severe, sometimes accompanied by syncope, dyspnea or signs of congestive heart failure or shock. Malignant ventricular arrhythmias may also occur (Pollak and Brady, 2012).

A variety of ECG features have been reported in patients with takotsubo cardiomyopathy. The ECG features are highly variable, depending upon the extent of left ventricular dysfunction and the time between symptom onset and presentation (Kosuge and Kimura, 2014; Kurisu and Kihara, 2012). Usually, patients present with localized (especially precordial lead) ST-segment elevations on their initial ECG *that are indistinguishable from acute STEMI* (Kosuge and Kimura, 2014; Nable and Lawner, 2015; Pollak and Brady, 2012; Kirusu, 2012; Sanchez-Jimenez, 2013). Not surprisingly, and especially given the troponin elevations, they will usually meet "cath-lab activation" or "emergent reperfusion" criteria (Senecal et al., 2011). When angiography is performed, it reveals ballooning of the apical segment along with akinesis or hyperkinesis in a variety of patterns. However, the angiogram reveals no culprit coronary artery obstructions.

241

Takotsubo cardiomyopathy, also referred to as the apical ballooning syndrome, stress cardiomyopathy or "broken heart" syndrome, is most common in postmenopausal women; the hallmark is a state of reversible myocardial ischemia and left ventricular dysfunction in the absence of a major coronary artery obstruction (Pelliccia et al., 2014; Kurisu and Kihara, 2012). Sometimes there is a discrete "trigger," such as psychological or physiological stress or an accumulation of repeated stresses. Catecholamine surges or neurologic or vasomotor triggers may be involved (Pelliccia et al., 2014; Nable and Lawner, 2015). Takotsubo cardiomyopathy is confirmed on cardiac echocardiography or angiography by the finding of apical ballooning, anterior and inferior hypokinesis or other classic wall motion abnormalities (Sanchez-Jimenez, 2013; Senecal et al., 2011; Pelliccia et al., 2014).

Examples of ST-segment elevations caused by takotsubo cardiomyopathy are included in the self-study ECGs in this chapter. Another case of takotsubo cardiomyopathy, manifesting deep T-wave inversions instead of ST-segment elevations, was presented in Chapter 6.

## Hyperkalemia

Widened QRS complexes, abnormally peaked T-waves and PR-segment prolongation (or absent P-waves indicating atrial asystole) are the hallmarks of hyperkalemia on the ECG. But striking ST-segment elevation may also occur, leading some to refer to hyperkalemia-induced ST-elevations using the old-fashioned term, "dialyzable current of injury" (Wang et al., 2003; Goldberger, 1980).

All emergency and critical care clinicians must be able to recognize hyperkalemia, and they must be confident enough to initiate lifesaving treatment based solely on the 12-lead ECG. Examples of hyperkalemia with ST-segment elevation are included in the self-study ECGs.

## Brugada Syndrome

The Brugada syndrome is not especially common. But, like arrhythmogenic right ventricular dysplasia (ARVD) and QT-prolongation, it is a relatively frequent cause of syncope and sudden cardiac death due to ventricular fibrillation. The Brugada syndrome and ARVD cause distinctive ECG abnormalities that must be recognized by emergency clinicians, especially when faced with young and apparently healthy patients who have had one or more syncopal episodes. As we noted in the Preface to this atlas, recognizing these ECG abnormalities in patients with syncope provides an opportunity to prevent sudden cardiac death.

The Brugada syndrome is a "sodium channelopathy," caused by one or more mutations to a sodium channel gene. The ECG is usually abnormal. The hallmark is the appearance of a right bundle branch block (or incomplete RBBB) *plus ST-segment elevation in one or more right precordial leads (V1–V3)* (Wagner and Strauss, 2014; Huang and Birnbaum, 2011; Nable

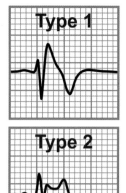

**Figure 7.2** The Brugada pattern.

and Lawner, 2015; Pollak and Brady, 2012; Veerakul and Nademanee, 2012).

Even if a distinct RBBB pattern is not present, the classic abnormality of a high takeoff of the ST-segment in lead V1 and V2 will usually be seen.

Depending on the shape of the ST-segment, the Brugada syndrome may be classified as Type 1 or Type 2 (or Type 3, which may be considered a hybrid of Types 1 and 2). Most distinct are Types 1 and 2 (see Figure 7.2):

- In Type 1 Brugada syndrome, the elevated ST-segment has a high take-off and emerges abruptly from the R or R' wave; then it immediately dives downward and terminates in an inverted T-wave.
- In Type 2 Brugada, the elevated ST-segment has a "saddle" appearance. The ST-segment is elevated with a mostly concave upward appearance (Nable and Lawner, 2015; Huang and Birnbaum, 2011; Pollak and Brady, 2012; Veerakul and Nademanee, 2012; Demangone, 2006).

The characteristic ST-elevations may come and go, especially if the sodium channelopathy is provoked by sodium channel blocking drugs.

Some patients with syncope or other symptoms may present with ECGs that are suggestive, but not diagnostic, of Brugada syndrome. The diagnostic yield may be increased by moving the right-sided precordial leads (V1, V2 and V3) to a higher position on the chest (in the third or second intercostal spaces), so that the exploring electrodes are more directly over the right ventricular outflow tract (RVOT). The RVOT is believed to be the arrhythmogenic site for the Brugada syndrome. In the electrophysiology laboratory, a procainamide challenge can also unmask Brugada and convert a borderline ECG into a classic Type 1 or Type 2 pattern (Veerakul and Nademanee, 2012).

See the following case for an example of the Brugada syndrome, which fooled the computer algorithm into suggesting "Acute MI."

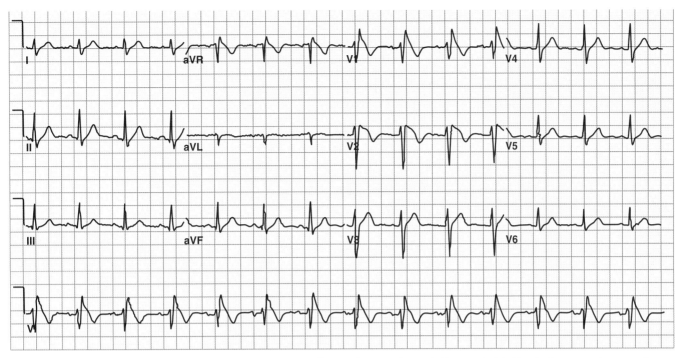

**ECG 7.7** A 57-year-old man was brought to the emergency department after a single syncopal episode. He was scheduled for elective surgery that same afternoon. The computer reading of the ECG was "normal sinus rhythm; incomplete right bundle branch block; ST-elevation anteriorly, cannot rule out acute anterior MI."

## The Electrocardiogram

Leads V1 and V2 represent a relatively common pseudo-infarct pattern – that is, a noncoronary cause of ST-segment elevation. Type 1 Brugada syndrome is present. The key features are: (a) an incomplete RBBB; (b) ST-segment elevation in V1 and V2 with a very high takeoff of the ST-segment from the R-wave (or R'-wave); and (c) a rapid, downwardly coved descent into an inverted T-wave.

## Clinical Course

Brugada syndrome places the patient at risk for syncope and sudden cardiac death. This patient had a family history of sudden cardiac death. His elective surgery was canceled, and he was referred for electrophysiologic testing and placement of an internal cardiac defibrillator.

## More Coronary Mimics: Tall T-Waves That Are *Not* Myocardial Infarction

The title of this chapter is "Confusing Conditions: ST-Segment Elevations and Tall T-Waves (Coronary Mimics)." Therefore, we need a separate discussion of the "prominent T-wave." These are T-waves, typically in the right precordial leads (V1–V3), that appear "tall," "peaked," "steepled," broad, bulky or, simply, "hyperacute." When a patient presents with chest pain, shortness of breath, dizziness, abdominal pain or other symptoms compatible with coronary insufficiency, the differential diagnosis of the prominent T-wave becomes critically important.

In normal, asymptomatic patients, the T-waves (which represent ventricular repolarization) should not exceed 0.5mV in the limb leads and 1.0 to 1.4 mV in the precordial leads; however, these upper limits vary with age, gender and race (Wagner and Strauss, 2014; Rautaharju et al., 2009). In normal adults, the T-wave amplitude is tallest (most positive) in precordial leads V2 and V3 (Rautaharju et al., 2009).

In symptomatic patients with tall, prominent T-waves leads in V1, V2, V3 and sometimes V4, the most important "rule out" diagnosis is anterior wall STEMI. However, in a 2002 review of "the prominent T-wave," Somers et al. began their discussion this way: "[There is] a large number of conditions in the differential diagnosis of prominent T-waves, including hyperkalemia, myocardial ischemia, left ventricular hypertrophy, benign early repolarization, bundle branch block, pericarditis, valvular heart disease, mitral stenosis, hemopericardium, ectopic ventricular rhythms, pacemaker rhythms, hypertrophic cardiomyopathy, Stokes-Adams episodes, cor pulmonale, central nervous system [hemorrhage], hyperthyroidism, exercise anemia, acidosis, and [even] tranylcypromine overdose" (Somers et al., 2002).

This list is long and unwieldy. Fortunately, Somers and others have correctly emphasized that it is wisest to focus on the hyperacute T-waves of early anterior wall STEMI plus three conditions that "most closely resemble the prominent T-waves of acute infarction": left ventricular hypertrophy, early repolarization and hyperkalemia (Somers et al., 2002; Goldberger, 1980; Nable and Lawner, 2015; Nikus et al., 2010; Birnbaum, 2014). LVH and ERP are common in patients with acute chest pain presenting to emergency departments. Somers et al. also advise that the term "hyperacute" should be reserved for the prominent T-waves that commonly appear in the early phases of anterior wall STEMI.

# Common Causes of Prominent T-Waves

*Hyperacute T-waves signaling acute anterior wall STEMI –* Prominent, large amplitude T-waves are one of the earliest ECG changes that may herald an acute ST-elevation myocardial infarction (Birnbaum, 2014; Nikus et al., 2010). Hyperacute T-waves occur early after left anterior descending artery (LAD) occlusion, often before the ST-segment is noticeably elevated. The hyperacute T-waves of early anterior wall STEMI can be tall and thin; or just as often, hyperacute T-waves may be broad and bulky with a splayed base. Often, unlike the peaked T-waves of hyperkalemia, the hyperacute T-waves of ACS are asymmetric (Somers et al., 2002; Nable and Lawner, 2015).

In symptomatic patients, increased amplitude of the T-waves may be the earliest warning sign of anterior wall STEMI. Most often, cardiac enzyme levels are not yet elevated, making recognition of the pattern of hyperacute T-waves even more critical. The hyperacute T-waves of acute STEMI are often associated with ST-segment straightening and QT-interval prolongation. But most importantly, these hyperacute T-waves are short-lived, evolving in minutes to hours into a more classic pattern of ST-segment elevation (Nikus et al., 2010). Refer to Chapter 3, Anterior Wall Myocardial Infarction, for further discussion and examples.

Chapter 3 also discusses a variation of hyperacute T-waves known as the "de Winter complex," which may signify occlusion of the left anterior descending artery or, at times, the left circumflex artery. The de Winter complex, found in the anterior precordial leads, stands out because it is more persistent than the classic, but transient, hyperacute T-waves seen in early STEMI. The de Winter pattern is characterized by ST-segment depressions at the J-point that are instantly upsloping and rapidly ascend into a tall, positive, "hyperacute" T-wave. ST-segment elevation is not present (Verouden et al., 2009; Birnbaum, 2014; de Winter et al., 2008; Lawner and Nable, et al., 2012).

## Hyperkalemia

The peaked T-waves of hyperkalemia tend to be tall, narrow and symmetric. Usually, the apex is pointed. As the serum potassium rises, more ominous ECG changes occur, especially QRS widening, PR prolongation, and diminution or complete loss of P-waves. ST-segment elevations can also appear in hyperkalemic patients, usually in combination with peaked T-waves and QRS widening (Pollak and Brady, 2012).

Of course, most patients with hyperkalemia do not present with chest pain. Emergency clinicians should recognize the patients most at risk for hyperkalemia, including those who have renal insufficiency or diabetes and those taking ACE inhibitors or beta-blocking drugs.

## Early Repolarization Pattern (ERP)

As described earlier in this chapter, ERP causes ST-segment elevations with an upward concavity that merges into a tall T-wave. This pattern is especially common in the precordial leads. Often, the J-point, which marks the end of the QRS complex and the start of the ST-segment, is notched.

## Left Ventricular Hypertrophy

The ECG findings of LVH were discussed earlier in this chapter and in Chapter 6. The characteristic ECG clues to LVH include: large amplitude R-waves in the leads facing the left ventricle (I, aVL, V5 and V6); deep S-waves in V1 and V2; characteristic ST-segment depressions in V5 and V6, associated with asymmetric T-wave inversions (the "strain" pattern); QRS widening; poor R-wave progression; left axis deviation; and left atrial enlargement. Leads V1 and V2 often demonstrate ST-segment elevation associated with tall T-waves.

When LVH causes right precordial ST-segment elevations and abnormally large amplitude T-waves, it may be impossible to distinguish these changes from acute anterior STEMI. As discussed in earlier chapters, comparison with old ECG tracings, serial ECGs and cardiac biomarkers and urgent echocardiography may help rule in or rule out acute myocardial infarction.

# Self-Study Electrocardiograms

**Case 7.1** A 53-year-old man presented with chest pain.

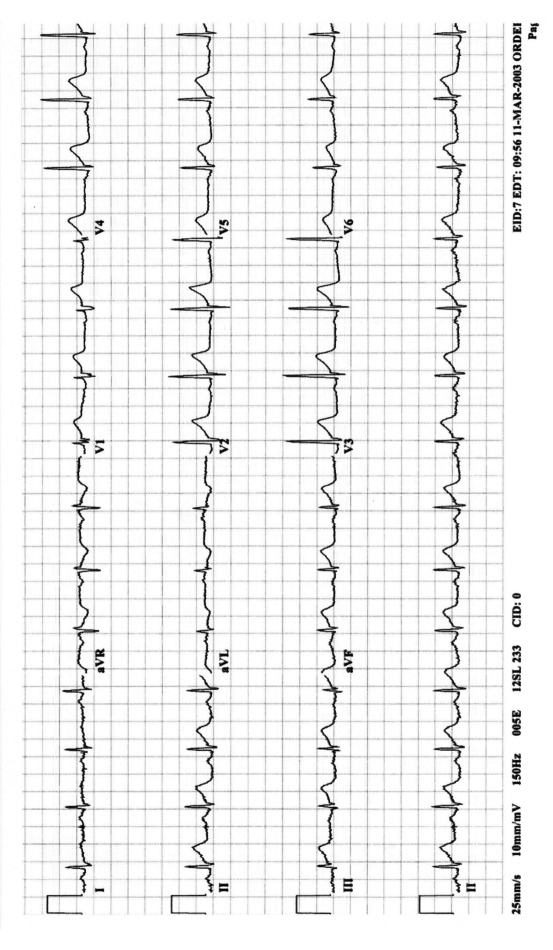

25mm/s    10mm/mV    150Hz    005E    12SL 233    CID: 0    EID:7 EDT: 09:56 11-MAR-2003 ORDEI

Pa<sub></sub>

**Case 7.2** A 19-year-old man presented with 1 hour of peri-umbilical pain and occasional diarrhea.

Male

Foom: W19

Opt:

| | | |
|---|---|---|
| Vent. rate | 44 | pbm |
| PR interval | 174 | ms |
| QRS duration | 116 | ms |
| QT/QTc | 474/405 | ms |
| P-R-T axes | 63 75 | 65 |

Techmician: 37646
Test ind: EVAL

Marked sinus bradycardia with marked sinus arrhythmia
ST elevation, consider anterolateral injury or acute infarct
ST elevation, consider inferior injury or acute infarct
** ** ACUTE MI ** **
Abnormal ECG

Order no: 119115857
Unconfirmed

Referred by:

Y:

Y:

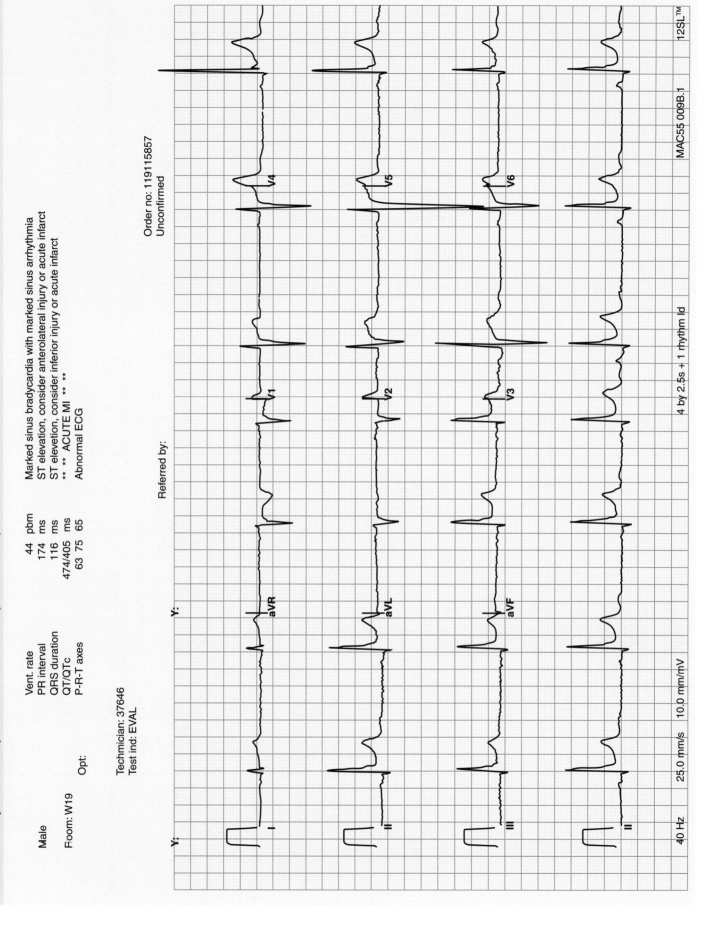

40 Hz    25.0 mm/s    10.0 mm/mV    4 by 2.5s + 1 rhythm ld    MAC55 009B.1    12SL™

**Case 7.3** A 22-year-old man was brought to the hospital after suffering a single syncopal episode. He had a history of chronic anxiety, posttraumatic stress disease and depression, and he reported frequent bouts of chest pain and palpitations.

Male    Unknown

Room:20
Loc:106

| | | |
|---|---|---|
| PR interval | 172 | ms |
| QRS duration | 96 | ms |
| QT/QTc | 464/467 | ms |
| P-R-T axes | 58  -24 | 11 |

ST elevation consider anterior injury or acute infarct
\* \* \* \* \* \* \* \* \* ACUTE MI \* \* \* \* \* \* \* \* \*

Abnormal ECG
When compared with ECG of 11:30.
No significant change was found

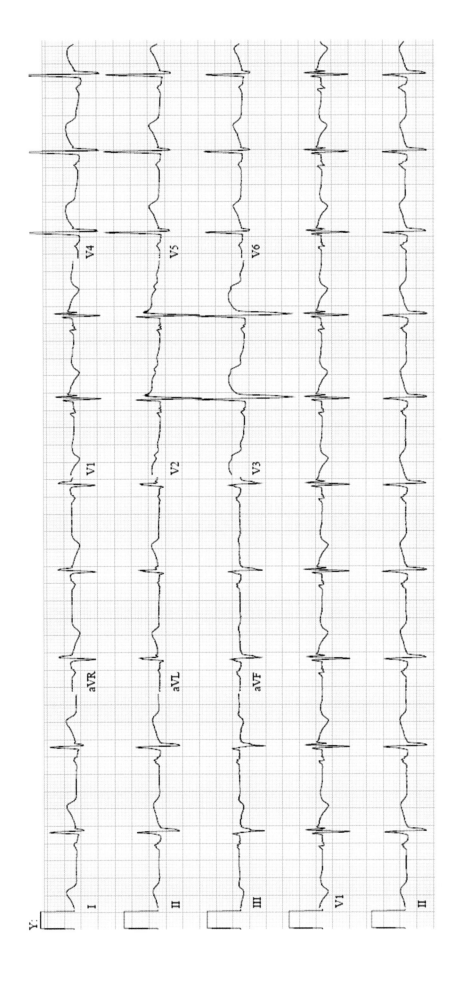

**Case 7.4** A 44-year-old man presented with chest pain and mild dyspnea.

**Case 7.5** A 21-year-old man with a history of asthma presented because of substernal chest discomfort. He had a cough and flulike illness over the past 2 days. His chest pain was not positional. He was afebrile on ED presentation. His initial troponin level was 2.65.

Male      Unknown

Room:371
Loc:1002

| | | |
|---|---|---|
| Vent. rate | 77 | BPM |
| PR interval | 154 | ms |
| QRS duration | 82 | ms |
| QT/QTc | 378/427 | ms |
| P-R-T axes | 8  78 | 52 |

Normal sinus rhythm
ST elevation consider inferolateral injury or acute infarct
**** ACUTE MI / STEMI ****
Abnormal ECG
No previous ECGs available

Technician:
Test ind:

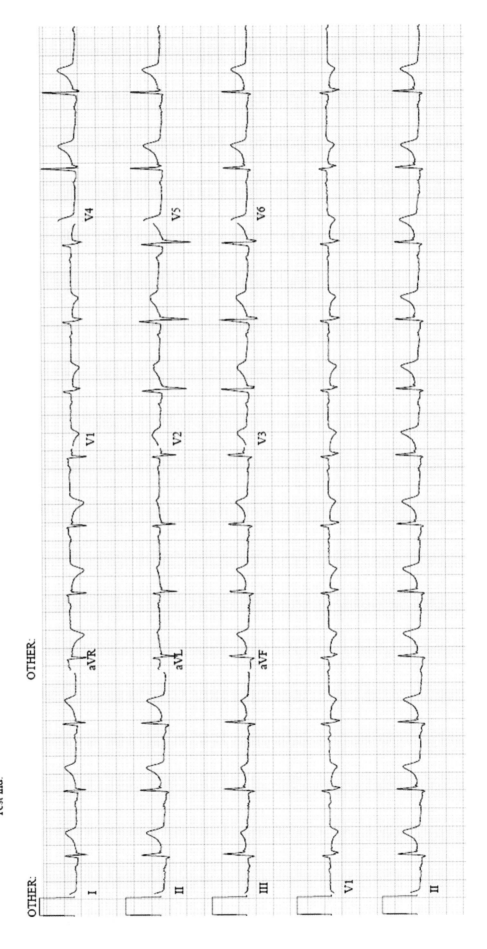

**Case 7.6** A 26-year-old man presented with chest pain. In the emergency department, he was smiling, alert and comfortable.

**Case 7.6 (Continued)** Same patient, 3 days later.

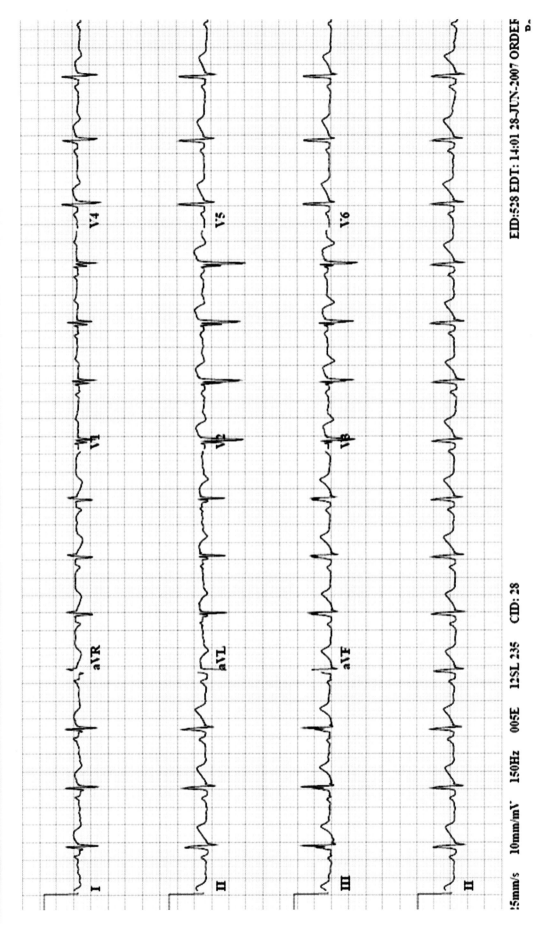

25mm/s    10mm/mV    150Hz    005E    12SL 235    CID: 28

EID:528 EDT: 14:01 28-JUN-2007 ORDER

**Case 7.7** A 25-year-old man was "found down" in a comatose state with twitching eyes. His history included diabetes and alcoholism. On presentation to the emergency department, he was hypotensive. His finger stick glucose was markedly elevated.

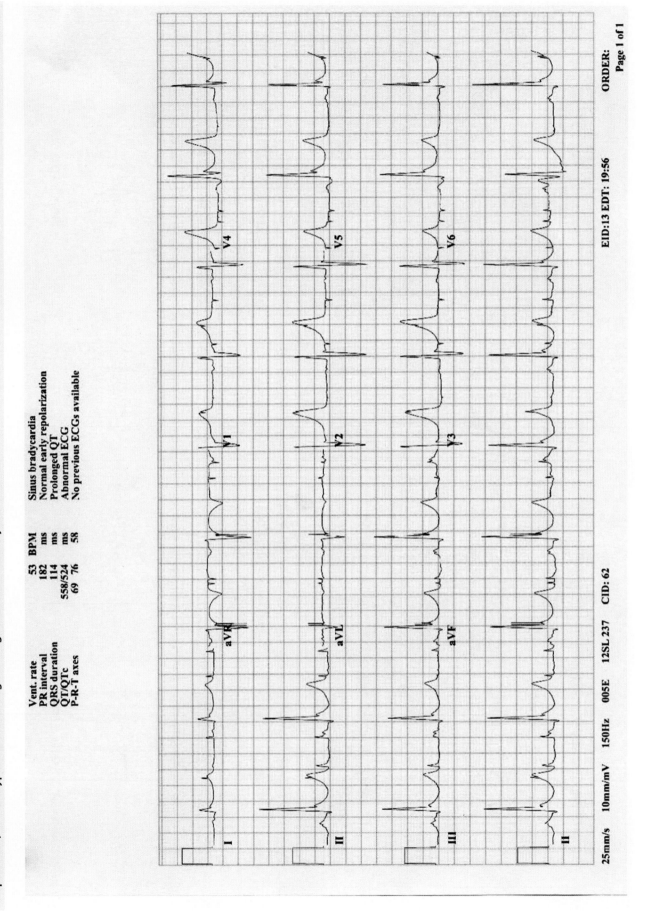

| Vent. rate | 53 | BPM | Sinus bradycardia |
| PR interval | 182 | ms | Normal early repolarization |
| QRS duration | 114 | ms | Prolonged QT |
| QT/QTc | 558/524 | ms | Abnormal ECG |
| P-R-T axes | 69 76 | 58 | No previous ECGs available |

25mm/s    10mm/mV    150Hz    005E    12SL 237    CID: 62    EID:13 EDT: 19:56    ORDER:

Page 1 of 1

**Case 7.8** A 41-year-old man presented with 2 days of heavy alcohol consumption and intermittent chest pain that radiated to his entire body.

**Case 7.9** A 27-year-old man presented after a bout of dizziness and near-syncope.

Male      Black

Room: W31

Opt:

PR interval            158   ms
QRS duration           98    ms
QT/QTc          338/406   ms
P-R-T axes       69  −9   49

ST elevation, consider anterolateral injury or acute infarct
** ** ACUTE MI ** **
Abnormal ECG

Techmician: 48140
Test ind:

Referred by:

Order no: 259595718
Unconfirmed

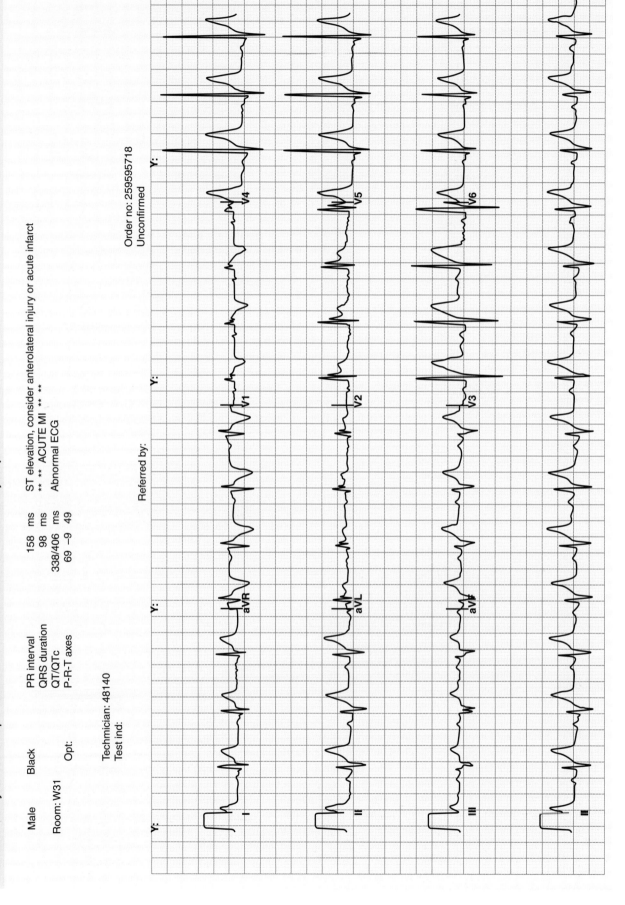

**Case 7.10** A 31-year-old man with hypertension, insulin-dependent diabetes and chronic gastroparesis presented with several hours of abdominal pain.

**Case 7.11** A 60-year-old man with a history of diabetes and hyperlipidemia presented with 1 hour of substernal chest pain. His initial serum troponin level was 0.01.

**Case 7.11 (Continued)** Same patient – baseline ECG (2 years earlier).

# Self-Study Electrocardiograms

## Case 7.1  A 53-year-old man presented with chest pain.

### The Electrocardiogram

The ECG is abnormal. The ST-segments are elevated in leads II, III and aVF. The ST-elevations are not dramatic and would not meet standard "cath lab activation" criteria in many hospitals and prehospital settings. The normal, upwardly concave pattern of the ST-segments is, more or less, preserved. The J-points are elevated. And benign-looking ST-segment elevations are also present in multiple precordial leads.

However, it is important not to get too carried away with the shape of the ST-segment or the "normal" J-point elevation, when evidence of a regional STEMI exists.

This is an inferior wall STEMI. Proof that the mild ST-segment elevations in the inferior leads are "real" resides in lead aVL, where there are ST-segment depressions that are especially noticeable, given the low amplitude of the R-wave. Once we acknowledge the presence of reciprocal ST-segment depressions, we will not make the mistake of calling this benign early repolarization or pericarditis or, simply, "normal."

### Clinical Course

The patient had continued chest pain while being cared for in the ED. He refused catheterization from the ED but was admitted to the hospital. The next day, his catheterization revealed a high-grade occlusion of the mid-RCA. His peak troponin was 48.

## Case 7.2  A 19-year-old man presented with 1 hour of peri-umbilical pain and occasional diarrhea.

### The Electrocardiogram

This patient did not have an acute myocardial infarction. The computer algorithm suggested the possibility of simultaneous injury to the anterior, lateral and inferior walls. While possible, this is unlikely. Of course this patient's age and his presenting symptoms (abdominal pain with diarrhea) also provide some reassurance. The absence of any reciprocal ST-segment depressions also helps exclude acute STEMI.

The ECG is most consistent with early repolarization. The ST-segments are elevated in multiple precordial and inferior leads; except for leads V2 and V3, the smooth upward concavity is preserved; the ST-segment elevations are upsloping; there are tall, upright (concordant) T-waves in almost every lead; and the J-points (especially in lead V4) have a characteristic notch. The bradycardia and prominent sinus arrhythmia are also consistent with ERP (and in fact the ST-elevations and J-point elevations are expected to be more dramatic at slower heart rates).

### Clinical Course

Four serial troponin measurements were zero, and repeated ECGs showed no evolution or other acute change.

## Case 7.3  A 22-year-old man was brought to the hospital after suffering a single syncopal episode. He had a history of chronic anxiety, posttraumatic stress disease and depression, and he reported frequent bouts of chest pain and palpitations.

### The Electrocardiogram

The patient underwent an extensive evaluation for syncope. He had a normal cardiac echocardiogram and MRI that revealed no wall motion abnormalities, no chamber enlargement and no abnormalities suggestive of arrhythmogenic right ventricular dysplasia (ARVD).

His 12-lead ECG was felt to be consistent with Type 1 Brugada syndrome. While not dramatic or conclusive, leads V1 and V2 have an abnormal RSR' pattern (incomplete RBBB), with a high takeoff of the ST-segment. The elevated ST-segment is downwardly coved and ends in the inverted T wave.

### Clinical Course

Additional history was positive for a family history of sudden cardiac death. He was admitted for further studies. He underwent an electrophysiologic (EP) study, including a procainamide challenge that was positive for "conversion of a borderline Brugada pattern to a more classic Type 1 pattern." An internal cardiac defibrillator was placed. He and his family members then underwent genetics testing. In this case, the emergency clinicians immediately recognized the electrocardiographic pattern of Brugada syndrome, elicited the family history of sudden cardiac death and admitted the patient for lifesaving diagnostic studies. This is how it should work.

## Case 7.4 A 44-year-old man presented with chest pain and mild dyspnea.

### The Electrocardiogram

There are mild ST-segment elevations across the precordial leads and also mild ST-segment elevations in the inferior limb leads. An acute myocardial infarction is unlikely (at least electrocardiographically) in the absence of any regional pattern or any reciprocal ST-segment depressions.

There are also PR-segment depressions (especially in lead II, V2 and V3) and very modest T-waves in V5 and V6, which suggest acute pericarditis.

Early repolarization is also possible, in light of the subtle J-point notching in precordial lead V4. However, in V6 the ratio of the ST-segment amplitude:T-wave amplitude is $\geq 0.25$ (approximately 0.50), strongly suggesting acute pericarditis.

### Clinical Course

This patient had a loud pericardial friction rub, confirming pericarditis. An echocardiogram was unremarkable, without evidence of a pericardial effusion or diffuse or regional wall motion abnormalities.

## Case 7.5 A 21-year-old man with a history of asthma presented because of substernal chest discomfort. He had a cough and flulike illness over the past 2 days. His chest pain was not positional. He was afebrile on ED presentation. His initial troponin level was 2.65.

### The Electrocardiogram

The ST-segment elevations in the inferior leads and in V6 were recognized immediately. An acute coronary syndrome was suspected despite his very young age. Aspirin was administered; and because the ST-segments were elevated in a distinct regional pattern (involving the inferior and lateral leads), he was taken to the catheterization laboratory. In view of his age and his history, acute myopericarditis was also considered.

### Clinical Course

The peak troponin was 13.1. An echocardiogram showed no regional or other wall motion abnormalities, and there was no pericardial effusion. Coronary angiogram showed normal coronary arteries.

Follow-up ECG s continued to demonstrate diffuse ST-segment elevations, consistent with pericarditis.

No errors were made in this case. Given his age and history of fever and viral symptoms and in light of the elevated serum troponin level, the most likely diagnosis is acute myocarditis. However, the echocardiogram showed no regional or global wall motion abnormalities. What is the lesson?

The initial ECG showed ST-segment elevations in a regional pattern; despite the absence of ST-segment depressions in the reciprocal leads (leads I and aVL), it was correct to interpret this ECG as consistent with an inferior and lateral STEMI. An acute STEMI is not impossible in a 21-year-old patient; in addition to coronary atherosclerosis, anomalous coronary arteries, embolic disease, vasculitis or another disease may be responsible. Catheterization was appropriate.

He was treated with ibuprofen and colchicine, and he recovered quickly. His hospital course was complicated only by brief periods of sinus tachycardia and occasional premature ventricular beats. The discharge diagnosis, based on his presentation, evolution of diffuse ECG changes and mild troponin elevations, was "acute myopericarditis."

## Case 7.6 A 26-year-old man presented with chest pain. In the emergency department, he was smiling, alert and comfortable.

### The Electrocardiogram

This is an important ECG, filled with pitfalls and traps. There are ST-segment elevations across the precordium, with a normal concave upward contour and tall T-waves. In fact, the T-waves, which are abnormally tall and broad (bulky) and asymmetric, must be considered "hyperacute." The ST-segments are also elevated in limb leads I and aVL (and these leads also show "J-point elevation").

Do the concave upward (smiley face) ST-elevations and obvious J-point elevations mean that the ECG is benign (for example, early repolarization or pericarditis)? Don't be fooled. As highlighted earlier in this chapter, "J-point elevations" and "concave upward ST-segment elevations" often provide only false reassurance.

This patient, even at age 26, is suffering from an acute anterior and high lateral ST-elevation myocardial infarction. The ST-elevations in the high lateral leads (I and aVL) are matched by dramatic reciprocal ST-segment depressions in III and aVF. Thus, any consideration of early repolarization syndrome or pericarditis or another benign pattern must end.

Now, it is suddenly clear why there are ST-segment elevations and broad, bulky and tall (yes, "hyperacute") T-waves in the anterior precordium: the LAD must be the culprit artery, and the occlusion is likely to be proximal to D1.

His ECG 3 days later is shown next.

## Case 7.6   Same patient, 3 days later.

### The Electrocardiogram

The follow-up ECG demonstrates evolution of the acute anterior-septal-high lateral STEMI, with loss of anterior wall and high lateral wall R-waves and persistent ST-segment elevations and T-wave inversions.

### Clinical Course

In the ED, he received aspirin, morphine and nitroglycerin, and the interventional cardiology team was consulted emergently. His initial troponin was 0.27. His peak troponin was 53.84. A screen for cocaine and other drugs was negative.

Angiography demonstrated a 100 percent thrombotic occlusion of the LAD, proximal to the first diagonal branch. In the catheterization laboratory, he required an intraortic balloon pump for hemodynamic support. Briefly, pulmonary edema developed. A bare metal stent was inserted. His echocardiogram prior to discharge demonstrated anteroapical hypokinesis.

## Case 7.7   A 25-year-old man was "found down" in a comatose state with twitching eyes. His history included diabetes and alcoholism. On presentation to the emergency department, he was hypotensive. His finger stick glucose was markedly elevated.

### The Electrocardiogram

The computer reading is descriptive but not diagnostic. Indeed, there is sinus bradycardia and a long QT interval. Electrical artifacts are also present. The computer suggests "normal early repolarization." But, in fact, the patient has severe hypothermia.

The notches on the terminal, descending limb of the QRS complexes are actually Osborn waves; they do not signify early repolarization. Because of the Osborn waves, the ST-segments appear elevated, mimicking ERP, STEMI or other conditions. The long QT interval and the sinus bradycardia are also consistent with hypothermia.

### Clinical Course

In this case, hypothermia was not suspected clinically. Initially, he was thought to have either diabetic ketoacidosis or hyperosmolar coma. A brain CT scan was ordered to rule out a central nervous system hemorrhage. Once his core temperature was measured (28.5 degrees), the diagnosis was clear, and core rewarming could begin.

## Case 7.8   A 41-year-old man presented with 2 days of heavy alcohol consumption and intermittent chest pain that radiated to his entire body.

### The Electrocardiogram

There is normal sinus rhythm. The diffuse, mild, concave upward ST-segment elevations in the precordial and limb leads are accompanied by J-point notching ("fish-hook" pattern), suggesting probable early repolarization pattern (ERP). There is no evidence of regional (anatomic) ST-segment elevation or any evidence of reciprocal ST-segment depression.

In the right clinical setting, acute pericarditis should also be considered, especially in light of the PR-segment depressions. In this case, inspection of V6 is helpful: the ratio of the amplitude of the ST-segment to the amplitude of the T-wave is < 0.25, suggesting early repolarization.

## Clinical Course

His chest x-ray, troponin and other routine studies were normal. His electrocardiographic diagnosis is ERP.

## Case 7.9   A 27-year-old man presented after a bout of dizziness and near-syncope.

### The Electrocardiogram

The patient's ECG demonstrates an RSR' pattern with ST-segment elevation isolated to lead V2. There is a high takeoff of the ST-segment. The elevated ST-segment has a saddle morphology. All this is suggestive of Type 2 Brugada syndrome. The ST-segment elevation in V2 represents a "coronary mimic" or "pseudo-infarction" pattern.

### Clinical Course

The patient reported a family history of sudden cardiac death. He was admitted to the hospital for electrophysiologic (EP) testing, which was negative for sustained inducible ventricular arrhythmias. His procainamide challenge was also negative. An intracardiac monitor was then inserted, and he was discharged in stable condition. His discharge diagnosis was "probable Type 2 Brugada Syndrome."

## Case 7.10   A 31-year-old man with hypertension, insulin-dependent diabetes and chronic gastroparesis presented with several hours of abdominal pain.

### The Electrocardiogram

This young man presented with severe diabetic ketoacidosis. On the ECG, the combination of peaked T-waves in the anterior precordial leads, with a narrow and symmetric base, are highly suggestive of hyperkalemia. Another critical clue to advanced hyperkalemia is the mild QRS widening (the QRS duration was just above the normal limit at 106 msec).

The differential diagnosis of peaked T-waves includes the hyperacute T-waves of early STEMI as well as the de Winter complex, ERP, LVH and other conditions.

### Clinical Course

His measured potassium was 7.4 mmol/L, his serum glucose was 1610 mg/dL, and his serum bicarbonate was 5.0 mmol/L with an anion gap = 36. His ECG returned to normal after treatment for his diabetic ketoacidosis and hyperkalemia.

## Case 7.11   A 60-year-old man with a history of diabetes and hyperlipidemia presented with 1 hour of substernal chest pain. His initial serum troponin level was 0.01.

### The Electrocardiogram

The rhythm is sinus, with a sinus arrhythmia. The QRS duration is prolonged (118 msec). The absent R-waves in V1 and V2 suggest an anteroseptal infarct of indeterminate age.

The most striking feature is the hyperacute T-waves across the anterior precordial leads. The T-waves are broad-based and "bulky"; they are also tall and appear to tower over the insignificant R-waves in leads V2 and V3. They have an altogether different appearance from the tall T-waves of hyperkalemia (although hyperkalemia cannot be excluded based solely on the shape of the tall T-waves). The tall and broad T-waves are the most significant findings, and this pattern should prompt action.

As emphasized in Chapter 3, Anterior Wall Myocardial Infarction, the presence of Q-waves in the precordial leads does *not* mean that the anterior infarction is old; in fact, in anterior wall STEMIs especially, R-waves are often diminished or absent and Q-waves are often present on the presenting ECG.

Also of critical importance, the ST-segment is elevated in lead aVL, and a broad Q-wave is beginning to form. The entire picture suggests an anteroseptal and high lateral STEMI, likely caused by an acute occlusion of the LAD, prior to the first diagonal branch.

Another reminder: hyperacute T-waves in the anterior precordial leads are an early warning of a critical LAD occlusion; often, as in this case, the troponin on presentation is negative.

### Clinical Course

Twelve hours after this patient's presentation, his troponin rose to 214.4. Emergent coronary angiography revealed a 100 percent proximal thrombotic occlusion of the LAD.

Two years earlier, his ECG was normal without any T-wave abnormalities, as shown in the next tracing.

## Case 7.11  Same patient – baseline ECG (2 years earlier).

This patient's most recent ECG was normal except for mild QT-interval prolongation. There is no evidence of an anteroseptal infarct on this ECG, and the T-waves are normal.

## References

Adhikarla C., Boga M., Wood A. D., Froelicher V. F. Natural history of the electrocardiographic pattern of early repolarization in ambulatory patients. *Am J Cardiol.* 2011; **108**:1831–1835.

Adler A., Rosso R., Viskin D. et al. What do we know about the "malignant form" of early repolarization? *J Am Coll Cardiol.* 2013; **62**:863–868.

Antzelevitch C., Yan G., Ackerman M. J. et al. J-wave syndromes expert consensus conference report: Emerging concepts and gaps in knowledge. *Europace.* 2017; **19**:665–694.

Antzelevitch C., Yan G., Viskin S. Rationale for the use of the terms J-wave syndromes and early repolarization. *J Am Coll Cardiol.* 2011; **57**:1587–1590.

Armstrong E. J., Kulkarni A. R., Bhave P. D. et al. Electrocardiographic criteria for ST-elevation myocardial infarction in patients with left ventricular hypertrophy. *Am J Cardiol.* 2012; **110**:977–983.

Benito B., Guasch E., Rivard L., Nattel S. Clinical and mechanistic issues in early repolarization. *J Am Coll Cardiol.* 2010; **56**:1177–1186.

Birnbaum Y., Nikus K., Kligfield P. et al. The role of the ECG in diagnosis, risk estimation and catheterization laboratory activation in patients with acute coronary syndromes: A consensus document. *Ann Noninvasive Electrocardiol.* 2014; **19**:412–425.

Birnbaum Y., Wilson J. M., Fiol M. et al. ECG diagnosis and classification of acute coronary syndromes. *Ann Noninvasive Electrocardiol.* 2014; **19**:4–14.

Brady W. J., Syverud S. A., Beagle C. W. et al. Electrocardiographic ST-segment elevation: The diagnosis of acute myocardial infarction by morphologic analysis of the ST-segment. *Acad Emerg Med.* 2001; **8**:961–967.

Cheitlin M. D., Armstrong W. F., Aurigemma G. P. et al. ACC/AHA/ASE 2003 guideline update for the clinical application of echocardiography: summary article. A report of the American College of Cardiology/American Heart Association Task Force on Practice Guidelines (ACC/AHA/ASE Committee to Update the 1997 Guidelines for the Clinical Application of Echocardiography). *Circulation.* 2003 **108**:1146–1162.

Chung S. L., Lei M. H., Chen C. C. et al. Characteristics and prognosis in patients with false-positive ST-elevation myocardial infarction in the ED. *Am J Emerg Med.* 2013; **31**:825–829.

Demangone D. ECG manifestations: Noncoronary heart disease. *Emerg Med Clin N Am.* 2006; **24**:113–131.

de Winter R. J., Verouden N. J., Wellens H. J. et al. A new ECG sign of proximal LAD occlusion. *N Engl M Med.* 2008; **359**:2071–2073.

Eastaugh J. A. The early repolarization syndrome. *J Emer Med.* 1985; **7**:257–262.

Ginzton L. E., Laks M. M. The differential diagnosis of acute pericarditis from the normal variant: new electrocardiographic criteria. *Circulation.* 1982; **65**:1004–1009.

Goldberger A. L. Recognition of ECG pseudo-infarct patterns. *Mod Concepts Cardiovasc Dis.* 1980; **49**(3):13–18.

His R. G., Lamb L. E., Allen M. F. Electrocardiographic findings in 67,375 asymptomatic subjects. *Am J Cardiol.* 1960; **6**:200–231.

Huang H. D., Birnbaum Y. ST elevation: Differentiation between ST-elevation myocardial infarction and nonischemic ST-elevation. *J Electrocardiol.* 2011; **44**:494e1–494e12.

Huston T. P., Puffer J. C., Rodney W. M. The athletic heart syndrome. *N Engl J Med.* 1985; **313**:24–32.

Imazio M., Cecchi E., Demichelis B. et al. Indicators of poor prognosis of acute pericarditis. *Circulation.* 2007; **115**:2739.

Imazio M., Spodick D. H., Brucato A. et al. Controversial issues in the management of pericardial diseases. *Circulation.* 2010; **121**:916–928.

Jayroe J. B., Spodick D. H., Nikus K. et al. Differentiating ST elevation myocardial infarction and nonischemic causes of ST elevation by analyzing the presenting electrocardiogram. *Am J Cardiol.* 2009; **103**:301–306.

Klatsky A. L., Oehm R., Cooper R. A. et al. The early repolarization normal variant electrocardiogram: correlates and consequences. *Am J Med.* 2003; **115**:171–177.

Klein A. L., Abbara S., Agler D. A. et al. American Society of Echocardiography Clinical Recommendations for multimodality cardiovascular imaging of patients with pericardial disease. *J Am Soc Echocardiogr.* 2013; **26**:965–1012.

Kosuge M., Kimura K. Electrocardiographic findings of takotsubo cardiomyopathy as compared with those of anterior acute myocardial infarction. *J Electrocardiol.* 2014; **46**:684–689.

Krantz M. J., Lowery C. M. Giant Osborn waves in hypothermia. Images in clinical medicine. *N Engl J Med.* 2005; **352**:184.

Kurisu S., Kihara Y. Takotsubo cardiomyopathy: clinical presentation and underlying mechanism. *J Cardiol.* 2012; **60**:429–437.

Lange R. A., Hillis L. D. Acute pericarditis. *N Engl J Med.* 2004; **351**:2195–2202.

Lawner B. J., Nable, J. V. Novel patterns of ischemia and STEMI equivalents. *Cardiol Clin.* 2012; **30**:591–599.

LeWinter M. M. Acute pericarditis. *N Engl J Med.* 2014; **371**:2410–2416.

McCabe J. M., Armstrong E. J., Kulkarni A. et al. Prevalence and factors associated with false-positive ST-segment elevation myocardial infarction diagnoses at primary percutaneous coronary intervention-capable centers. *Arch Intern Med.* 2012; **172**:864–871.

Meizlish J. L., Berger H. J., Plankey M. et al. Functional left ventricular aneurysm formation after acute anterior transmural myocardial infarction: incidence, natural history and prognostic implications. *N Engl J Med.* 1984; **311**:1001–1006.

Mustafa S., Shaikh N., Gowda R. M., Khan I. A. Electrocardiographic features of hypothermia. *Cardiology.* 2005; **103**:118–119.

Nable J. V., Lawner B. J. Chameleons: Electrocardiogram imitators of ST-segment elevation myocardial infarction. *Emerg Med Clin N Am.* 2015; **33**:529–537.

Nikus K., Pahlm O., Wagner G. et al. Electrocardiographic classification of acute coronary syndromes: A review by a committee of the International Society for Holter and Non-invasive Cardiology. *J Electrocardio.* 2010; **43**:91–103.

O'Gara P. T., Kushner F. G., Ascheim D. D. et al. 2013 ACCF/AHA guideline for the management of ST-elevation myocardial infarction. *J Am Coll Cardiol.* 2013; **61**:e78–e140.

Osborn J. Experimental hypothermia: respiratory and blood pH changes in relation to cardiac function. *Am J Physiol.* 1953; **175**:389.

Patton K. K., Ellinor P. T., Ezekowitz M. Electrocardiographic early repolarization: A scientific statement from the American Heart Association. *Circulation.* 2016; **133**:1520–1529.

Pelliccia F., Greco C., Vitale C. et al. Takotsubo syndrome (stress cardiomyopathy): An intriguing clinical condition in search of its identity. *Am J Med.* 2014; **127**:699–704.

Pollak P., Brady W. Electrocardiographic patterns mimicking ST-segment elevation myocardial infarction. *Cardiol. Clin.* 2012; **30**:601–615.

Rautaharju P. M., Surawicz B., Gettes L. S. AHA/ACCF/HRS recommendations for the standardization and interpretation of the electrocardiogram. Part IV: The ST segment, T and U waves and the QT interval. *J Am Coll Cardiol.* 2009; **53**:982–991.

Rosso R., Kogan E., Belhassen B. et al. J-point elevation in survivors of primary ventricular fibrillation and matched control subjects. *J Am Coll Cardiol.* 2008; **52**:1231–1238.

Rutsky E. A., Rostand S. G. Pericarditis in end-stage renal disease: Clinical characteristics and management. *Semin Dial.* 1989; **2**:25.

Salinsky E. P., Worrilow C. C. ST-segment elevation myocardial infarction vs. hypothermia-induced electrocardiographic

changes: A case report and brief review of the literature. *J Emerg Med.* 2014; **46**:e107–e111.

Sanchez-Jimenez E. F. Initial clinical presentation of takotsubo cardiomyopathy with a focus on electrocardiographic changes: A literature review of cases. *World J Cardiol.* 2013; **5**:228–241.

Senecal E. L., Rosenfield K., Caldera A. E., Passeri J. J. Case 36:2011: A 93-year-old woman with shortness of breath and chest pain. *N Engl J Med.* 2011; **365**:2021–2028.

Sgarbossa E. B., Pinski S.L., Barbagelata A. et al. Electrocardiographic diagnosis of evolving acute myocardial infarction in the presence of left bundle branch block. *N Engl J Med.* 1996; **334**:481–487.

Smith S. Upwardly concave ST segment morphology is common in acute left anterior descending coronary occlusion. *J Emerg Med.* 2006; **31**:69–77.

Smith S. W., Khalil A., Henry T. D. et al. Electrocardiographic differentiation of early repolarization from subtle anterior ST-segment elevation myocardial infarction. *Ann Emerg Med.* 2012; **60**:45–56.

Solomon A., Barish R. A., Browne B., Tso E. The electrocardiographic features of hypothermia. *J Emerg Med.* 1988; **7**:169–173.

Somers M. P., Brady W. J., Perron A. D., Mattu A. The prominent T-wave: Electrocardiographic differential diagnosis. *Am J Emerg Med.* 2002; **20**:243–251.

Spodick D. H. Acute pericarditis: Current concepts and practice. *JAMA.* 2003; **289**:1150–1153.

Arrhythmias during acute pericarditis. A prospective study of 100 consecutive cases. *JAMA.* 1976; **235**:39–41.

Spodick D. H. Differential characteristics of the electrocardiogram in early repolarization

and acute pericarditis. *N Engl J Med.* 1976; **295**:523–526.

Tabas J. A., Rodgriguez R. M., Seligman H. K., Goldschlager N. F. Electrocardiographic criteria for detecting acute myocardial infarction in patients with left bundle branch block: A meta-analysis. *Ann Emerg Med.* 2008; **52**:329–336.

Tikkanen J. T., Anttonen O., Junttila M. J. et al. Long-term outcome associated with early repolarization in electrocardiography. *N Engl J Med.* 2009; **361**:2529–2537.

Tran V., Huang H. D., Diez J. G. et al. Differentiating ST-elevation myocardial infarction from nonischemic ST-elevation in patients with chest pain. *Am J Cardiol.* 2011; **108**:1096–1101.

Vassallo S. U., Delaney K. A., Hoffman R. S. et al. A prospective evaluation of the electrocardiographic manifestations of hypothermia. *Acad Emerg Med.* 1999; **6**:1121–1126.

Veerakul G., Nademanee K. Brugada syndrome: Two decades of progress. *Circ J.* 2012; **76**:2713–2722.

Verouden N. J., Koch K. T., Peters R. J. et al. Persistent precordial "hyperacute" T-waves signify proximal left anterior descending artery occlusion. *Heart.* 2009; **95**:1701–1706.

Wagner G. S., Strauss D. G. *Marriott's practical electrocardiography.* Twelfth edition. Philadelphia, PA: Lippincott, Williams & Wilkins, 2014.

Wang K., Asinger R. W., Marriott H. J. L. ST-segment elevation in conditions other than acute myocardial infarction. *N Engl J Med.* 2003; **349**:2128–2135.

Wu S. H., Lin X. X., Cheng Y. J. et al. Early repolarization pattern and risk for arrhythmia death: A meta-analysis. *J Am Coll Cardiol.* 2013; **61**:645–650.

263

# Critical Cases at 3 A.M.

We should first endeavor to better understand the working of the heart in all its details, and the cause of a large variety of abnormalities. This will enable us, in a possibly still distant future and based upon a clear insight and improved knowledge, to give relief to the suffering of our patients.
—*Willem Einthoven (1906)*

In the Preface to this atlas, I began with a self-evident observation – that the ECG plays a pivotal role in patient care. I wrote that the ECG is "where the money is" for a wide variety of chief complaints, including chest pain, dyspnea, syncope, electrolyte abnormalities, shock, cardiac arrest, arrhythmias, poisonings and other critical emergencies. And then, belaboring the point, I wrote that "more often than not, the ECG rules in or out one or more life-threatening conditions and changes management."

*Critical Cases in Electrocardiography* has focused on "don't-miss" tracings (especially those that are essential in managing patients with chest pain or dyspnea). But in fact, most of the examples in this atlas were missed – by the emergency clinicians, the consulting specialists, the computer algorithm or, often enough, all of the above. It goes without saying that I have missed many of these diagnoses too.

As famed electrocardiographer and teacher Marriott wrote, "There are two main categories of urgent electrocardiograms: Those that present you with a clear-cut, unambivalent picture that justifies definitive diagnosis, decision and action; and those that are not diagnostic but suggest a disaster that may be unforgiving if you fail to think of it" (Marriott, 1997).

*Critical Cases in Electrocardiography* has emphasized everyday emergencies. As I wrote in the Preface, my focus is "clinical diagnosis, late at night in the emergency department or critical care unit, in the service of seriously ill patients."

It is time to review. This final chapter, Critical Cases at 3 A.M., is a collection of ECG tracings from patients with chest pain, shortness of breath, syncope and other cardiovascular complaints. A few have been presented in earlier chapters. Almost all of the ECGs were misinterpreted, at least at first, by the treating clinicians. I suspect that you will not miss any.

# Self-Study Electrocardiograms

**Case 8.1** A 75-year-old female had a syncopal episode at the airport. She had no memory of the event. There was no report of chest pain. On arrival in the emergency department, she was asymptomatic; her examination was normal except for a forehead laceration.

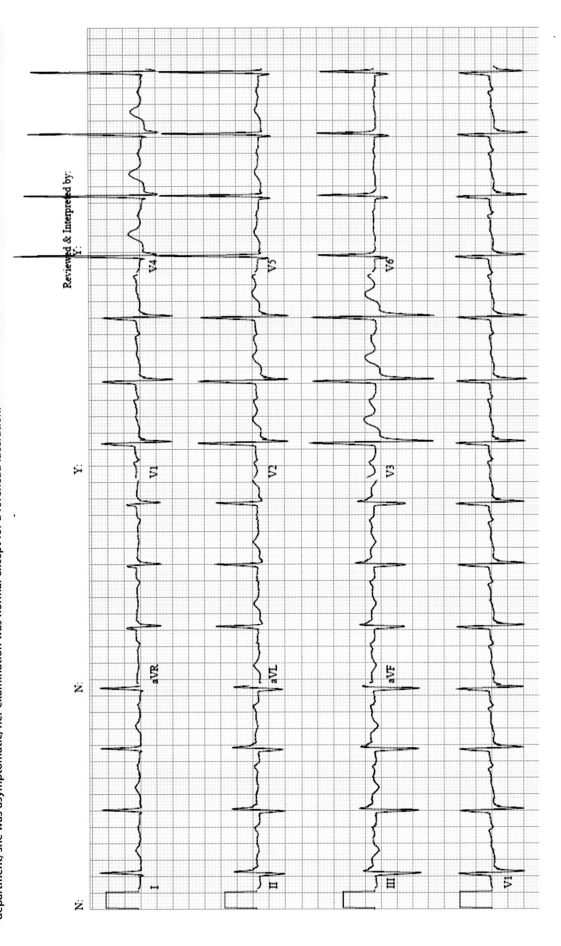

**Case 8.2** A 69-year-old female with a history of prior aortic dissection presented to the emergency department with chest pain for 4 hours, accompanied by mild nausea. She was transported by paramedics as a "cardiac alert." She received aspirin, nitroglycerin and an analgesic in the field, with complete resolution of her chest pain. Her blood pressure on arrival to the ED was 163/75.

Female    Unknown

Room:369
Loc:1002

| | | |
|---|---|---|
| PR interval | 150 | ms |
| QRS duration | 130 | ms |
| QT/QTc | 454/513 | ms |
| P-R-T axes | 73 117 | 65 |

Sinus rhythm with marked sinus arrhythmia
Right atrial enlargement
Right bundle branch block
Left posterior fascicular block
 Bifascicular block
Cannot rule out Anterior infarct , age undetermined
Inferolateral injury pattern
** ** ** ** * ACUTE MI * ** ** ** **

Abnormal ECG ...

Technician:
Test ind:

Referred by:  SELF
             Y:

Y:

Reviewed & Interpreted by:
             Y:

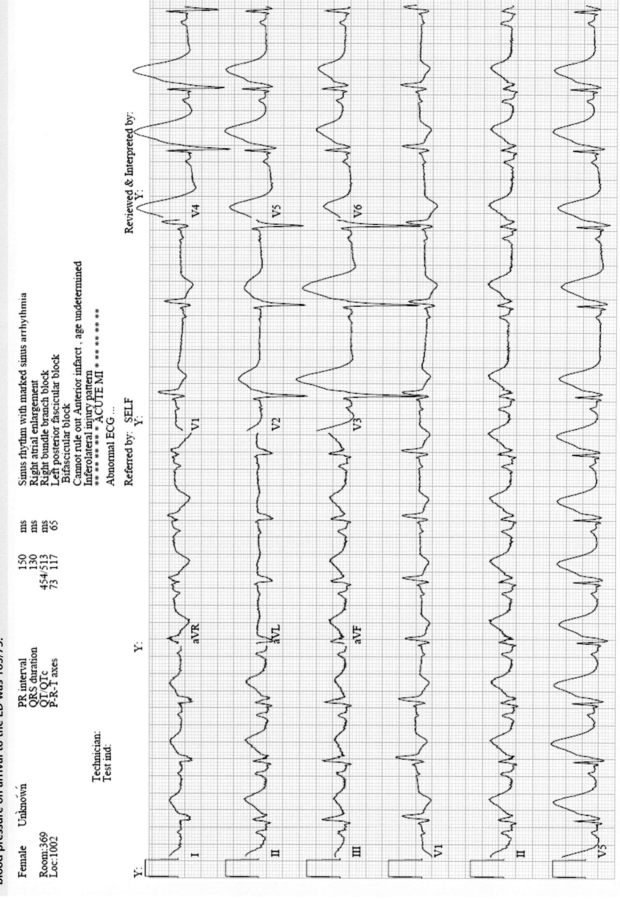

I    aVR    V1    V4

II    aVL    V2    V5

III    aVF    V3    V6

V1

II

V5

**Case 8.3** A 21-year-old female had substernal chest pain followed by a syncopal event while running between gates at the airport.

**Case 8.4** A 79-year-old female awoke at 2 A.M. with epigastric and chest pain, diaphoresis and dyspnea. She reported a history of hypertension.

**Case 8.5** A 64-year-old man presented with chest pain, headache and altered mental status.

| | | | |
|---|---|---|---|
| Vent. rate | 63 | BPM | Normal sinus rhythm |
| PR interval | 166 | ms | Nonspecific ST and T wave abnormality |
| QRS duration | 88 | ms | Prolonged QT |
| QT/QTc | 458/468 | ms | Abnormal ECG |
| P-R-T axes | 48 54 | 82 | |

**Case 8.6** A 63-year-old man presented with chest pain and dyspnea. He had a white blood cell count of 18,000, and his chest x-ray suggested an acute pneumonia. His initial ED diagnosis was "pneumonia, with possible early sepsis." His initial troponin level was 0.3. The note from the ED team read, "He appears to have pneumonia. In addition, his ECG shows a RBBB and possible anterior wall ischemia. With indeterminate troponin, we will treat him for ACS and non-STEMI."

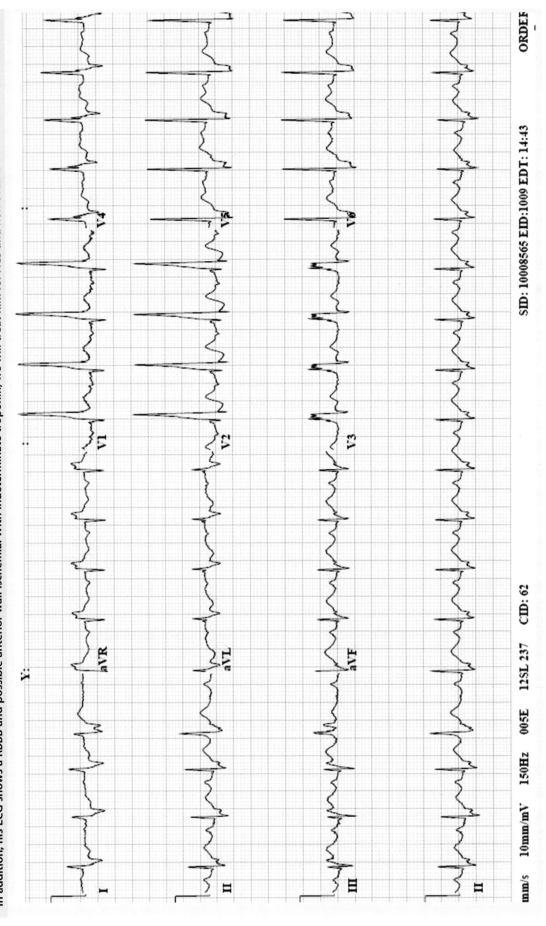

mm/s    10mm/mV    150Hz    005E    12SL 237    CID: 62    SID: 10008565 EID:1009 EDT: 14:43    ORDEF

**Case 8.7** A 79-year-old man presented with three episodes of syncope over a 2-week period. The most recent syncopal episode occurred the morning of his emergency department visit while he was sitting on his couch.

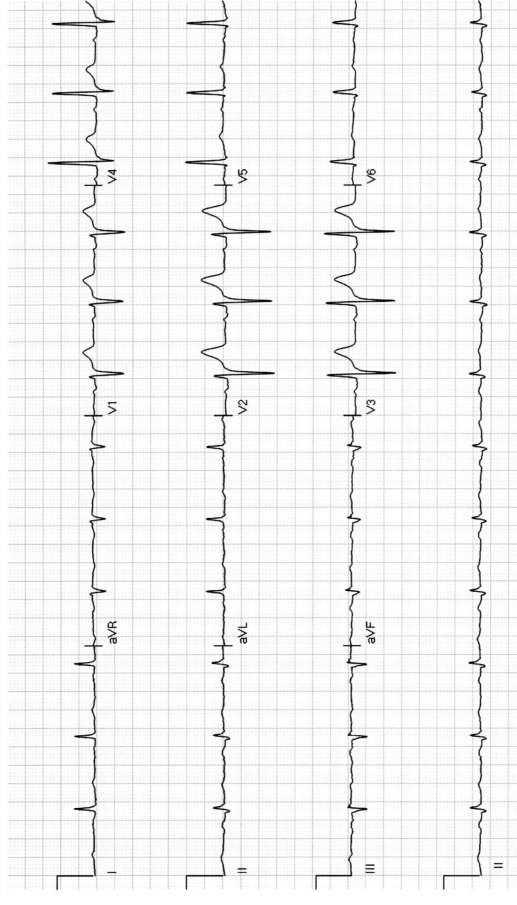

**Case 8.8** A 47-year-old man presented with stuttering chest pain, with radiation to both arms and his right jaw. Aspirin was administered by the paramedics, and his chest pain resolved. Patient was a former smoker, but there was no other medical history. The initial troponin level was 0.11.

Room:Y23
Loc:1001

| | | BPM |
|---|---|---|
| Vent. rate | 82 | BPM |
| PR interval | 126 | ms |
| QRS duration | 84 | ms |
| QT/QTc | 344/401 | ms |
| P-R-T axes | 13 71 | 70 |

Normal sinus rhythm
Normal ECG
No previous ECGs available

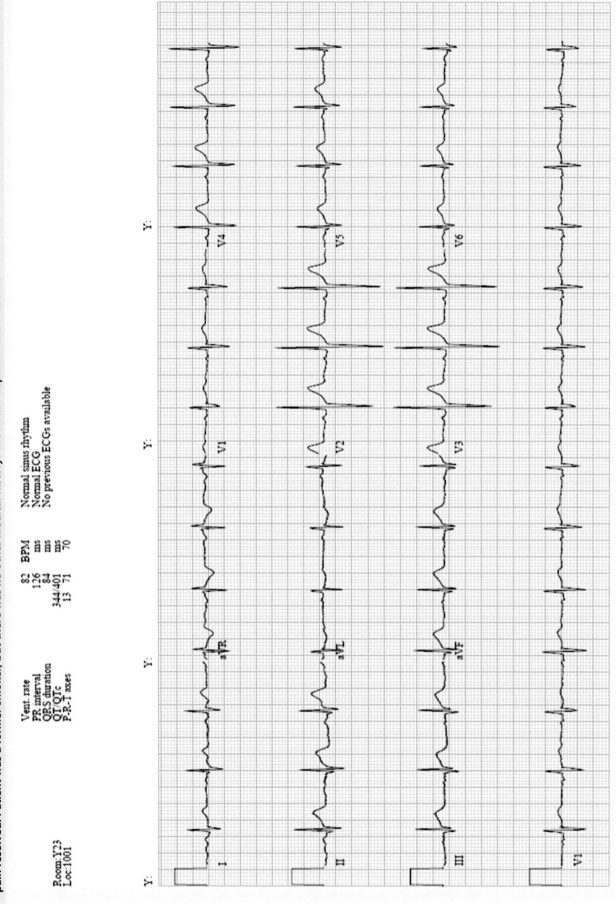

**Case 8.9** A 59-year-old man presented with several hours of chest discomfort, nausea and hiccups. He had a recent diagnosis of GERD.

**Case 8.10** A 40-year-old man presented with 3 hours of substernal chest pain after playing a strenuous game of basketball.

**Case 8.11** A 67-year-old man with a history of anemia and prostate carcinoma presented with chest pain, nausea and shortness of breath. His triage BP was 101/70.

**Case 8.11** The same patient – 54 minutes later.

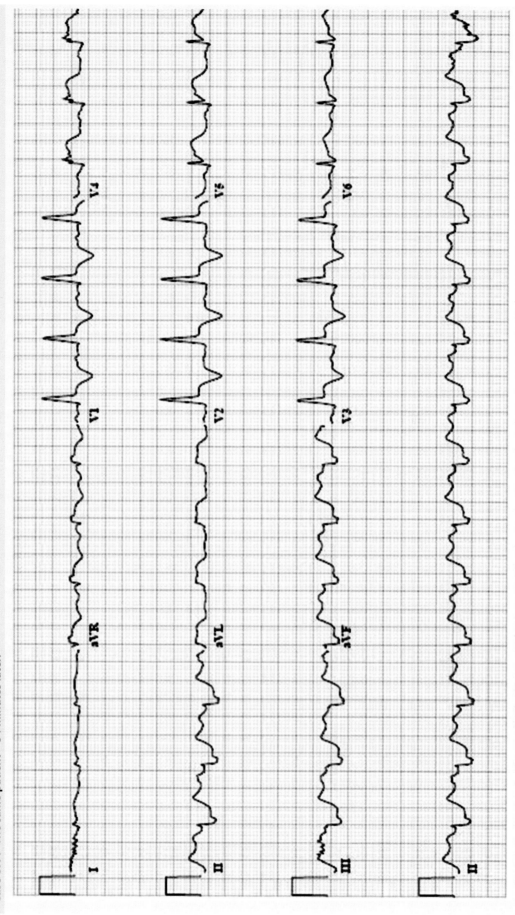

**Case 8.12** A 63-year-old man presented with 2 hours of left chest pressure. He reported intermittent "indigestion" the night before his visit. After obtaining initial laboratory studies and the ECG, he was admitted to the coronary care unit with a diagnosis of "unstable angina, possible inferior ischemia."

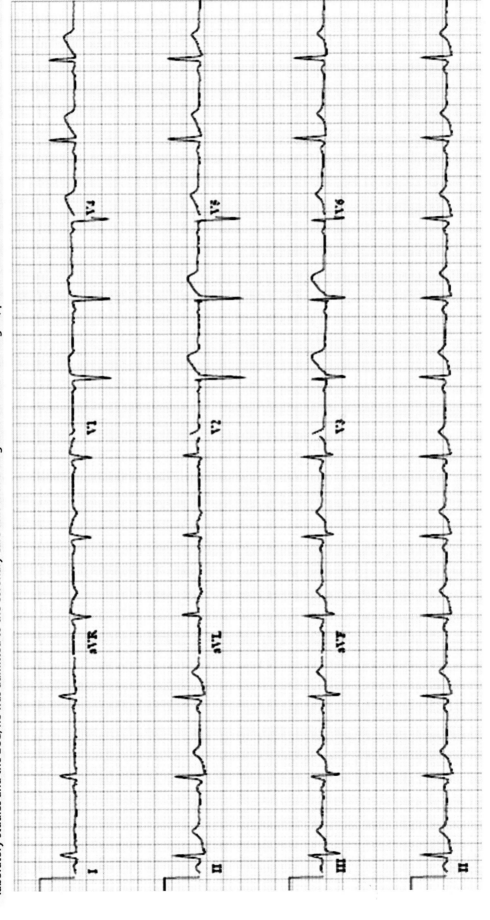

**Case 8.12** The same patient – the following morning.

**Case 8.13** A 42-year-old man presented with severe, resting substernal chest pain ("like a ton of bricks"). He also endorsed mild dyspnea and diaphoresis.

**Case 8.14** A 68-year-old man was on an antiretroviral regimen for HIV/AIDS. He presented with substernal chest pain at rest, reporting two similar episodes with mild exertion over the past 2 weeks. He was asymptomatic in the emergency department.

**Case 8.15** A 64-year-old female with a history of COPD but no history of coronary artery disease presented with 5 days of stuttering chest pain that radiated to both arms. In the emergency department, she had bilateral rales on lung examination. She received heparin and nitroglycerin for a presumed diagnosis of "unstable angina, possible non-STEMI." The computer reading is shown.

Loc: 0

| | | |
|---|---|---|
| Veat. rate | 127 BPM | Atrial fibrillation with rapid veatricular respease |
| PR interval | * ms | Marked ST abnormality, possible anteroseptal subendocardial injury |
| QRS duration | 88 ms | Abnormal ECG |
| QT/QTc | 296/430 ms | No previous ECGs available |
| P-R-T axes | * 55 143 | |

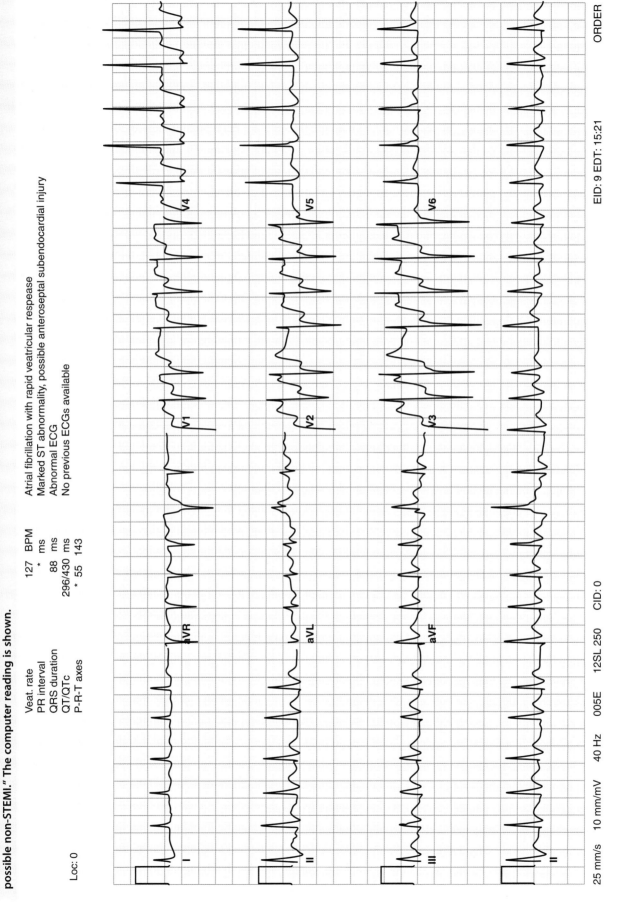

25 mm/s    10 mm/mV    40 Hz    005E    12SL 250    CID: 0    EID: 9 EDT: 15:21    ORDER

**Case 8.16** A 59-year-old man presented in cardiac arrest. He had a history of coronary artery disease. His wife reported he had complained of left arm numbness and shortness of breath and then collapsed. Paramedics found him in ventricular fibrillation. In the ED, despite receiving more than an hour of chest compressions and multiple rounds of cardiac medications, he could not be resuscitated. This rhythm strip was obtained after a third defibrillation shock.

**Case 8.16** Same patient, 12-lead ECG taken during the resuscitation.

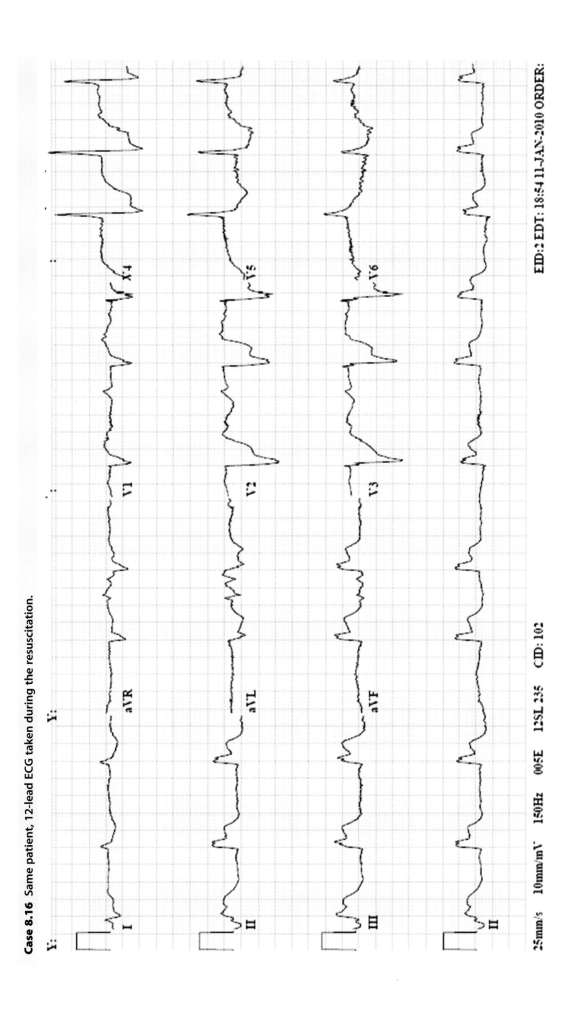

25mm/s    10mm/mV    150Hz    005E    12SL 235    CID: 102

EID: 2 EDT: 18:54 11-JAN-2010 ORDER:

**Case 8.17** A 72-year-old man with no history of coronary artery disease had severe chest pain while running at the airport. He reported a history of pulmonary fibrosis, and he used home oxygen. His initial troponin was 0.01.

| | | | |
|---|---|---|---|
| Vent.rate | 62 | BPM | Sinus rhythm with 1st degree A-V block |
| PR interval | 262 | ms | Right bundle branch block |
| QRS duration | 132 | ms | Inferior infarct, age undetermined |
| QT/QTc | 450/456 | ms | Abnormal ECG |
| P-R-T axes | 27  256 | -22 | No previous ECGs available |

Referred by:

OTHER:

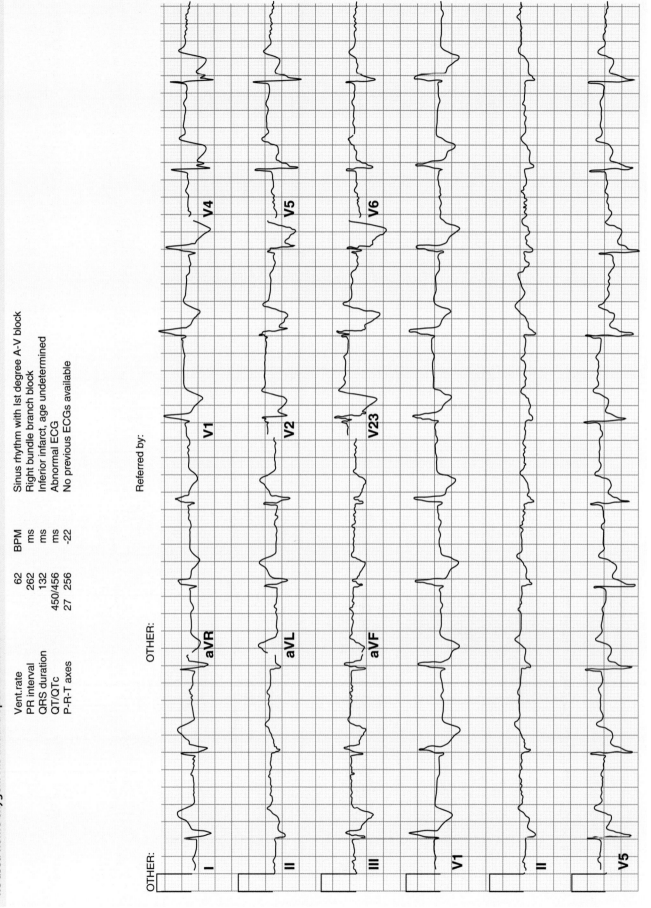

OTHER:

I  aVR  V1  V4

II  aVL  V2  V5

III  aVF  V23  V6

V1

II

V5

**Case 8.18** A 47-year-old man presented with sharp chest pain. He had a history of pericarditis 2 years earlier.

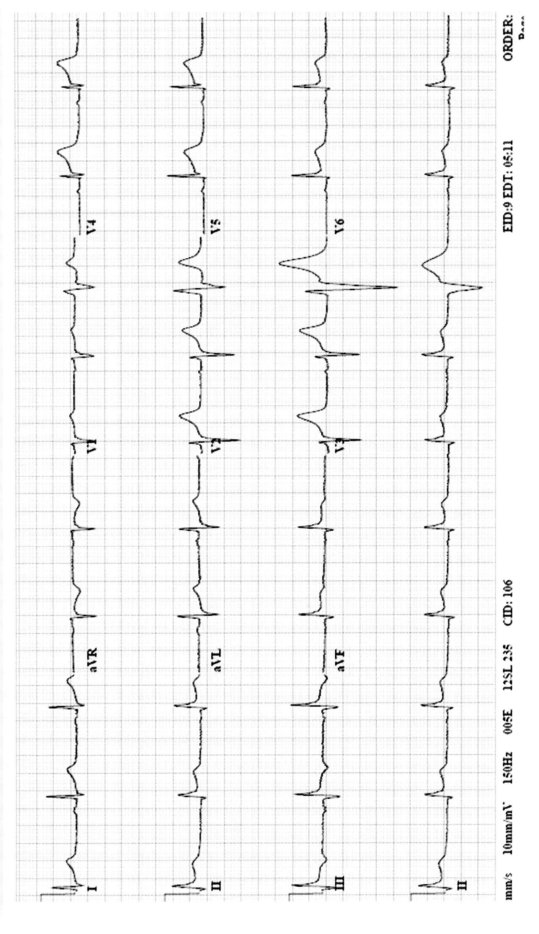

mm/s    10mm/mV    150Hz    005E    12SL 235    CID: 106    EID:9 EDT: 05:11    ORDER:

**Case 8.19** A 57-year-old female presented with leg stiffness and shortness of breath. On examination, she was well appearing. However, her oxygen saturation was only 90 percent on 5 liters of nasal oxygen, and she had signs of deep venous thrombophlebitis of the left leg.

**Case 8.20** A 36-year-old man presented with hallucinations and fatigue.

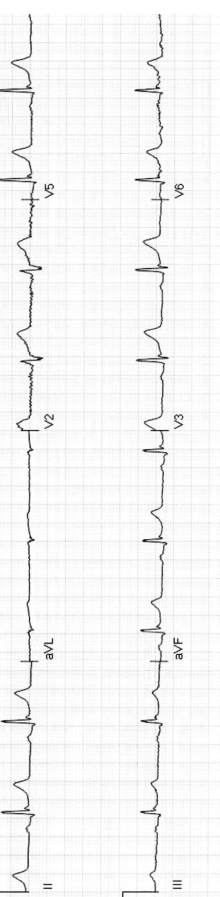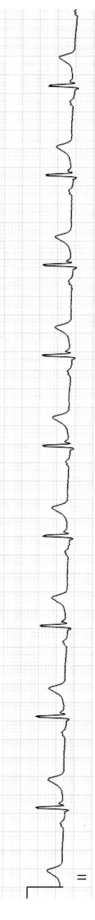

**Case 8.21** A 67-year-old female had a history of chronic alcohol use and frequent emergency department visits for chest and back pain and other symptoms. She presented with worsening chest pain over 5 days. Her triage troponin level was 0.40.

**Case 8.22** A 33-year-old man presented with an acute asthma attack. This electrocardiogram was obtained because he had a tachycardia at triage.

| | | |
|---|---|---|
| Vent. rate | 102 | BPM |
| PR interval | 150 | ms |
| QRS duration | 96 | ms |
| QT/QTc | 326/425 | ms |
| P-R-T axes | 68 –36 | 65 |

Sinus tachycardia
Left axis deviation
ST elevation consider anterior injury or acute infarct
** ** ** ** * ACUTE MI * ** ** ** **
Abnormal ECG
No prvious ECGs available

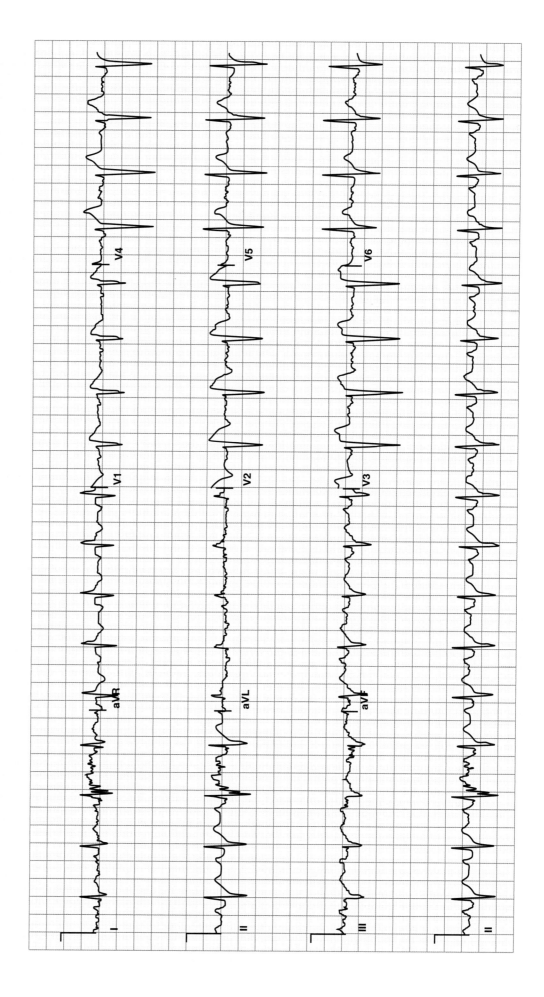

**Case 8.23** A 35-year-old female noted shortness of breath and anxiety while visiting her newborn in the neonatal intensive care unit.

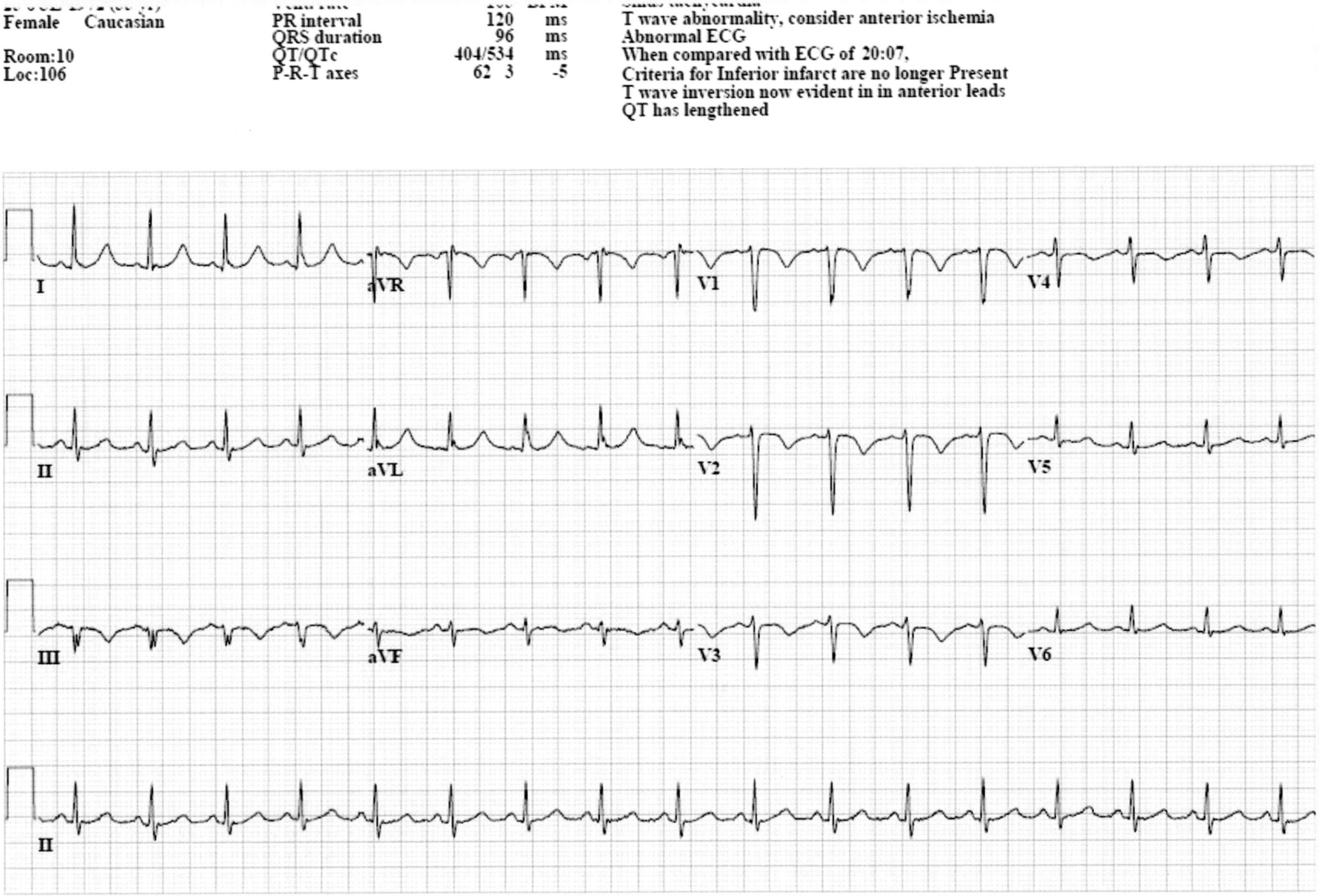

Female Caucasian
Room:10
Loc:106
PR interval 120 ms
QRS duration 96 ms
QT/QTc 404/534 ms
P-R-T axes 62 3 -5
T wave abnormality, consider anterior ischemia
Abnormal ECG
When compared with ECG of 20:07,
Criteria for Inferior infarct are no longer Present
T wave inversion now evident in in anterior leads
QT has lengthened
I
aVR
V1
V4
II
aVL
V2
V5
III
aVF
V3
V6
II

**Case 8.24** A 54-year-old man without any significant medical history presented with new-onset shortness of breath. He reported progressive fatigue and weakness over the past month, and on the day of his visit, he noted marked exertional dyspnea while shopping. In the ED, he was tachypneic (RR = 30), and he was in respiratory distress. His lung examination revealed decreased breath sounds and dullness to percussion at the left base. Rales were noted in the middle left lung field. He was felt to have an acute coronary syndrome; his first troponin was elevated at 8.0.

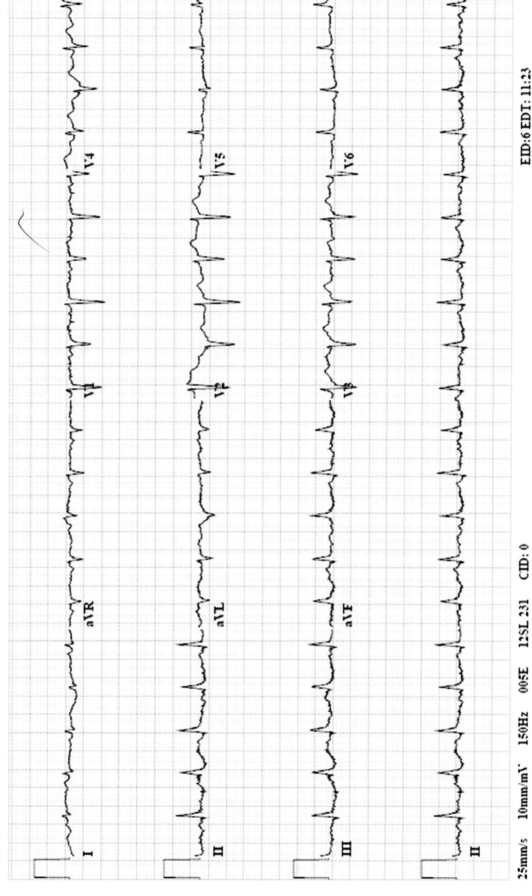

25mm/s  10mm/mV  150Hz  005E  12SL 231  CID: 0  EID:6 EDT: 11:23

**Case 8.25** A 53-year-old female with diabetes and chronic renal insufficiency presented with shortness of breath, chest pain, pulmonary edema, hypoxia and hypotension.

**Case 8.26** A 52-year-old man presented with shortness of breath and generalized weakness. His initial blood pressure was 118/84. His respirations were 18 and unlabored. He was not in any respiratory distress. He had a history of lung carcinoma, chronic hoarseness and a prior episode of deep venous thrombosis (DVT), and he was taking warfarin.

Caucasian

| | | |
|---|---|---|
| Vent. rate | 128 | BPM |
| PR interval | 126 | ms |
| QRS duration | 72 | ms |
| QT/QTc | 282/411 | ms |
| P-R-T axes | 59  34 | 45 |

Sinus tachycardia
Otherwise normal ECG
When compared with ECG of 14:36,
No significant change was found

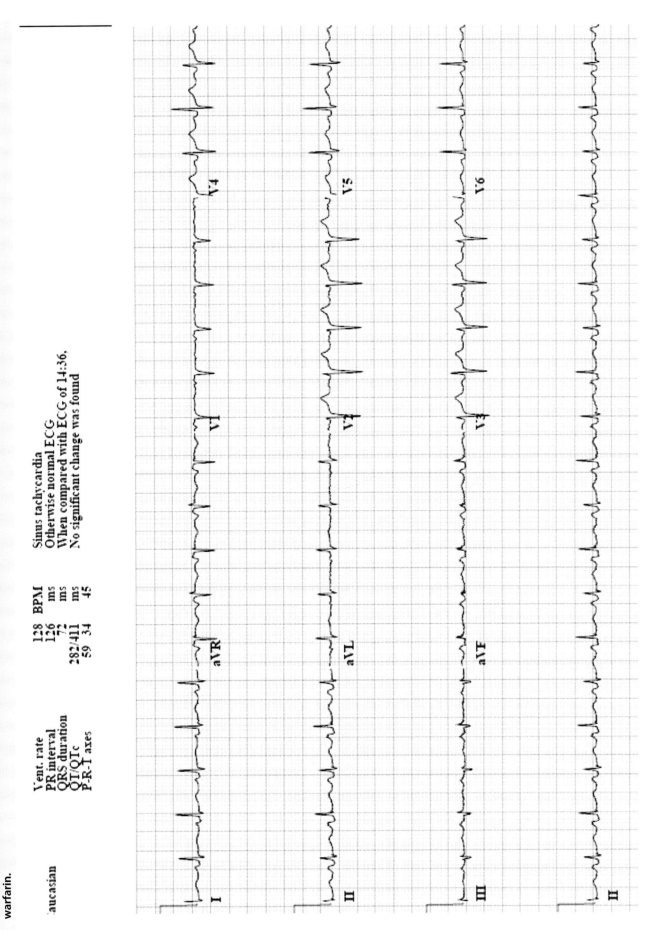

**Case 8.27** A 41-year-old man presented with intermittent chest pain over 1 day, worsening in the previous 30 minutes. The pain radiated down both arms but was reproduced by changes in body position and direct chest wall palpation. He was pain-free in the emergency department. His initial diagnosis was chest pain, likely musculoskeletal muscle strain.

Room:OTF
Loc:1002

| | | |
|---|---|---|
| Vent. rate | 66 | BPM |
| PR interval | 132 | ms |
| QRS duration | 94 | ms |
| QT/QTc | 388/406 | |
| P-R-T axes | 59 28 | 21 |

Normal sinus rhythm
Normal ECG
No previous ECGs available

Technician:
Test ind:

COMMENT:

Referred by:

Reviewed & Interpreted by:

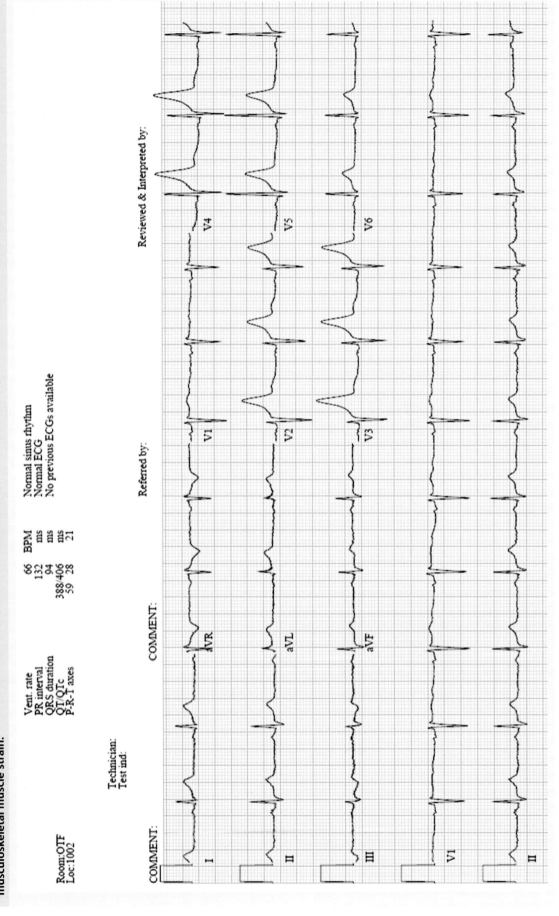

COMMENT:

I

II

III

V1

II

aVR

aVL

aVF

V1

V2

V3

V4

V5

V6

**Case 8.27** Same patient, 40 minutes after the first ECG.

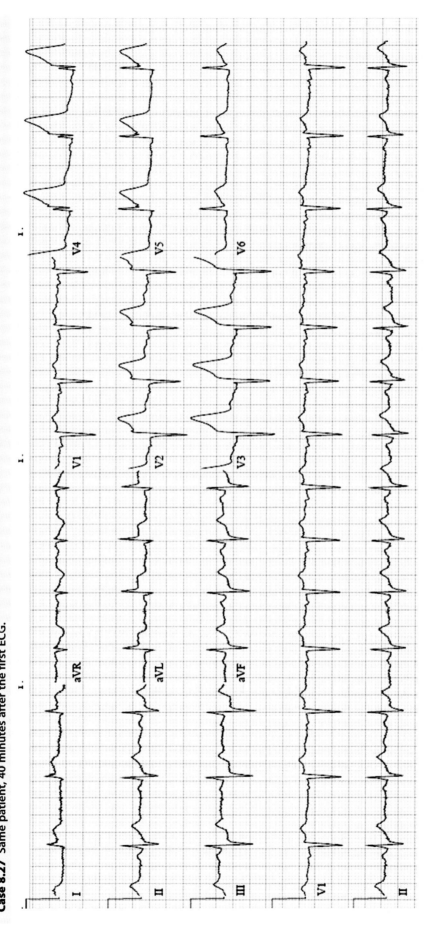

**Case 8.28** A 73-year-old female with a history of hypertension presented with epigastric pain starting at 1 A.M. Her pain was relieved by sublingual nitroglycerin. Her initial troponin level was 0.04.

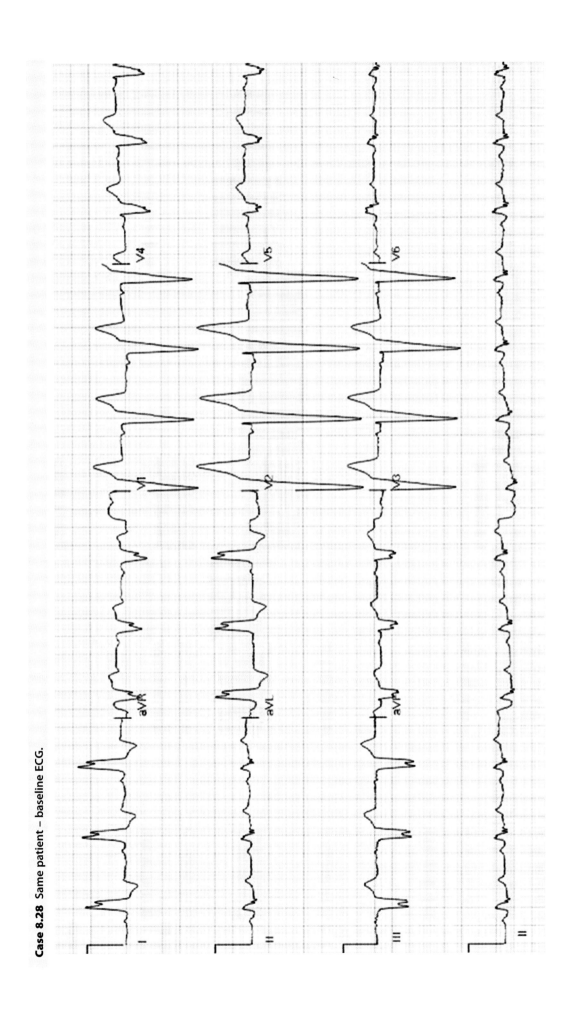

**Case 8.28** Same patient – baseline ECG.

**Case 8.29** A 72-year-old female presented with chest and epigastric pain. The initial troponin levels in the emergency department were 0.01 (negative) and 0.10 (indeterminate). She had recurring episodes of pain; heparin was administered.

**Case 8.30** A 22-year-old female presented to an urgent care clinic with a complaint of shortness of breath and pleuritic chest pain. The ECG was obtained while she was in the waiting room. After a prolonged wait, she left the clinic.

**Case 8.31** A 47-year-old man with a history of hypertension presented after a prolonged episode of chest pain. He experienced temporary relief with sublingual nitroglycerin.

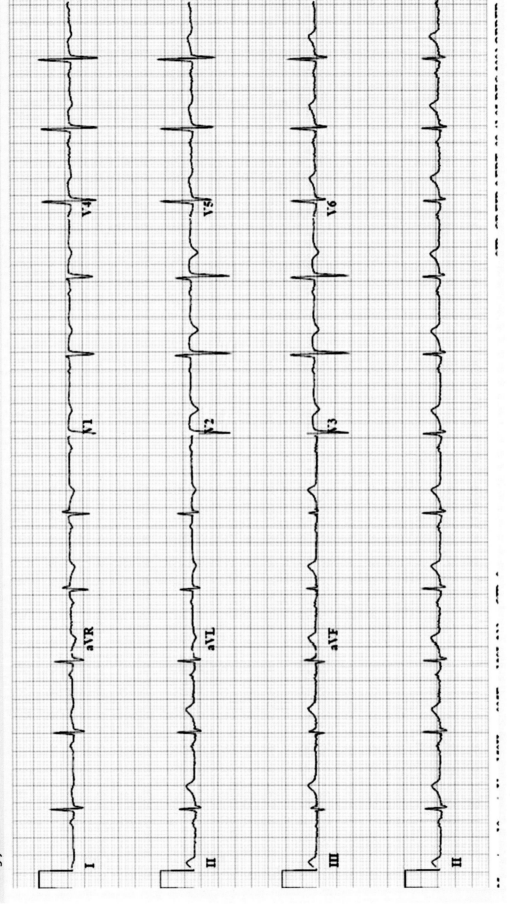

**Case 8.32** A 75-year-old man presented with 5 days of increasing chest pain and shortness of breath. He had a history of hypertension, congestive heart failure and prostate cancer. The ECG computer algorithm suggested the following: "marked T-wave abnormality, consider anterior ischemia."

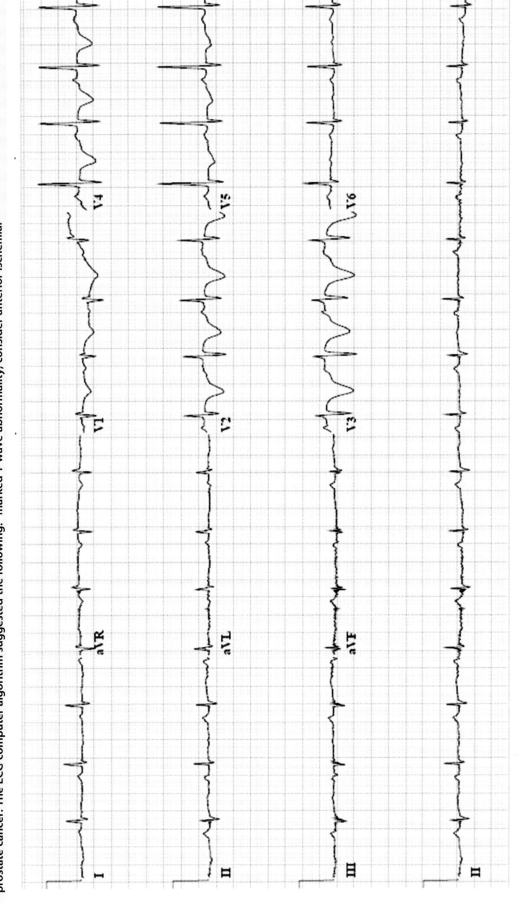

**Case 8.33** A 58-year-old female with a history of diabetes and hypertension presented with shortness of breath, weakness and confusion along with subjective fevers. In the emergency department, she was noted to be "ill-appearing and lethargic, with anasarca."

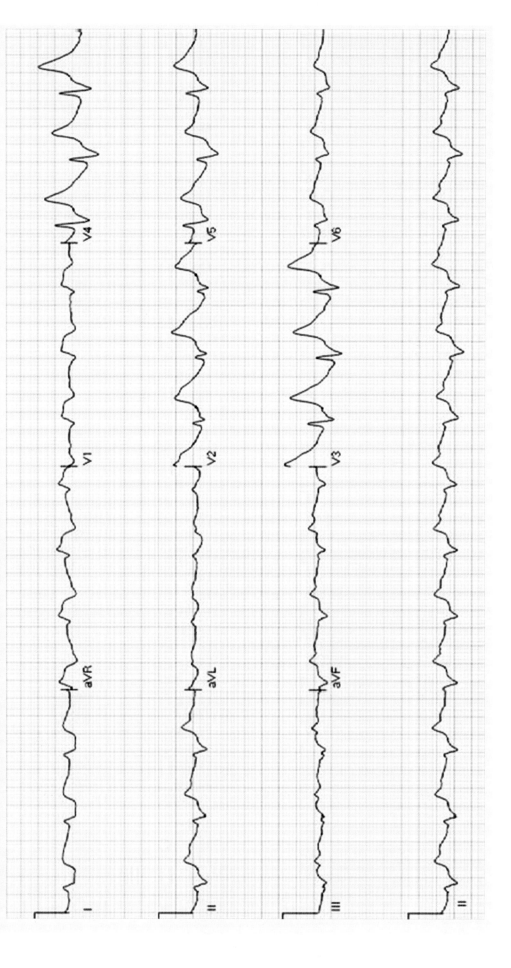

**Case 8.34** A 59-year-old man with a history of diabetes presented with chest and epigastric pain for 2–3 days. He endorsed shortness of breath, dizziness and bilateral ankle swelling.

**Case 8.35** A 66-year-old female returning from Mexico complained of nausea, vomiting, weakness and vision changes (halos and spots).

**Case 8.36** An older man presented with altered mentation, possibly after a fall. No other clinical information was available.

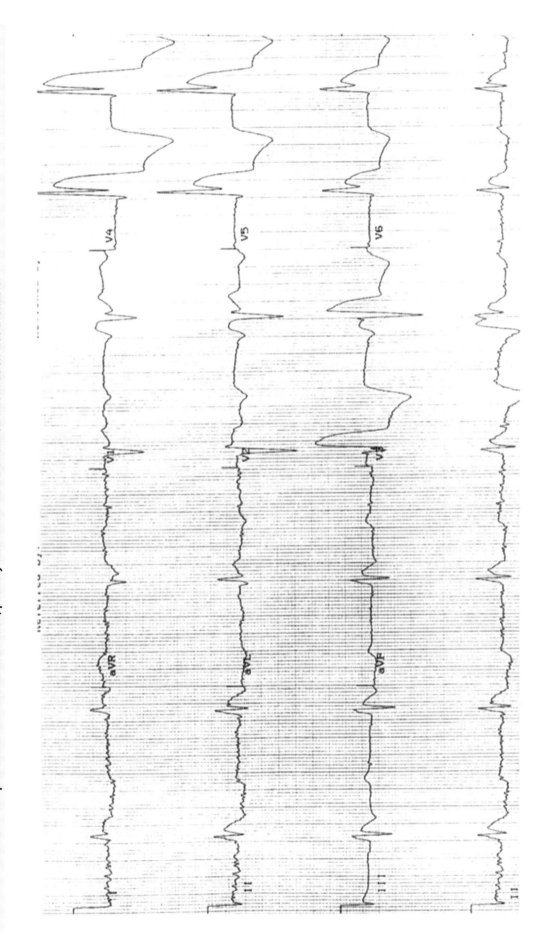

**Case 8.37** A 75-year-old man presented with chest pressure that radiated to both arms, waxing and waning over 2–3 days. The initial troponin level was 3.93.

**Case 8.37** Same patient – ECG recorded 3 hours after the patient's initial presentation.

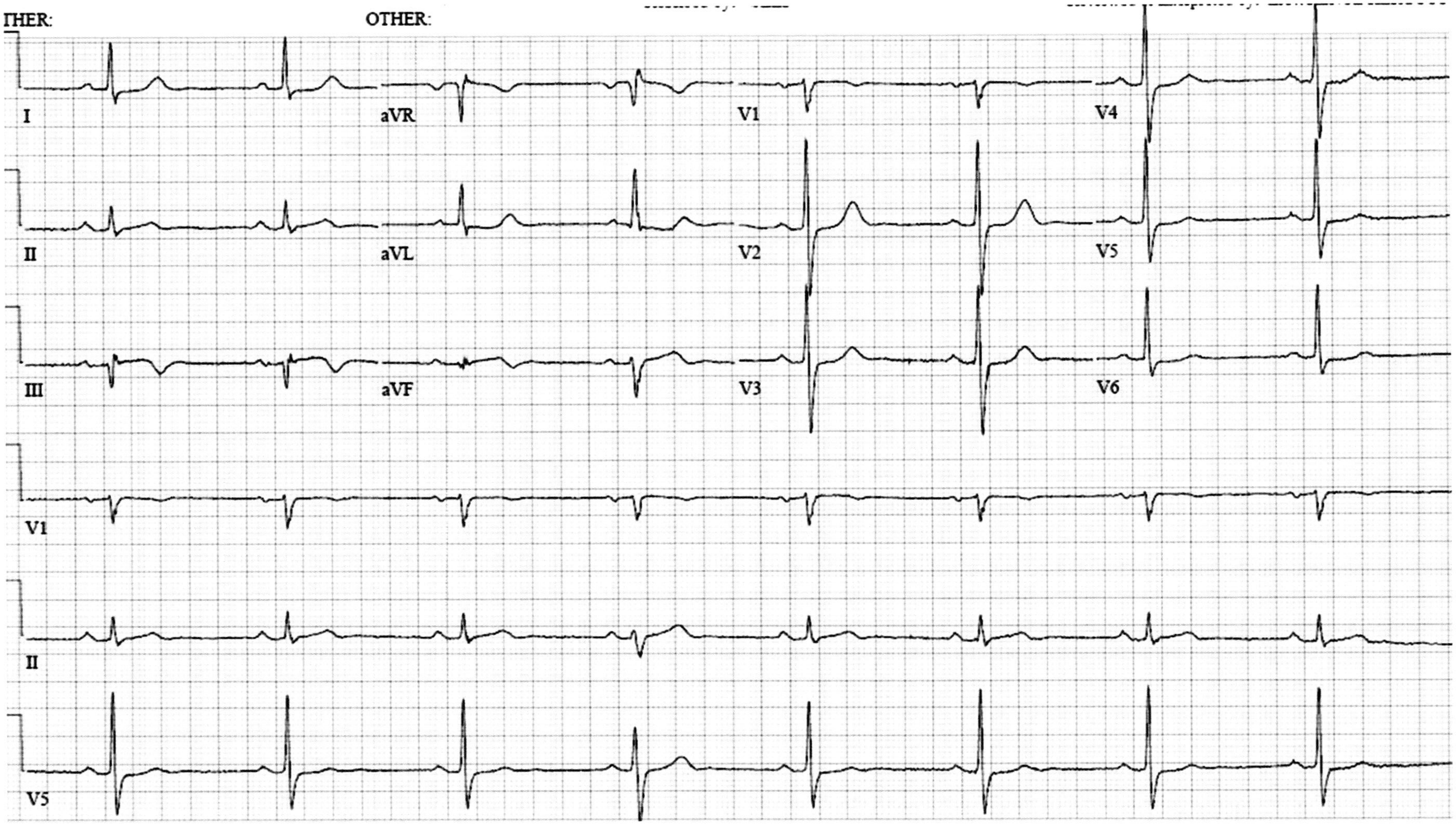

THER:

OTHER:

I  aVR  V1  V4

II  aVL  V2  V5

III  aVF  V3  V6

V1

II

V5

**Case 8.38** A 39-year-old man with a history of bilateral shoulder tendonitis and hypertension presented with 3 days of intermittent shoulder, back and chest pain. He had bilateral upper extremity pain that "moved into his chest." For the past 3 days he had been engaged in heavy lifting, which made the pain worse. He reported having a "negative evaluation of his heart" 1 year earlier. On presentation, his vital signs were normal. His examination was remarkable only for tenderness to palpation over both deltoids. He had normal and symmetric radial and femoral pulses bilaterally.

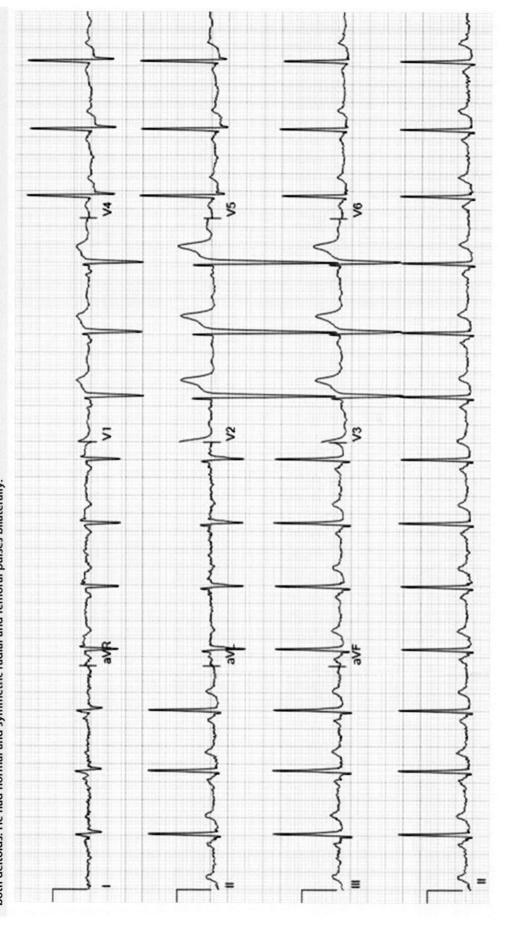

**Case 8.38** Same patient – 2 hours later.

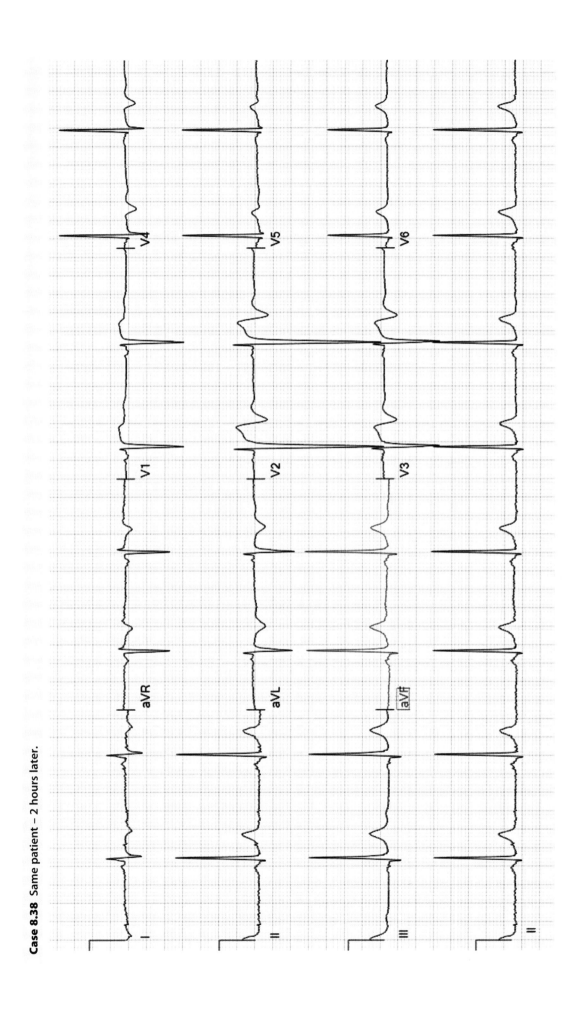

# Self-Study Notes

**Case 8.1** A 75-year-old female had a syncopal episode at the airport. She had no memory of the event. There was no report of chest pain. On arrival in the emergency department, she was asymptomatic; her examination was normal except for a forehead laceration.

## The Electrocardiogram

The ECG shows LVH by voltage criteria. The emergency medicine and cardiology teams both interpreted this tracing as showing only "LVH with strain." However, this cannot be simply "LVH with strain."

- First, the left-sided leads (I, aVL, V5 and V6) do not show the repolarization changes that we are accustomed to seeing with LVH (downsloping ST-segment depressions with asymmetric T-wave inversions).
- Second, there are clear changes of an acute inferior wall STEMI in the inferior leads, along with subtle ST-segment depression in aVL. While LVH routinely causes ST-segment depressions in left-facing leads, including aVL, the T-waves would be expected to be inverted if this were simply "LVH with strain."
- Third, there is definite ST-segment *depression* in precordial leads V2–V3, along with very upright T-waves. The R-waves in V1 and V2 are also abnormally tall; these findings indicate posterior wall involvement (extension of the inferior STEMI into the posterior wall). As discussed in Chapters 2 and 6, the "repolarization abnormalities" in patients with LVH include ST-segment *elevation*, not depression, in the right precordial leads.

Thus, her electrocardiographic diagnosis is clear: LVH is present, but there is also an acute inferior wall STEMI with extension into the posterior wall.

## Clinical Course

This patient was admitted to the hospital for monitoring, evaluation of her syncopal episode and "rule-out acute coronary syndrome." She had a second syncopal episode approximately 12 hours after her admission; she was found to have bradycardia with complete heart block. She was taken to the angiography suite, where she had a 99 percent distal occlusion of the right coronary artery.

**Case 8.2** A 69-year-old female with a history of prior aortic dissection presented to the emergency department with chest pain for 4 hours, accompanied by mild nausea. She was transported by paramedics as a "cardiac alert." She received aspirin, nitroglycerin and an analgesic in the field, with complete resolution of her chest pain. Her blood pressure on arrival to the ED was 163/75.

## The Electrocardiogram

The ECG demonstrates widespread ST-segment elevations, consistent with an extensive anterior, lateral and high lateral STEMI. The patient was transported to the catheterization laboratory emergently for coronary angiography.

## Clinical Course

The patient remained stable in the ED and in the cath lab. Her initial troponin levels were 0.01 and 4.08. The peak troponin level was 10.54. Catheterization revealed minimal, nonobstructive coronary artery disease. However, she had a hyperdyamic base and severe apical akinesis, consistent with takotsubo ballooning cardiomyopathy. Her ejection fraction was moderately reduced (and on follow-up echocardiography, her left ventricular ejection fraction was estimated at 30–35 percent). Urinary toxicologic screens and thyroid function tests were normal. A cardiac MRI study demonstrated severe hypokinesis and ballooning of the mid- and apical LV.

The patient reported no acute or recent stressors. During her hospital stay, she experienced a 45-minute episode of word-finding difficulty, likely caused by cardiac thromboemboli. A follow-up echocardiogram demonstrated a small LV thrombus. She was anticoagulated and improved steadily; she was discharged on hospital day 7.

There were no errors in the care of this patient. It is presented because it represents a "coronary mimic."

## Case 8.3   A 21-year-old female had substernal chest pain followed by a syncopal event while running between gates at the airport.

### The Electrocardiogram

The computer algorithm suggested only "sinus tachycardia" and "T-wave abnormality, consider anterior ischemia." The ECG shows a right axis deviation, but this is not abnormal in a 21-year-old patient. In the limb leads, the low-voltage QRS complexes are also noteworthy and should raise the possibility of acute myocarditis. However, important clues to another diagnosis are present.

There is an S1-Q3-T3 pattern as well as T-wave inversions in both the anterior and inferior leads. Based solely on the ECG, acute pulmonary embolism with right heart strain is highly likely.

### Clinical Course

This patient also endorsed moderate left lower extremity cramping over the preceding two weeks. Her history was also positive for placement of a NuvaRing* 1 week earlier.

A CT-PE study demonstrated a "large pulmonary artery saddle embolus with extensive clot extending into all lobar distributions, and with evidence of right heart strain." There was also evidence of right heart strain on the bedside echocardiogram.

## Case 8.4   A 79-year-old female awoke at 2 A.M. with epigastric and chest pain, diaphoresis and dyspnea. She reported a history of hypertension.

### The Electrocardiogram

Her presenting ECG demonstrates an acute inferior and lateral wall STEMI. The ST-segment elevations in the inferior leads (and the reciprocal ST-segment depressions in I and aVL) and the ST-segment elevations in the lateral precordial leads are not subtle, but they are trying to hide next to the unifocal PVCs. Do not be distracted.

Her ECG also demonstrates Q-waves (and absent R-wave voltage) in the anterior precordial leads due to an anterior wall STEMI that she suffered 4 years earlier.

## Clinical Course

The patient suffered a VF arrest shortly after arrival in the emergency department. After a single shock and intravenous amiodarone, she regained an organized, perfusing rhythm. She was taken emergently to the catheterization laboratory, which demonstrated a 99 percent thrombotic occlusion of the proximal RCA.

## Case 8.5   A 64-year-old man presented with chest pain, headache and altered mental status.

### The Electrocardiogram

The computer algorithm suggests only "nonspecific ST and T wave abnormality" plus a prolonged QT. However, there is more.

The T-waves are hyperacute (they are abnormally tall, broad-based and "bulky" and asymmetric). The T-wave in precordial lead V1 is much taller than the T-wave in V6. These are classic hyperacute T-waves, signaling acute coronary artery occlusion in the earliest stages. There is already straightening and elevation of the ST-segments in V1–V3. ST-segment straightening and hyperacute T-waves occur commonly in the earliest stages of an anterior wall STEMI. The QT-interval prolongation is also suggestive acute ischemia.

### Clinical Course

The emergency medicine team recognized the broad T-waves and ST-segment elevations. Prior to admitting him, they ordered a brain CT scan, which was normal. He was admitted to the cardiology service and underwent angiography, which revealed three-vessel disease, with extensive collaterals and high-grade obstructions in the left anterior descending, right coronary and left circumflex arteries the next day. Three days later he underwent successful coronary artery bypass grafting.

Case 8.6    A 63-year-old man presented with chest pain and dyspnea. He had a white blood cell count of 18,000, and his chest x-ray suggested an acute pneumonia. His initial ED diagnosis was "pneumonia, with possible early sepsis." His initial troponin level was 0.3. The note from the ED team read, "He appears to have pneumonia. In addition, his ECG shows a RBBB and possible anterior wall ischemia. With indeterminate troponin, we will treat him for ACS and non-STEMI."

**The Electrocardiogram**

The ED team missed the diagnosis of acute inferior wall STEMI because of the RBBB. However, the cardiology team recognized the abnormal ST-segments in lead III, accompanied by diagnostic reciprocal ST-segment depressions in leads I and aVL. As discussed in Chapter 2, lead III is the most sensitive lead for making the diagnosis of inferior STEMI caused by RCA occlusion.

The ST-segment elevation in lead III cannot be attributed to the RBBB alone because the ST-segments should be normal in the presence of a RBBB. In most cases, it should be easy to diagnose an acute inferior STEMI in the presence of a RBBB.

The ST-segment elevation in lead V1 is also a critical finding; as discussed in Chapter 2, this signifies RVMI.

**Clinical Course**

The patient's catheterization revealed a 100 percent proximal RCA occlusion. On echocardiogram, his left ventricular function was essentially normal, but his entire right ventricle, as predicted, was dilated and akinetic.

Case 8.7    A 79-year-old man presented with three episodes of syncope over a 2-week period. The most recent syncopal episode occurred the morning of his emergency department visit while he was sitting on his couch.

**The Electrocardiogram**

The ECG demonstrates an old (technically, an "indeterminate age") inferior wall myocardial infarction. Pathologic Q-waves are present in leads III and aVF. In patients with syncope, there is a close association between ECG evidence of an old infarction (pathologic Q-waves) and ventricular tachycardia as the cause of the syncope.

**Clinical Course**

Based on this ECG finding (as well as this patient's age and the repeated episodes of syncope while sitting), he was admitted. An electrophysiologic study was performed that demonstrated inducible VT. An AICD was implanted, and the patient did well.

Case 8.8    A 47-year-old man presented with stuttering chest pain, with radiation to both arms and his right jaw. Aspirin was administered by the paramedics, and his chest pain resolved. Patient was a former smoker, but there was no other medical history. The initial troponin level was 0.11.

**The Electrocardiogram**

The computer reading simply says, "Normal ECG." In fact, the ECG is not at all normal. There is ST-segment straightening and noticeable ST-segment elevation in leads II, III and aVF. Proof that these changes are real resides in the usual place: There is a sagging ST-segment in aVL. The ST-segment depression in aVL may appear minor, but the ST-segment depression is quite significant, given the very low amplitude of the R-wave. The correct diagnosis is inferior wall STEMI.

**Clinical Course**

The patient was observed in the ED. His chest pain returned, and he was taken emergently to the catheterization laboratory, where the main finding was a 100 percent occlusion of the distal RCA. The peak troponin was 42.

## Case 8.9   A 59-year-old man presented with several hours of chest discomfort, nausea and hiccups. He had a recent diagnosis of GERD.

### The Electrocardiogram

The ECG demonstrates an extensive STEMI involving the anteroseptal, lateral and high lateral leads. The ST-segment depressions in the inferior leads are reciprocal to the high lateral (I and aVL) acute STEMI. There is also a RBBB and left anterior fascicular block (bifascicular block). This is a high-risk ECG – the patient is at risk of developing pump failure and complete heart block.

This ECG pattern is familiar and indicates a proximal LAD occlusion before the first diagonal branch and before the septal perforators.

### Clinical Course

This patient had a 100 percent ostial LAD occlusion; he expired shortly after catheterization.

## Case 8.10   A 40-year-old man presented with 3 hours of substernal chest pain after playing a strenuous game of basketball.

### The Electrocardiogram

The ECG has several important abnormalities. The most obvious is the presence of abnormally tall T-waves in leads V1–V3. These T-waves appear "hyperacute." The T-wave in lead V1 should never be this tall (never taller than the T-wave in lead V6). In this tracing, the T-waves are very narrow and peaked, also raising the possibility of hyperkalemia.

Also, there is ST-segment depression in six different leads (V4–V6 and in leads I, II and aVL). These might be interpreted as showing just "ischemia." However, the ST-segment is markedly elevated in lead aVR. The presence of ST-segment elevation in lead aVR and ST-depressions in multiple inferior and lateral leads ("concentric" ischemia) suggests an LAD or left main coronary artery (LCMA) occlusion. This is a STEMI equivalent.

### Clinical Course

The serum potassium was normal. Emergent catheterization revealed a 100 percent ostial LAD occlusion.

This tracing illustrates the importance of ST-elevations in aVR as a "STEMI equivalent." Lead aVR monitors the heart from the upper right side, as if it is exploring the region of the heart between leads I and II. In essence, the ST-segment elevations in aVR are reciprocal to the ST-segment depressions in the left lateral and inferolateral leads (limb leads I, II and aVL and precordial leads V4–V6).

Q-waves (QS-patterns) are also present in leads V1–V3; while it is more common for Q-waves to appear 1 or more days after an acute STEMI, Q-waves frequently appear in the first hours of an evolving anterior wall STEMI. In fact, in anterior wall STEMI, Q-waves are often well developed on the presenting ECG. As emphasized in Chapter 3, these early (near-immediate) Q-waves do not mean that the STEMI is many hours or days old nor that irreversible myocardial cell necrosis has occurred nor that the at-risk myocardium cannot be salvaged via reperfusion interventions.

## Case 8.11   A 67-year-old man with a history of anemia and prostate carcinoma presented with chest pain, nausea and shortness of breath. His triage BP was 101/70.

### The Electrocardiogram

This patient presented with symptoms that are obviously concerning for an acute coronary syndrome. His systolic BP is low.

At first glance, his ECG is not dramatic. But on closer inspection, the pattern is familiar. His anterior precordial leads demonstrate ST-segment straightening (V2 and V3). The T-waves are broad and bulky; the bases are widely splayed, like Marriott's "wishbone effect."

And once we examine the limb leads, the case is closed. Most obvious are the inferior wall ST-segment depressions. And immediately, we see that these ST-segment depressions are reciprocal to the subtle ST-segment elevations in leads aVL and I. The pattern is immediately recognizable. This is an acute anterior and high lateral STEMI in its earliest stages.

It is likely that he is in early cardiogenic shock. And we can predict the culprit coronary vessel – it is likely to be an acute LAD occlusion proximal to D-1.

A repeat ECG was obtained less than 1 hour later (see next tracing).

## Case 8.11  The same patient – 54 minutes later.

### Clinical Course

His follow-up ECG demonstrates an evolving anterior, septal, lateral and high lateral STEMI with a new RBBB and LAFB (bifascicular block). As predicted, "the LAD was totally occluded in the proximal segment before the takeoff of the septal perforators and before D-1."

## Case 8.12  A 63-year-old man presented with 2 hours of left chest pressure. He reported intermittent "indigestion" the night before his visit. After obtaining initial laboratory studies and the ECG, he was admitted to the coronary care unit with a diagnosis of "unstable angina, possible inferior ischemia."

### The Electrocardiogram

It is easy to underread and underappreciate this patient's presenting ECG. "Possible inferior ischemia" is not the correct diagnosis.

Once we see the ST-segment depressions in the inferior leads, it is critical to examine the electrically opposite leads. And, indeed, there is mild ST-segment elevation in lead aVL. Yes, the ST-elevation in aVL is subtle, but it is more than sufficient, given the low amplitude of the R-wave in this lead. This alone is sufficient to make a diagnosis of high lateral STEMI, which may be caused by occlusion of the LAD proximal to D-1, D-1 itself or the LCA (or its obtuse marginal branch).

In this case, there is another clue to the correct culprit vessel. There are abnormally broad and bulky T-waves in leads V2 and V3. There is also ST-segment straightening in leads V1–V4. Although not diagnostic, these anterior ST-T-wave changes are consistent with an early presentation of anterior wall STEMI.

### Clinical Course

After a delay of more than 6 hours, he underwent coronary angiography, which revealed, as predicted, that he had complete occlusion of the proximal LAD. His ECG obtained the morning after admission demonstrates evolution of his anterior and high lateral STEMI (see next tracing).

## Case 8.12  The same patient – the following morning.

The anteroseptal, lateral and high lateral STEMI is now obvious. He has lost all R-wave voltage in I and aVL and in leads V1–V4, consistent with his STEMI. This patient was followed for a number of years for heart failure, with an ejection fraction of about 25 percent.

## Case 8.13  A 42-year-old man presented with severe, resting substernal chest pain ("like a ton of bricks"). He also endorsed mild dyspnea and diaphoresis.

### The Electrocardiogram

Could this young, previously healthy man have acute pericarditis? Could he have benign early repolarization? The answer to both questions is, unequivocally, "no."

Sure, he has ST-segment elevations that are concave upward. But they are regional, affecting predominantly the high lateral leads (I and aVL). And, of course, there are marked reciprocal ST-segment depressions in the inferior leads. The correct diagnosis is acute high lateral STEMI.

### Clinical Course

His initial troponin was 0.5, but it later peaked at 86.9. The culprit artery occlusion in an isolated high lateral STEMI is usually the first diagonal branch of the LAD (D1) or the circumflex artery or one of its proximal branches. In this case, catheterization confirmed an acute proximal circumflex artery obstruction.

## Case 8.14  A 68-year-old man was on an antiretroviral regimen for HIV/AIDS. He presented with substernal chest pain at rest, reporting two similar episodes with mild exertion over the past 2 weeks. He was asymptomatic in the emergency department.

### The Electrocardiogram

In precordial leads V3 and V4, the ST-segments are nearly normal. However, the T-wave is biphasic, ending in a terminal deflection. This is Wellens' syndrome (Type A). Often, this pattern is seen in patients who are no longer symptomatic and in the absence of troponin elevations. In many cases, Wellens' syndrome is indicative of a critical proximal LAD occlusion that has undergone reperfusion but that remains at risk for rethrombosis.

### Clinical Course

Several hours after his presentation, he was taken to the catheterization laboratory, where the culprit lesion was, in fact, a subtotal proximal LAD occlusion. A stent was placed, and his electrocardiogram never showed evolutionary changes of an anteroseptal STEMI. However, his troponin level peaked at 81, and his echocardiogram showed a "moderately reduced left ventricular ejection fraction (35–40 percent) and wall motion abnormalities suggesting an anterior wall infarction in the territory of the LAD."

## Case 8.15  A 64-year-old female with a history of COPD but no history of coronary artery disease presented with 5 days of stuttering chest pain that radiated to both arms. In the emergency department, she had bilateral rales on lung examination. She received heparin and nitroglycerin for a presumed diagnosis of "unstable angina, possible non-STEMI." The computer reading is shown.

### The Electrocardiogram

The computer reading is incorrect, and it is our job to overrule it. Atrial fibrillation is present. But it is doubtful that the ECG represents "anteroseptal subendocardial injury."

In fact, the ECG is highly suggestive of a true (isolated) posterior wall STEMI. The right precordial leads show marked ST-segment depressions with "bolt upright" T-waves. This pattern should not be misclassified as "anterior wall ischemia." Posterior leads could have added to the diagnostic sensitivity. Point-of-care echocardiography might also have been helpful.

### Clinical Course

The patient was given metoprolol, heparin and sublingual nitroglycerin in the emergency department, and she was then admitted with a diagnosis of "acute coronary syndrome (non-STEMI)."

Her troponin peaked at 107. She developed a loud mitral insufficiency murmur and florid pulmonary edema, likely due to papillary muscle insufficiency. The emergency department records made no mention of a mitral insufficiency murmur. Her catheterization revealed an acute subtotal clot obstructing the LCA.

The electrocardiographic lesson is clear. ST-segment depressions in the right precordial leads do not always indicate subendocardial ischemia or a NSTEMI. This pattern is also highly suggestive of a posterior STEMI, especially when the T-waves in V1–V3 are upright.

As discussed in Chapter 4, Posterior Wall Myocardial Infarction, true posterior STEMIs are often missed; they are usually misclassified as "anterior wall ischemia" or "non-ST elevation MI." Catheterization is often delayed by hours or days. Delayed reperfusion is associated with worse outcomes. We should not automatically declare "NSTEMI" when caring for these patients.

## Case 8.16 A 59-year-old man presented in cardiac arrest. He had a history of coronary artery disease. His wife reported he had complained of left arm numbness and shortness of breath and then collapsed. Paramedics found him in ventricular fibrillation. In the ED, despite receiving more than an hour of chest compressions and multiple rounds of cardiac medications, he could not be resuscitated. This rhythm strip was obtained after a third defibrillation shock.

### The Electrocardiogram

The rhythm strip was interpreted as showing an idioventricular rhythm, possibly a reperfusion dysthymia. He was also treated with intravenous calcium, insulin and glucose for possible hyperkalemia.

In fact, these complexes demonstrate a current of injury, suggesting a STEMI. The QRS complexes are not diffusely "wide and ugly"; rather, there is a normal, sharp upstroke to the complexes followed by ST-segment elevation. The underlying rhythm is atrial fibrillation. Had a STEMI been considered, thrombolytic agents could have been administered, although it is impossible to know whether the patient would have survived. Eventually, a 12-lead ECG was obtained.

## Case 8.16 Same patient, 12-lead ECG taken during the resuscitation.

### The Electrocardiogram

The 12-lead ECG, obtained during this patient's prolonged resuscitation, demonstrates the acute inferior and posterior STEMI and atrial fibrillation. It is easy to see how this might be misinterpreted as showing, instead, an idioventricular rhythm, hyperkalemia calcium channel or beta blocker overdose or any other cause of a slow, wide complex rhythm.

The absence of R-waves in V1–V3 also suggests an anteroseptal infarction of indeterminate age (and, indeed, this was demonstrated on ECG tracings taken 2 years earlier).

## Case 8.17 A 72-year-old man with no history of coronary artery disease had severe chest pain while running at the airport. He reported a history of pulmonary fibrosis, and he used home oxygen. His initial troponin was 0.01.

### The Electrocardiogram

The computer algorithm correctly read the first-degree AV block and the right bundle branch block along with the inferior wall infarction of indeterminate age. But the computer missed the acute posterior wall STEMI.

The pattern in leads V2 and V3 is familiar. There are marked ST-segment depressions and unusually tall ("bolt upright") T-waves in these leads; this "reciprocal sign" is consistent with posterior wall STEMI. The ST-segment depressions and tall T-waves in V2 and V3 are far out of proportion to what might be expected with a RBBB alone.

There is also an acute high lateral STEMI. The ST-segments are elevated in leads I and aVL, accompanied by marked ST-segment depressions in III and aVF. High lateral STEMIs commonly accompany posterior wall STEMIs.

### Clinical Course

Despite the normal troponin level, the posterior and high lateral wall STEMI was recognized immediately by the emergency department team. Catheterization revealed a 100 percent occlusion of the proximal LCA, prior to the takeoff of the first obtuse marginal (OM) branch. As highlighted in Chapter 4, LCA occlusion frequently results in posterior STEMI; the large OM perfuses the high later wall. Thus, the ECG pattern of high lateral and posterior wall injury is easily explained.

The peak troponin was 25.8. He recovered completely after placement of a drug-eluting stent in the LCA.

## Case 8.18 A 47-year-old man presented with sharp chest pain. He had a history of pericarditis 2 years earlier.

### The Electrocardiogram

The patient's chest pain was felt to be "atypical" for an acute coronary syndrome. His ECG was initially interpreted as showing acute pericarditis. Indeed, the ST-segments are diffusely elevated across most of the precordial leads and in the inferior leads, with preservation of the normal upward concavity in most of the leads. But as we have emphasized, upwardly concave ST-segments often provide only false reassurance.

Why is acute pericarditis (or early repolarization) highly unlikely in this case? First, the ST-segment elevations are actually in a regional (anatomic) distribution; they are not "global." They are most prominent in the inferior leads (II, III and aVF) and the lateral precordial leads (V4–V6). The ST-segments in lead aVL may be slightly depressed (reciprocal to the inferior wall ST-segment elevations). Notably, there is no PR-segment depression anywhere that might suggest pericarditis. The only other abnormality is the single PVC.

## Clinical Course

His initial troponin was 5.6. Immediately, he underwent coronary angiography, which revealed a 100 percent mid-RCA occlusion. His right-sided leads were also positive for acute right ventricular infarction.

## Case 8.19 A 57-year-old female presented with leg stiffness and shortness of breath. On examination, she was well appearing. However, her oxygen saturation was only 90 percent on 5 liters of nasal oxygen, and she had signs of deep venous thrombophlebitis of the left leg.

### The Electrocardiogram

She has an abnormal S-wave in lead I (abnormal right axis deviation), sinus tachycardia, right precordial T-wave inversions and a small rSR' in precordial lead V1 ("incomplete RBBB").

The computer algorithm could not put these together, suggesting only "right axis deviation, possible right ventricular enlargement; and T-wave abnormality, consider anterior ischemia." We have come to expect that. The clinician has to put the clues together.

### Clinical Course

Given the history, leg examination and hypoxemia, the case is not so challenging. Her history and physical examination were highly suggestive of an acute DVT and pulmonary thromboembolism. But the ECG findings are still important, and in another setting (without the hypoxemia), we might miss them.

She underwent an immediate CTPE study, which demonstrated: "Extensive clot in the right and left main pulmonary arteries, extending bilaterally into the lower lobes, with mild pulmonary hypertension." Her echocardiogram revealed a flattened septum, indicative of right ventricular pressure and volume overload, moderate dilatation of the right ventricle and right atrium, and mild tricuspid regurgitation.

## Case 8.20 A 36-year-old man presented with hallucinations and fatigue.

### The Electrocardiogram

The ECG shows only early repolarization, with classic diffuse ST-segment elevations and "fish-hook" notching of the J-points in the anterior precordial (V3–V4) and inferior limb leads. A careful examination of the ECG shows no regional (anatomic) localization of the ST-segment elevations nor any sign of reciprocal ST-segment depressions.

### Clinical Course

The hallucinations and fatigue were evaluated in the emergency department. He improved after intravenous hydration and was admitted to the hospital. His troponin level was 0.00, and his electrolytes and toxicologic studies were unremarkable. His ECG remained stable.

## Case 8.21 A 67-year-old female had a history of chronic alcohol use and frequent emergency department visits for chest and back pain and other symptoms. She presented with worsening chest pain over 5 days. Her triage troponin level was 0.40.

### The Electrocardiogram

The computer correctly read the sinus bradycardia, borderline limb lead criteria for left ventricular hypertrophy and the AV dissociation. The computer also queried "anterior ischemia" and "lateral ischemia." But the computer algorithm was unable to decipher the other changes present on this ECG.

First, there is an acute inferior wall STEMI. The ST-segment is straightened and mildly elevated in lead III, and there is reciprocal ST-segment depression in aVL. The ST-segment depressions in V1–V3 indicate extension of the infarction into the posterior wall. A repeat ECG 15 minutes later was interpreted correctly by the computer algorithm. The tall, terminal R-wave in aVR was unexplained.

One would predict that the culprit vessel is the RCA, based on the ST-elevations that are taller in lead III compared with lead II, suggesting a rightward and inferior direction to the injury vector. The AV block is not surprising, given that in 90 percent of individuals, the RCA gives off the posterior descending branch, which in turn supplies the AV nodal artery.

### Clinical Course

Her repeat troponin level was 22. The angiography report concluded: "The RCA is a dominant, large caliber vessel which gives rise to acute marginal and RV branches before continuing in the AV groove. It gives off a large PDA. The proximal and mid-RCA have multifocal 70 percent stenosing lesions that appear to be ruptured plaques."

## Case 8.22   A 33-year-old man presented with an acute asthma attack. This electrocardiogram was obtained because he had a tachycardia at triage.

### The Electrocardiogram

According to the computer interpretation, the patient has an acute anterior wall ST-elevation myocardial infarction. Indeed, ST-segment elevations are present in the right precordial leads, which could represent an acute anteroseptal STEMI. In fact, the ECG demonstrates a "coronary mimic" (or pseudo-infarct pattern). This patient has the Brugada syndrome and is at risk for sudden cardiac death.

As highlighted in Chapter 7, Confusing Conditions: ST-Segment Elevations and Tall T-Waves (Coronary Mimics), the hallmark of the Brugada syndrome is a RBBB-like pattern (or incomplete RBBB) in leads V1 or V2. Specifically, there is a high takeoff of the ST-segment from the T-wave. The ST-segment is elevated as it is here. In Type 1 Brugada, the ST-segment emerges suddenly from the R-wave (or R' wave) and then descends rapidly into an inverted T-wave. In Type 2 Brugada, the ST-segment remains elevated and has a "saddle" appearance. This ECG is most consistent with a Type 1 pattern.

The Brugada pattern represents a genetically based sodium channelopathy. The ECG features may come and go, especially if the sodium channelopathy is provoked by sodium channel blocking drugs. As highlighted in Chapter 7, when the ECG is equivocal, the diagnostic features of Brugada may be unmasked by recording the right-sided precordial leads (V1–V3) one to two intercostal spaces higher on the chest so that the leads are more directly over the right ventricular outflow track, where the arrhythmogenic substrate for the Brugada syndrome resides. In the hospital, administering a procainamide challenge can also unmask the sodium channelopathy, resulting in a more diagnostic ECG.

### Clinical Course

This patient had no family history of sudden cardiac death. He was admitted directly from the emergency department for electrophysiologic testing and AICD placement.

Brugada syndrome is not particularly common; however, it is a relatively frequent cause of syncope and sudden cardiac death due to ventricular fibrillation, even among young and healthy patients. Therefore, it must not be overlooked by the emergency electrocardiographer.

## Case 8.23   A 35-year-old female noted shortness of breath and anxiety while visiting her newborn in the neonatal intensive care unit.

### The Electrocardiogram

This patient's ECG is highly suggestive of an acute pulmonary embolism. Although the computer is unable to decipher the meaning of the right precordial T-wave inversions (or the concurrent T-wave inversions in the inferior leads), we immediately recognize that this pattern is suggestive of acute pulmonary embolism. Sinus tachycardia is also present.

### Clinical Course

This patient was 2 weeks post-partum normal vaginal delivery at 32 weeks. Her CT-PE study demonstrated large, bilateral saddle pulmonary emboli. A baseline ECG 3 weeks earlier was normal without T-wave inversions.

The differential diagnosis of shortness of breath during and after pregnancy is broad. In addition to the routine causes, we must consider pulmonary embolism, amniotic fluid embolism, peripartum cardiomyopathy with congestive heart failure, congestive heart failure caused by preeclampsia and severe hypertension, and mitral stenosis (more common in earlier decades).

**Case 8.24   A 54-year-old man without any significant medical history presented with new-onset shortness of breath. He reported progressive fatigue and weakness over the past month, and on the day of his visit, he noted marked exertional dyspnea while shopping. In the ED, he was tachypneic (RR = 30), and he was in respiratory distress. His lung examination revealed decreased breath sounds and dullness to percussion at the left base. Rales were noted in the middle left lung field. He was felt to have an acute coronary syndrome; his first troponin was elevated at 8.0.**

### The Electrocardiogram

The ECG is abnormal. There is sinus tachycardia and diffuse low voltage across the limb and precordial leads. The differential diagnosis of low-voltage QRS complexes in a patient with acute dyspnea includes pericardial tamponade, myocarditis, chronic emphysema and infiltrative myocardial disease (in addition to noncardiac causes such as obesity). In this case, the diagnosis of pericardial tamponade is suggested by the finding of electrical alternans, most evident in the lead II rhythm strip and in lead V1.

The lung findings (rales and consolidation findings in the lower, posterior, left lung field) were probably attributable to the posterior location of the pericardial effusion (Ewart's sign). Ewart's sign is dullness to percussion, egophony and bronchial breath sounds below the tip of the left scapula, attributed to posterior localization of a large pericardial effusion causing lung consolidation.

**Case 8.25   A 53-year-old female with diabetes and chronic renal insufficiency presented with shortness of breath, chest pain, pulmonary edema, hypoxia and hypotension.**

### The Electrocardiogram

The computer algorithm made numerous observations: "Sinus tachycardia; possible left atrial enlargement; left axis deviation; ST-T-wave abnormalities, possible lateral ischemia; and anterior infarct, possibly acute." The summary computer interpretation was: "******ACUTE MI*******."

However, the emergency medicine clinicians immediately focused on the combination of tall, peaked and narrow-based T-waves, which could be the hyperacute T-waves of ischemia or hyperkalemia. The widened QRS complex (QRS duration = 122 msec) makes hyperkalemia likely.

Hyperkalemia can cause ST-segment elevation, typically (as in this case) in the setting of peaked T-waves and QRS widening.

### Clinical Course

Treatment was initiated based on this ECG alone. This patient, who had missed three or more scheduled dialysis visits, had a serum potassium of 7.2. Her creatinine was 10.4. After receiving calcium, sodium bicarbonate, insulin and glucose, all her ECG changes resolved, and her clinical status began to improve. She underwent emergent hemodialysis. Follow-up ECGs showed a normal QRS duration, normal ST-segments, shortening of the PR interval and normal T-waves.

**Case 8.26   A 52-year-old man presented with shortness of breath and generalized weakness. His initial blood pressure was 118/84. His respirations were 18 and unlabored. He was not in any respiratory distress. He had a history of lung carcinoma, chronic hoarseness and a prior episode of deep venous thrombosis (DVT), and he was taking warfarin.**

### The Electrocardiogram

The computer suggests "sinus tachycardia, otherwise normal ECG." Fortunately, the emergency physicians paid no attention and made the correct diagnosis from this ECG.

The combination of sinus tachycardia, low-voltage QRS complexes and electrical alternans is highly suggestive of pericardial tamponade. The electrical alternans is most evident in lead II (and in the lead II rhythm strip) and in leads V4 and V5.

## Clinical Course

The point-of-care ultrasound revealed a large, concentric pericardial effusion with mild tamponade physiology. Pericardiocentesis demonstrated that he had a 750 cc malignant pericardial effusion.

Shortness of breath and a low BP in the setting of lung cancer may not always indicate acute pulmonary embolism. Pericardial effusion is also high on the list. The ECG may provide the first diagnostic clues.

## Case 8.27 A 41-year-old man presented with intermittent chest pain over 1 day, worsening in the previous 30 minutes. The pain radiated down both arms but was reproduced by changes in body position and direct chest wall palpation. He was pain-free in the emergency department. His initial diagnosis was chest pain, likely musculoskeletal muscle strain.

### The Electrocardiogram

The ECG was initially interpreted as "within normal limits." There was some debate about whether his precordial T-waves were "hyperacute." Therefore, he was observed in the ED. Forty minutes later, he had an acute episode of severe chest pain, accompanied by diaphoresis. His repeat ECG follows.

## Case 8.27 Same patient, 40 minutes after the first ECG.

### The Electrocardiogram

The second ECG demonstrates an acute anterior, lateral and high lateral STEMI.

Reexamine the initial 12-lead ECG. The first question is whether the T-waves in precordial leads V2, V3 and V4 are hyperacute. It is not always easy to tell. However, these T-waves are probably abnormal: they are tall, they are broad-based, they are asymmetric, and they tower over the diminished R-waves in these leads. Whenever hyperacute T-waves are suspected, it is critical to repeat the ECG at 15-minute intervals. As discussed in Chapter 7, hyperacute T-waves are often the first abnormality to appear after acute coronary artery occlusion; they are usually a temporary abnormality.

But even on the original ECG, there is much more to see. A high lateral STEMI is already present, enough to activate the catheterization team. There is marked ST-segment depression in lead III; and in the reciprocal lead (aVL), the ST-segments are noticeably elevated. Now, we know that the hyperacute T-waves in the right precordial leads are real. And we recognize this pattern: the combination of *hyperacute T-waves in the right precordial leads plus early, subtle changes of a high lateral STEMI*. We know what this means: the patient almost certainly has an obstructing thrombus in the LAD, proximal to the first diagonal branch.

### Clinical Course

Following the second ECG, the patient was taken immediately to the catheterization laboratory. Not surprisingly, "the LAD was 100 percent occluded in its proximal segment." A bare metal stent was inserted. His peak troponin level (on the second day) was 167. An echocardiogram showed akinesis of the apex and the anteroseptal wall, with hypokinesis of the anterior wall. The study suggested evolution of a small apical thrombus.

## Case 8.28 A 73-year-old female with a history of hypertension presented with epigastric pain starting at 1 A.M. Her pain was relieved by sublingual nitroglycerin. Her initial troponin level was 0.04.

### The Electrocardiogram

The ECG shows a normal sinus tachycardia; the long pause is caused by a blocked premature atrial contraction (PAC). A left bundle branch block (LBBB) is also present. There are ST-segment elevations and tall T-waves in the right precordial leads (V1–V3).

Do the ST-segment elevations in the right precordial leads (V1–V3) indicate a STEMI? Or just the patient's LBBB? Given this patient's symptoms, how should we proceed?

Perhaps the first step is to apply the Sgarbossa criteria. One of the well-known criteria is *excessively discordant ST-elevations (≥ 5 mm) in leads with a negative QRS complex*. In this case, the ST-segment elevation in lead V2 (measured at the J-point) is almost exactly 5 mm. Strictly speaking, this is only borderline, and it may not meet the Sgarbossa threshold. And, in any case, this criterion (5 mm or more of discordant ST-elevation) is not highly specific. But it still suggests the possibility of an acute anterior wall STEMI. Leads V5 and V6 also show deep ST-segment depressions (although these are not included in the Sgarbossa algorithm).

There are additional steps that may help in ruling in or out an acute anterior wall STEMI. One is to compare this ECG with old tracings. Another is to perform emergent bedside echocardiography.

## Clinical Course

A previous ECG was obtained (see next figure). The ST-segments on the baseline tracing are much less elevated in V1, V2 and V3. This is a significant finding.

A bedside echocardiogram was then performed. It was a limited study, but it demonstrated large anterior wall and apical hypokinesis, with an estimated ejection fraction of 10–15 percent. She went immediately to the angiography suite, where she had a totally occluded LAD immediately after the first and second diagonal branches. Her troponin was never higher than 2.1. Her follow-up echocardiogram showed persistent anterior, lateral, apical, septal and posterior wall hypokinesis with an improved ejection fraction of 35 percent.

## Case 8.28  Same patient – baseline ECG.

### The Electrocardiogram

The old ECG demonstrates a typical LBBB; here there are discordant ST-segment elevations in the right precordial leads, but the ST-segment elevations never exceed 4 mm.

## Case 8.29  A 72-year-old female presented with chest and epigastric pain. The initial troponin levels in the emergency department were 0.01 (negative) and 0.10 (indeterminate). She had recurring episodes of pain; heparin was administered.

### The Electrocardiogram

Would you call for immediate activation of the catheterization laboratory?

The most notable abnormality (apart from the atrial fibrillation) is the ST-segment depression in the inferior leads (III and aVF). This immediately calls our attention to the ST-segments in leads I and aVL, which are mildly elevated. Of course, the ST-segment elevation in aVL is more dramatic and diagnostic in the context of the very low-amplitude R-wave.

This is a STEMI involving the high lateral leads. The ECG also shows poor R-wave progression across the precordial leads, consistent with an old (more properly, "indeterminate age") anterior wall infarction.

### Clinical Course

The peak troponin was 80.1. The interventional cardiology team was called. She underwent immediate angiography, which revealed, predictably, normal coronary arteries except for occlusion of a large first diagonal branch (D-1). The occlusions were felt to be indicative of an embolic event, secondary to her chronic atrial fibrillation.

## Case 8.30  A 22-year-old female presented to an urgent care clinic with a complaint of shortness of breath and pleuritic chest pain. The ECG was obtained while she was in the waiting room. After a prolonged wait, she left the clinic.

### The Electrocardiogram

The ECG is remarkable for sinus tachycardia and marked low-voltage QRS complexes in the limb leads. This combination should immediately suggest myocarditis, especially in a young patient. Pericardial tamponade also presents with these ECG findings.

### Clinical Course

After a long stay in the waiting room, she left and returned home. About 4 hours later, she sustained a cardiac arrest. Resuscitation attempts were unsuccessful. An autopsy was performed, which confirmed that she had acute, fulminant myocarditis.

## Case 8.31  A 47-year-old man with a history of hypertension presented after a prolonged episode of chest pain. He experienced temporary relief with sublingual nitroglycerin.

### The Electrocardiogram

The ECG is normal except for the anterior T-wave inversions. The T-wave is also inverted in aVL. The differential diagnosis should include anterior wall ischemia or, with an elevated troponin, a non-STEMI. Acute pulmonary embolism should also be considered whenever there are T-wave inversions in leads V1–V3. Intracerebral hemorrhage would be quite unlikely given his history. Various forms of cardiomyopathy, including takotsubo syndrome, could be considered, along with hypokalemia (although the QT interval is not prolonged).

In this case, the symmetric T-wave inversions in a regional distribution (anterior and high lateral walls) suggest ischemia.

## Clinical Course

The initial troponin level was 1.6. His chest pain resolved after treatment with intravenous nitroglycerin and heparin. He was sent for urgent coronary angiography, which revealed a 90 percent proximal thrombotic LAD occlusion. Given the T-wave inversion involving the high lateral lead (aVL), it was not surprising that the LAD was occluded proximal to the origin of the first diagonal branch (see Chapter 3).

His final clinical and electrocardiographic diagnosis was acute NSTEMI (with a troponin leak) involving the anterior and high lateral wall.

## Case 8.32    A 75-year-old man presented with 5 days of increasing chest pain and shortness of breath. He had a history of hypertension, congestive heart failure and prostate cancer. The ECG computer algorithm suggested the following: "marked T-wave abnormality, consider anterior ischemia."

### The Electrocardiogram

The ECG is consistent with an inferior wall infarction of indeterminate age. However, the most significant abnormality is the presence of deep T-wave inversions in the anterior precordium. The computer suggested only one possibility: "Anterior ischemia."

Fortunately, the treating physicians considered other diagnoses as well. Of course, they were concerned about anterior wall ischemia. But given the anterior precordial T-wave inversions (and his history of cancer), they also included acute pulmonary embolism in the differential diagnosis.

As discussed in Chapter 5, T-wave inversions in the anterior precordial leads are the most common ECG abnormality in patients with acute, hemodynamically significant PE after sinus tachycardia. In this case, there are two additional ECG clues that suggest acute PE. The first is the very small, barely noticeable S-wave in lead I; it catches our attention only because we are looking for it – and because we know that any right axis deviation may be abnormal in a patient in his 70s. Also, there is an rSR' in lead V1; this findings may signify acute right heart strain.

### Clinical Course

The initial serum troponin level was normal. The d-dimer was 5,100. Because his creatinine was elevated, a ventilation-perfusion scan was performed, which demonstrated a "massive pulmonary embolism."

Emergent bedside echocardiography can also help differentiate anterior wall ischemia from acute pulmonary embolism. This patient's echocardiogram demonstrated severe right heart strain and other changes of a large clot burden. Refer back to Chapter 5 for additional examples of acute pulmonary emboli and for discussion of the electrocardiographic changes that signify higher pulmonary artery pressures, more extensive pulmonary vascular occlusion and a higher risk of cardiovascular collapse and early mortality.

## Case 8.33    A 58-year-old female with a history of diabetes and hypertension presented with shortness of breath, weakness and confusion along with subjective fevers. In the emergency department, she was noted to be "ill-appearing and lethargic, with anasarca."

### The Electrocardiogram

Sometimes we refer to this presentation as "wide and ugly QRS complexes in a patient who is critically ill."

There are ST-segment elevations in leads V1, V2 and aVR. But do these signify a STEMI?

What is more compelling is the other "company": the QRS is markedly widened, in a pattern that does not resemble a classic right or left bundle branch block. The T-waves are very prominent (peaked). And while the rhythm is uncertain, it appears that there are low-amplitude P-waves with a markedly prolonged PR-interval (best seen in the lead II rhythm strip). Prolongation of the PR-interval or complete absence of the P-waves (atrial asystole) is common in severe hyperkalemia.

The diagnosis is hyperkalemia. Treatment must begin based on this ECG alone.

## Clinical Course

She was intubated in the emergency department for airway protection. Treatment was initiated with intravenous calcium gluconate, sodium bicarbonate and insulin and glucose. Her first serum potassium level was 8.0. Her ECG rapidly improved, with a return to a normal sinus rhythm and a normal, narrow QRS complex. She had a history of end-stage renal disease and was on dialysis; she underwent emergent hemodialysis immediately after admission to the hospital.

## Case 8.34  A 59-year-old man with a history of diabetes presented with chest and epigastric pain for 2–3 days. He endorsed shortness of breath, dizziness and bilateral ankle swelling.

### The Electrocardiogram

There is an extensive, acute anteroseptal STEMI and also a right bundle branch block (RBBB) and a left anterior fascicular block (LAFB). The ST-segments are elevated in all the precordial leads (V1–V6).

This is a familiar picture. The ECG suggests an acute occlusion of the LAD proximal to the septal perforator branches. Q-waves are already forming in the anterior precordial leads. However, as emphasized in Chapter 3, in an anterior STEMI, early Q-waves appear commonly; these Q-waves do not necessarily signify an old infarction or that the myocardial injury is irreversible or that reperfusion therapies are not indicated.

Sinus tachycardia is also present. In the setting of an acute STEMI, sinus tachycardia is often an arrhythmia of pump failure. Indeed, the ED clinicians observed that he was hypotensive (systolic blood pressure = 90 mm Hg), had cool extremities, was slightly confused and had a lactic acidosis, all consistent with rapidly worsening cardiogenic shock.

### Clinical Course

His initial troponin level was 11.26. Obviously, he was transported immediately to the catheterization laboratory. He had a 100 percent thrombotic occlusion of the proximal LAD; there was also severe stenosis of the left circumflex artery. After aspiration thrombectomy of the clotted proximal LAD, overlapping bare metal stents were placed. He also had a stent placed in the mid-LCA. An intra-aortic balloon pump was inserted because of cardiogenic shock. Dobutamine was also administered, and he was admitted for further care.

His peak troponin level was 30.81. He developed a large left ventricular thrombus, and he had bouts of atrial fibrillation. He was discharged home after a 2-week hospitalization.

## Case 8.35  A 66-year-old female returning from Mexico complained of nausea, vomiting, weakness and vision changes (halos and spots).

### The Electrocardiogram

The lead II rhythm strip demonstrates a sinus rhythm with second-degree heart block (Mobitz Type I). The etiology of the AV nodal block becomes obvious after examining the shape of the diffuse ST-segment depressions. The ST-segments are smooth, coved and upwardly concave; they resemble Salvador Dalí's mustache (or the cables of a suspension bridge). The sagging ST-segments are consistent with digitalis effect; the AV nodal block indicates digitalis toxicity.

### Clinical Course

Her serum digoxin level was 4.7. Her creatinine was 2.7. She was treated with digoxin immune Fab (Digibind®), and her heart block and bradycardia slowly improved. This tracing illustrates both digitalis "effect" as well as signs of digitalis toxicity.

## Case 8.36  An older man presented with altered mentation, possibly after a fall. No other clinical information was available.

### The Electrocardiogram

There is some artifact that could be related to electrical noise or a tremor. Or it could represent shivering. The rhythm is probably junctional, although slow, regularized atrial fibrillation cannot be excluded.

And the diffuse, dome-shaped ST-segment elevations? It would be easy to mistake these Osborn waves for an acute ST-elevation myocardial infarction.

## Clinical Course

No other clinical history was available. This patient's core temperature was 31 degrees Centigrade. He was successfully managed with core rewarming techniques.

## Case 8.37   A 75-year-old man presented with chest pressure that radiated to both arms, waxing and waning over 2–3 days. The initial troponin level was 3.93.

### The Electrocardiogram

Sinus bradycardia is present, along with mild ST-elevation in lead III and T-wave inversions in III and aVF. The ECG was repeated every 15–30 minutes without any noticeable change.

The question that the ED and cardiology teams asked was is there a STEMI? The decision was made to admit this patient to the coronary care unit for medical management. However, evidence of a STEMI and indications for immediate reperfusion may already be present. There is a 1 mm ST-segment elevation in lead III, accompanied by a barely detectable reciprocal ST-segment depression in the opposite lead (aVL). ST-segment straightening and T-wave inversions are present in leads III and aVF.

As Marriott might say, at the very least "this patient needs to be kept under wraps."

### Clinical Course

After admission, the patient continued to have chest pressure with radiation to his arms and jaw despite receiving nitroglycerin and heparin infusions. Within 8 hours, his troponin level peaked at 113.3.

Six hours after his presentation to the ED, he was taken to the catheterization laboratory, where he had a 100 percent thrombotic occlusion of the middle portion of the left circumflex artery. He underwent a successful aspiration thrombectomy, followed by placement of a drug-eluting stent. His transthoracic echocardiography was normal.

Just prior to his catheterization, a follow-up ECG was recorded (next ECG).

## Case 8.37   Same patient – ECG recorded 3 hours after the patient's initial presentation.

### The Electrocardiogram

The inferior wall STEMI is somewhat more obvious on this tracing. The ST-segment elevation in lead III is now unmistakable, and there is still ST-segment straightening and T-wave inversion in III and aVF. The ST-segments are now clearly depressed in leads I and aVL.

This patient's discharge diagnosis was "non-STEMI"; however, it is clear that he suffered an inferior wall STEMI due to a complete occlusion of a major coronary artery.

The initial ECG abnormalities were subtle. But as Marriott wrote, "There are two main categories of urgent electrocardiograms: Those that present you with a clear-cut, unambivalent picture that justifies definitive diagnosis, decision and action; and those that are not diagnostic but suggest a disaster that may be unforgiving if you fail to think of it" (Marriott, 1997).

## Case 8.38   A 39-year-old man with a history of bilateral shoulder tendonitis and hypertension presented with 3 days of intermittent shoulder, back and chest pain. He had bilateral upper extremity pain that "moved into his chest." For the past 3 days he had been engaged in heavy lifting, which made the pain worse. He reported having a "negative evaluation of his heart" 1 year earlier. On presentation, his vital signs were normal. His examination was remarkable only for tenderness to palpation over both deltoids. He had normal and symmetric radial and femoral pulses bilaterally.

### The Electrocardiogram

The initial ECG was read as "compatible with LVH with repolarization abnormalities." The initial diagnosis was "atypical chest wall and shoulder pain." The troponin was negative. A chest x-ray and shoulder x-rays were ordered.

The patient's ECG does meet voltage criteria for left ventricular hypertrophy. However, there are ST-segment depressions in precordial leads V4–V6 that *are suggestive of regional sub-endocardial ischemia* rather than LVH with "strain." As highlighted in Chapter 6 and throughout this atlas, the repolarization abnormalities associated with LVH usually have three characteristic features: the ST-segments in the left-facing leads are downsloping; the downsloping ST-segments then merge imperceptibly into an *inverted* T-wave; and the T-wave inversions are asymmetric, with a noticeably sharper upstroke (return to baseline). In this case, the ST-segment depressions are flat, *and the T-waves are upright*. Lateral wall ischemia is more likely. The S-wave in lead I is probably normal for his age. In addition, the careful electrocardiographer will notice the ST-segment elevations in lead aVR, which raises the possibility of severe left main, left anterior descending or three-vessel coronary disease. Finally, the T-waves in the right precordial leads are prominent. Whether they are "hyperacute" is a tough call, especially when LVH is present. However, it is noteworthy that the T-wave is abnormally tall in lead V1. (Recall from Chapter 7 that the T-wave in lead V1 should never be taller than the T-wave in V6.)

LVH is a notorious confounder that can lead to false-positive readings of cardiac ischemia or infarction when none exists. Old ECG tracings can be invaluable but were not available in this case. Bedside echocardiography might have been helpful in deciding whether there was cardiac ischemia (regional wall motion abnormalities) or only LVH with strain. Of note, in this case, the computer algorithm sounded a warning: "ST depression, consider subendocardial injury. Abnormal ECG."

### Clinical Course

The patient's chest x-ray and shoulder x-rays were completely normal. While in radiology, he suddenly became diaphoretic and reported severe, crushing chest pain that radiated to his back. He underwent a CT-angiogram that showed no aortic dissection. A repeat troponin level was mildly elevated (3.14). Two hours after his presentation, a repeat ECG was ordered (see next ECG).

## Case 8.38  Same patient – 2 hours later.

### The Electrocardiogram

Dynamic changes have occurred. The ST-segment depressions in the lateral precordial leads have resolved. A Wellens' Type A pattern (with biphasic T-waves) is now present in precordial leads V2 and V3, warning of severe occlusion or unstable plaques in the left anterior descending artery. In fact, a STEMI may already be present, given the ST-segment elevation that is present in V2. Lateral limb leads I and aVL now demonstrate more prominent T-wave inversions.

### Clinical Course

The catheterization team was notified, and plans were made for immediate angiography. The troponin continued to trend upward. A bedside echocardiogram demonstrated severe anterolateral hypokinesis. Heparin, a IIb/IIIa agent and nitroglycerin were administered prior to catheterization. The principal error in this case was the failure to appreciate the flat ST-segment depressions suggestive of regional subendocardial ischemia (unstable angina or non-STEMI) on the first tracing (and the ST-segment elevations in aVR). The other critical error was the failure to repeat the ECG in 15–30 minutes (not two hours later). Perhaps not surprising, given the dynamic ECG changes and the initial ST-segment elevation in lead aVR, his catheterization revealed a 99 percent occlusion of the proximal LAD, 90 percent stenosis of the ostial first obtuse marginal and an 80 percent ulcerative distal RCA stenosis. The patient had successful coronary artery bypass surgery the next day.

## References

Einthoven W. Le Telecardiogramme. *Archives Internationale de Physiologie.* 1906; 4:132–164. Translation by

Dr. Henry Blackburn. *Am Heart J.* 1957; 53: 602–615. Quotation from Willem Einthoven.

Marriott H. J. L. *Emergency electrocardiography.* Naples, FL: Trinity Press, 1997.

# Index

# Critical Cases in Electrocardiography

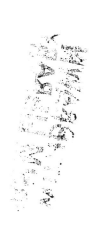